Gastroenterology

Editors

DARIO D'OVIDIO
JOÃO BRANDÃO

VETERINARY CLINICS OF NORTH AMERICA: EXOTIC ANIMAL PRACTICE

www.vetexotic.theclinics.com

Consulting Editor
JÖRG MAYER

May 2025 • Volume 28 • Number 2

ELSEVIER

1600 John F. Kennedy Boulevard • Suite 1800 • Philadelphia, Pennsylvania, 19103-2899
http://www.vetexotic.theclinics.com

VETERINARY CLINICS OF NORTH AMERICA: EXOTIC ANIMAL PRACTICE Volume 28, Number 2
May 2025 ISSN 1094-9194, ISBN-13: 978-0-443-34617-0

Editor: Stacy Eastman
Developmental Editor: Varun Gopal

Publication information: *Veterinary Clinics of North America: Exotic Animal Practice* (ISSN 1094-9194) is published in January, May, and September by Elsevier, 230 Park Avenue, Suite 800, New York, NY 10169. Periodicals postage paid at New York, NY and additional mailing offices. USA POSTMASTER: Send address changes to *Veterinary Clinics of North America: Exotic Animal Practice*, Elsevier Customer Service Department, 3251 Riverport Lane, Maryland Heights, MO 63043, USA. Subscription prices are $311.00 per year for US individuals, $100.00 per year for US students and residents, $362.00 per year for Canadian individuals, $377.00 per year for international individuals, $100.00 per year for Canadian students/residents, and $165.00 per year for international students/residents. For institutional access pricing please contact Customer Service via the contact information below. To receive student/resident rate, orders must be accompanied by name of affiliated institution, date of term, and the *signature* of program/residency coordinator on institution letterhead. Orders will be billed at individual rate until proof of status is received. Foreign air speed delivery is included in all *Clinics* subscription prices. All prices are subject to change without notice. Orders, claims, and journal inquiries: Please visit our Support Hub page https://service.elsevier.com for assistance.

Reprints. For copies of 100 or more of articles in this publication, please contact the Commercial Reprints Department, Elsevier Inc., 360 Park Avenue South, New York, New York 10010-1710. Tel.: 212-633-3874; Fax: 212-633-3820; E-mail: reprints@elsevier.com.

Veterinary Clinics of North America: Exotic Animal Practice is covered in *MEDLINE/PubMed (Index Medicus)*.

Contributors

CONSULTING EDITOR

JÖRG MAYER, Dr. med. vet., M.Sc., DABVP (ECM), DECZM (Small Mammals), DACZM
Diplomate, American Board of Veterinary Practitioners (Exotic Companion Mammals); Diplomate, European College of Zoological Medicine (Small Mammals); Diplomate, American College of Zoological Medicine; Associate Professor of Zoological Medicine, Department of Small Animal Medicine and Surgery, University of Georgia College of Veterinary Medicine, Athens, Georgia, USA

EDITORS

DARIO D'OVIDIO, DVM, MS, SpecPACS, PhD, DECZM (Small Mammals)
Diplomate, European College of Zoological Medicine (Small Mammals); Private Practitioner, Arzano, Naples, Italy; CDVet, Rome, Italy

JOÃO BRANDÃO, LMV, MS, DECZM (Avian), DACZM
Diplomate, European College of Zoological Medicine (Avian); Diplomate, American College of Zoological Medicine; Department of Veterinary Clinical Sciences, College of Veterinary Medicine, Oklahoma State University, Stillwater, Oklahoma, USA

AUTHORS

CHIARA ADAMI, DMV, FRCVS, FHAE, PhD
Diplomate of the American College of Veterinary Anesthesia and Analgesia; Diplomate of the European College of Veterinary Anaesthesia and Analgesia; RCVS Specialist in Anaesthesia and Analgesia, Professor, Department of Veterinary Medicine, University of Cambridge, Cambridge, United Kingdom

KARINE BÉLAND, DMV, IPSAV, DES, MSc
Diplomate of the American College of Zoological Medicine; Clinical Teacher in Zoological Medicine, Centre Hospitalier Universitaire Vétérinaire, Université de Montréal, St Hyacinthe, Canada

NORIN CHAI, DVM, MSc, PhD
Diplomate of the European College of Zoological Medicine (Zoo Health Management); President, Yaboumba, Paris, France

LUCILE CHASSANG, DVM, IPSAV
Assistant Professor, Zoo, Exotic and Wildlife Medicine, Western College of Veterinary Medicine, University of Saskatchewan, Saskatoon, Canada; Small Animal Clinical Sciences Department, Saskatoon, Saskatchewan, Canada

DARIO D'OVIDIO, DVM, MS, SpecPACS, PhD
Diplomate, European College of Zoological Medicine (Small Mammals), Private Practitioner, Arzano, Naples, Italy; CDVet, Rome, Italy

ISABELLE DESPREZ, DVM
Diplomate of the European College of Zoological Medicine (Small Mammal); Diplomate of the American Board of Veterinary Practitioners (Exotic Companion Mammal); Associate Professor, Zoo, Exotic and Wildlife Medicine, Western College of Veterinary Medicine, University of Saskatchewan, Saskatoon, Canada; Small Animal Clinical Sciences Department, Saskatoon, Saskatchewan, Canada

ROBERT J.T. DONELEY, BVSc, FANZCVS (Avian Medicine)
Professor, Avian and Exotic Pet Medicine, UQ Veterinary Medical Centre, The University of Queensland, UQ Gatton, Gatton, Queensland, Australia

LUCIA GOMEZ PRIETO, DVM, MRCVS
ECZM (Avian) Resident, Great Western Exotics, Swindon, Wiltshire, United Kingdom

METTE L. HALCK, DVM, DVM
Danish Specialist (Small Mammal), Department of Veterinary Clinical Sciences, University of Copenhagen, København, Denmark; University Hospital for Companion Animals, Frederiksberg, Denmark

JOANNA HEDLEY, BVM&S, MRCVS
RCVS Diploma in Zoological Medicine (Reptilian); Diplomate of the European College of Zoological Medicine (Herpetology); Senior Lecturer in Exotic Species and Small Mammal Medicine and Surgery, Beaumont Sainsbury Animal Hospital, Royal Veterinary College, London, United Kingdom

CAITLIN M. HEPPS KEENEY, DVM
Diplomate of the American College of Zoological Medicine; Staff Veterinarian, Columbus Zoo and Aquarium, Powell, Ohio, USA

ASHTON HOLLWARTH, BSc, BVMS, CertAVP (Zoo Med), ANZCVS (Avian Medicine & Surgery), MRCVS
Diplomate of the European College of Zoological Medicine (Avian); Avian and Exotics Veterinary Surgeon, Great Western Exotics, Swindon, Wiltshire, United Kingdom

JESSICA M. HORNBY, BVetMed, PGDip(VCP), MVetMed, MRCVS
Clinical Assistant Professor in Small Animal Practice (Exotics and Small mammals), School of Veterinary Medicine and Science, University of Nottingham, Sutton Bonington Campus, Leicestershire, United Kingdom

VLADIMÍR JEKL, MVDr, PhD
Diplomate European College of Zoological Medicine (Small Mammal Medicine and Surgery); EBVS European Recognized Veterinary Specialist in Zoologic Medicine (Small Mammal Medicine and Surgery), Associate Professor, Department of Pharmacology and Pharmacy, Faculty of Veterinary Medicine, Veterinary University Brno, Jekl & Hauptman Veterinary Clinic – Focused on Exotic Companion Mammal Care, Brno, Czech Republic

JULIANNE E. McCREADY, DVM, DVSc
Diplomate of the American College of Zoological Medicine; Assistant Professor, Zoological Medicine Service, Department of Veterinary Clinical Sciences, College of Veterinary Medicine, Oklahoma State University, Stillwater, Oklahoma, USA

DAVID MODRY, MVDr, PhD
Univ Prof cde, Professor, Department of Veterinary Sciences and CINeZ, FAPPZ, Czech University of Life Sciences Prague, Czech Republic; Deptartment of Botany and Zoology,

Faculty of Science, Masaryk University, Brno, Czech Republic; Parasitological Institute of
CAS, Biology Center, České Budějovice, Czech Republic

OLIVIA A. PETRITZ, DVM
Diplomate of the American College of Zoological Medicine; Associate Professor of Avian
and Exotic Animal Medicine, Department of Clinical Sciences, North Carolina State
University, College of Veterinary Medicine, Raleigh, North Carolina, USA

JULIETTE RAULIC, DMV, IPSAV, DES
Diplomate of the American College of Zoological Medicine; Clinical Teacher in Zoological
Medicine, Centre Hospitalier Universitaire Vétérinaire, Université de Montréal, St
Hyacinthe, Canada

NICO J. SCHOEMAKER, DVM, PhD
Diplomate European College of Zoological Medicine (Avian, Small Mammal); Assistant
Professor, Division of Zoological Medicine, Department of Clinical Sciences, Faculty of
Veterinary Medicine, Utrecht University, Utrecht, The Netherlands

YVONNE R.A. VAN ZEELAND, DVM, MVR, PhD
Diplomate European College of Zoological Medicine (Avian, Small Mammal); Assistant
Professor, Division of Zoological Medicine, Department of Clinical Sciences, Faculty of
Veterinary Medicine, Utrecht University, Utrecht, The Netherlands

CLAIRE VERGNEAU-GROSSET, DMV, IPSAV, CES
Diplomate of the American College of Zoological Medicine; Associate Professor,
Zoological Medicine, Department of Clinical Sciences, Faculté de Médecine Vétérinaire,
Université de Montréal, St Hyacinthe, Canada

Contents

Gastrointestinal (GI) disorders are a common cause of emergency presentation in rabbits. Gastrointestinal stasis is a syndrome that is frequently caused by various primary conditions (including but not limited to affections of the GI tract itself). Over the last years, clinical features, diagnosis, management, and prognosis of GI disorders—such as GI obstructions, appendicitis, rabbit hemorrhagic virus disease, or liver lobe torsion—have been studied. Recent data about diseases of the stomach, intestine, liver, and pancreas in rabbits are reviewed in this article.

Ferrets (*Mustela putorius furo*) commonly present with gastrointestinal disease, which can be of noninfectious and infectious origin. Clinical signs are often nonspecific, and can include lethargy, anorexia, vomiting, diarrhea, and melena. Obtaining a detailed history, followed by a thorough physical examination and systematic diagnostic approach are the key to obtaining a correct diagnosis. This review provides an overview of ferret gastrointestinal anatomy and physiology, and diagnostic approach to gastrointestinal problems in ferrets, followed by relevant gastrointestinal diseases related to the different sections of the gastrointestinal tract, including their work up and treatment.

Gastrointestinal (GI) diseases are frequently diagnosed in rodents. Clinical signs are usually nonspecific and include anorexia, weight loss, chronic wasting, abdominal discomfort, gas accumulation in the intestine and stomach, and diarrhea. Malabsorption associated with GI dysfunction or gastroenteritis quickly leads to negative energy balance and metabolic acidosis. Therefore, all disorders of the GI tract should be treated as soon as possible. The article describes selected disorders of the GI tract in guinea pigs (*Cavia porcellus*), chinchillas (*Chinchilla lanigera*), degus (*Octodon degus*), and rats (*Rattus norvegicus*).

Reptile and amphibian veterinarians are frequently presented with patients exhibiting clinical signs suggestive of gastrointestinal (GI) disease. Understanding the normal structure and function of the GI tract is essential to aid appropriate diagnosis. This article will concentrate on the approach to a patient with GI signs and the problems affecting the GI tract from the esophagus to the colon.

Fish represent the most common companion exotic animal in the United States and Canada in number of individuals and hold the third place after dogs and cats in terms of the number of households. Beyond companion animals, fish gastrointestinal diseases are particularly relevant for the aquaculture industry as feeding represents about 50% to 70% of the costs associated with fish production. Thus, nutrient malabsorption may have dramatic consequences both for the fish health and body condition score, but also for farmers. In this review, the authors discuss the anatomy, physiology, and pathology of the digestive system of fish.

This review explores the application of gastrointestinal endoscopy in exotic animals, a field with unique challenges due to the diverse anatomic and physiologic characteristics of species such as small mammals, birds, reptiles, and amphibians. The study outlines its indications, including diagnostic and therapeutic purposes, and discusses the specific equipment and techniques required. Despite the technical difficulties and anesthesia risks associated with these procedures, gastrointestinal endoscopy remains a valuable tool in exotic animal medicine. Like in other diagnostic methods, the large number of species demands special knowledge of the anatomic characteristics.

Gastrointestinal (GI) disorders are very common in exotic animals, such as reptiles, birds, mammals, and can be extremely painful. This review aims to provide the reader with a better understanding of the different pain mechanisms and manifestations across orders and species in order to provide the most updated information on pain recognition and management for GI conditions in exotic animals.

Exotic pet ownership has steadily increased over the last decade, and with increased numbers of these species in close contact with humans, the risk of gastrointestinal zoonoses has also increased. Non-typhoidal serovars of *Salmonella enterica* are one of the most prevalent and important zoonoses of exotic pets, and reptile and backyard poultry are common asymptomatic carriers of these bacteria. Outbreaks of reptile-associated salmonellosis have occurred yearly in the United States since 2019 but contact with backyard poultry has actually been associated with more Salmonella outbreaks in the United States than any other animal species to date.

Imaging of an exotic animal with gastroenteric disease is often essential to make a diagnosis. The selection of a modality and its effective use needs careful consideration in each case. Obtaining a high-quality image and its interpretation are an acquired skill. This article describes how to obtain a high-quality image, and then presents guidelines for its interpretation.

Gastrointestinal disease is a common presenting complaint in avian patients as owners can readily identify clinical signs associated with disorders of the gastrointestinal system. In birds, vastly different diets, environments, and feeding strategies have resulted in vast anatomic and physiologic differences between families. Practitioners treating avian patients should be familiar with the normal gastrointestinal anatomy and physiology of the species they are treating as well as how these species differences affect the diet and husbandry of captive and noncaptive avian patients.

A vast range of infectious and noninfectious diseases can affect avian patients. Practitioners should be familiar with common presenting signs of these diseases in order to steer diagnostic testing and treatment.

This article reviews treatment of gastrointestinal (GI) disorders in exotic companion mammal species, birds, reptiles, amphibians, and fish. Treatment of GI stasis involves fluids, nutrition, and analgesia; there is minimal evidence suggesting prokinetics are useful. Research has evaluated the efficacy of various appetite stimulants in several exotic animal species. Although rabbits and rodents cannot vomit, maropitant may be beneficial by providing visceral analgesia. Gastroprotectants may be indicated for patients at risk for GI ulceration, such as anorexic psittacine birds. Immunosuppressives may be indicated for GI neoplasia and inflammatory bowel disease.

Antimicrobials should be used judiciously when managing gastrointestinal disorders in exotic animals. Oral administration of antibiotics targeting Gram-positive flora must be avoided in hindgut fermenters. Immunosuppressives may be indicated for certain infectious diseases, such as chronic enteric coronavirus in ferrets and avian ganglioneuritis in parrots.

VETERINARY CLINICS OF NORTH AMERICA: EXOTIC ANIMAL PRACTICE

SERIES OF RELATED INTEREST

Veterinary Clinics: Small Animal Practice
https://www.vetsmall.theclinics.com/
Advances in Small Animal Care
https://www.advancesinsmallanimalcare.com

THE CLINICS ARE NOW AVAILABLE ONLINE!
Access your subscription at:
www.theclinics.com

Preface

Zoological Companion Animal Gastroenterology

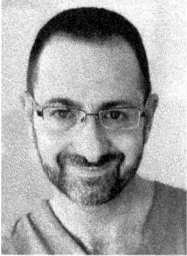

Dario d'Ovidio, DVM, MS, SpecPACS, PhD, DECZM (Small Mammals)

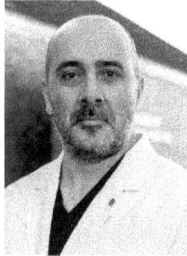

João Brandão, LMV, MS, DECZM (Avian), DACZM

Editors

Zoological companion animal medicine has seen tremendous advancement in the last few decades. As nontraditional or zoological companion animals have become more prevalent, our understanding of their diseases has also evolved. Gastrointestinal (GI) diseases are one of the most common reasons for owners/caregivers to seek veterinary care. This may be because the clinical signs of GI disease can be readily noticed by their owners, which in turn justifies such a high prevalence. Since 2014, when the last gastroenterology-dedicated issue was published in *Veterinary Clinics of North America: Exotic Animal Practice*, this field has experienced significant advances, transforming the diagnosis and treatment of many GI diseases, from the use of endoscopy to the recent advancements in microbiology, histopathology, and imaging necessary to achieve a definitive diagnosis. However, there are still many aspects that need to be implemented and grow rapidly in order to give us new options for the understanding and treatment of these disease processes.

We feel honored to serve as guest editors of this issue, the purpose of which is to give an overview on the main infectious (including zoonoses) and noninfectious conditions affecting fish, amphibians, reptiles, birds, and exotic companion mammals kept in captivity, provide the most up-to-date information on diagnostic tests that can be used in zoological companion animals as well as describe the new therapeutic options currently available for the therapy of these conditions.

When developing this issue, we sought to identify leading experts from around the world with extensive experience in this field. Several of the articles are focused on the species group so that information specific to it is readily available to the reader. These articles are complemented with others focusing on diagnostic modalities, such as diagnostic imaging or endoscopy, and therapeutic options across the species.

Vet Clin Exot Anim 28 (2025) xi–xii
https://doi.org/10.1016/j.cvex.2024.12.001
1094-9194/25/© 2024 Elsevier Inc. All rights are reserved, including those for text and data mining, AI training, and similar technologies.

vetexotic.theclinics.com

We are pleased to include a zoonotic disease-specific article, as we feel that this is an important subject that should be available to the readership. The information included in it is essential for a One Health approach in regard to pet ownership, and we hope it will give clinicians a readily available source of information that will help them educate their clients and prevent zoonotic diseases. Last, but not least, clinicians cannot ignore the potential pain associated with GI diseases and how we should address such conditions. The welfare of our patients is paramount for the success of treatment. Therefore, a dedicated article on analgesia reviews the current understanding of pain management as it pertains to the GI tract.

We wish to acknowledge all the authors for their efforts and valuable contribution to this issue and for sharing their experience and knowledge. We also would like to thank Elsevier and its editorial team, and Dr Jörg Mayer for giving us this opportunity. Finally, we hope that in reading these articles clinicians will find new useful information and ideas that might help diagnose and treat GI disorders in zoological companion animals.

Dario d'Ovidio, DVM, MS, SpecPACS, PhD, DECZM (Small Mammals)
Diplomate, European College of Zoological Medicine
(Small Mammals); Private Practitioner
Via Colombo 118
Arzano, Naples 80022, Italy

João Brandão, LMV, MS, DECZM (Avian), DACZM
Diplomate, European College of Zoological Medicine (Avian);
Diplomate, American College of Zoological Medicine
Department of Veterinary Clinical Sciences
College of Veterinary Medicine
Oklahoma State University
2065 West Farm Road
Stillwater, OK 74078, USA

E-mail addresses:
dariodovidio@yahoo.it (D. d'Ovidio)
jbrandao@okstate.edu (J. Brandão)

Rabbit Gastroenterology

Isabelle Desprez, DVM, Dipl ECZM (SM), Dipl ABVP (ECM)[a,b,*],
Lucile Chassang, DVM, IPSAV[a,b]

KEYWORDS

- Oryctolagus cuniculus • Rabbits • Gastrointestinal

KEY POINTS

- Gastrointestinal (GI) disorders are a common cause of emergency presentation in rabbits.
- Gastrointestinal stasis (GIS) and obstructions can initially present similarly and must be differentiated for appropriate management.
- Most GI diseases are noninfectious, and clinical signs are generally unspecific. However, specific infectious disorders such as rabbit hemorrhagic disease are important to consider in differential diagnoses.
- Appendicitis, liver lobe torsion, and GI obstruction should be included in the differential diagnosis of GIS and may require surgical management.

INTRODUCTION

Disorders of the digestive tract are among the most common presenting complaints in pet rabbits. A retrospective study conducted in a referral hospital in Brazil identified the gastrointestinal (GI) body system, including oral cavity, as the second most commonly affected, accounting for 23.6% of presenting complaints.[1] Another retrospective study conducted in the United Kingdom identified anorexia and ileus as the second and fourth identified cause for mortality, respectively, while the GI/abdominal group term (excluding oral cavity) was the third most commonly represented, accounting for 9.5% of recorded diagnoses.[2] Finally, a questionnaire-based study surveying veterinarians in the United Kingdom reported GI (excluding oral cavity) as the third most common body system for presenting complaints, representing 15.2% of them.[3] This study also compared the perception that veterinarians had on the available information and compared it to the published literature, finding that veterinarians are under the impression that there is less available information on rabbit GI diseases compared to what actually is available.

[a] Zoo, Exotic and Wildlife Medicine, Western College of Veterinary Medicine, University of Saskatchewan, Saskatoon, Canada; [b] Small Animal Clinical Sciences Department, 52 Campus Drive, Saskatoon, Saskatchewan S7N 5B4, Canada
* Corresponding author. Small Animal Clinical Sciences Department, 52 Campus Drive, Saskatoon, Saskatchewan S7N 5B4, Canada.
E-mail address: isabelle.desprez@gmail.com

Vet Clin Exot Anim 28 (2025) 209–225
https://doi.org/10.1016/j.cvex.2024.11.001
1094-9194/25/© 2024 Elsevier Inc. All rights reserved, including those for text and data mining, AI training, and similar technologies.

Abbreviations	
BG	blood glucose
CT	computed tomography
GI	gastrointestinal
GIS	gastrointestinal stasis
HU	Hounsfield units
LLT	liver lobe torsion
LVU	lumbar vertebral units
RHD	rabbit hemorrhagic disease
SIRS	systemic inflammatory reaction syndrome

The objective of this article is to summarize the essential information published on rabbit GI diseases over the past decade. Anatomy and physiology of the rabbit GI tract have been previously described and can be found elsewhere.[4–7]

RABBIT GASTROINTESTINAL STASIS SYNDROME

GIS syndrome is a common presentation and cause for consultation in pet rabbits. Whereas it is often considered as a final diagnosis, GIS is the description of a common group of symptoms, and the primary cause should be determined whenever possible.

A retrospective cohort study conducted in a referral center in the United Kingdom showed that 25.1% of the rabbits presented within a 5-year period experienced GIS, with approximately a third of these GIS rabbits experiencing multiple episodes during the collection period.[8] A similar prevalence of GIS was reported in a retrospective study conducted in the United States, in which the majority of the rabbits were examined on an emergency basis.[9] The proportion of rabbits presented for multiple episodes of GIS in this study was comparable to the previous one. In both studies, dwarf and lop rabbits appeared overrepresented and may therefore be at a higher risk of developing GIS.[8,9] Sex, hair coat length, or time of the year do not appear to be predisposing factors for GIS, and based on reported mean and median ages for occurrence, the syndrome most commonly occurs in young adults.[8,9] The syndrome is typically due to reduced GI motility, and identifying the underlying cause may prove challenging. Any cause of reduced food intake (eg, pain, anxiety, environmental or dietary changes, dental disease, other illness, among others) could in turn cause reduced GI motility and lead to GIS.[10,11] The reduction in GI motility then triggers a cascade of events, typically including decreased fecal output, dehydration of the GI content leading to the formation of trichobezoar in the stomach, and disruption of cecal fermentation and flora.[10,11] These events will then worsen the initial anorexia, creating a vicious cycle. In a single case report, dysmotility has been hypothesized as a possible cause for an intussusception.[12]

Clinical presentation is nonspecific and variable. It may include reduced to absent food intake and fecal output, lethargy/depression, hunched posture, and bruxism.[11,13] Diagnosis is based on a thorough history collection, aiming at identifying a potential underlying cause that could potentially be treated or resolved, physical examination findings, and diagnostic tests aiming at assessing the overall health status of the patient and the potential presence of an underlying disease or comorbidity. The size and consistency of the stomach are important in differentiating GIS from gastric dilatation. In case of GIS, the content of the stomach should be dehydrated ingesta that typically feels doughy and should retain a finger indent upon compression (play doh texture).[10] The stomach may palpate quite firm, depending on the severity of dehydration, but little to no gas or fluid should be palpated in the stomach, while the cecum and intestines may contain gas. Decreased gut sounds may also be noticed.[9] Hypothermia may also be present and was found to be associated with higher odds of death or euthanasia in 1 study.[9]

Complete blood count, serum/plasma biochemistry, and abdominal radiographs are routinely recommended to assess rabbits suffering from GIS.[6,9–11,14] While hematology tends to be unremarkable or unspecific, hyperglycemia (evaluated using a point-of-care glucometers) has been noted in 50% of the rabbits suffering from GIS in 1 study,[9] and reported as moderately elevated in 51 rabbits with GIS in another study.[15] This is in contrast with other sources[10] indicating that only signs of dehydration would be present on the biochemical profile of rabbits suffering from GIS. Moderate to marked elevation of circulating creatinine concentration was also observed in 16% of the rabbits diagnosed with GIS in 1 study, while 18% had mild azotemia.[9] However, none of these findings is specific for GIS.

Abdominal radiographs are recommended to differentiate GIS from GI obstruction.[6,10,11] The typical reported appearance of a GIS stomach includes an ingesta-type content that may be denser than in a normal stomach and may be surrounded by a gas rim.[10,16] The stomach size is typically smaller in cases of GIS, compared to obstruction, the caudal aspect of the stomach typically not reaching L2 on lateral radiographs.[16] Gas distension of the cecum or large intestine may also be present.[16]

Typical treatment for GIS includes fluid therapy, which can be administered intravenously or subcutaneously, depending on the degree of dehydration noticed on physical examination. Administration of oral fluids or enemas could also be considered if alternate routes of fluid administration are needed (eg, IV catheter difficult to maintain, poor absorption of subcutaneous fluids). GIS often induces mild to severe abdominal pain, and analgesia should be part of the treatment plan. Commonly used analgesics include opioids, meloxicam, lidocaine, or metamizole (also known as dipyrone).[10,11,17,18] Support feeding is the third part of the treatment of GIS and should be implemented as soon as the rabbit is able to swallow, is normothermic, and hydrated. Although syringe-feeding is usually well-tolerated, if a rabbit is particularly resistant or if prolonged support feeding is required, a nasogastric tube could be placed. The use of prokinetics, such as metoclopramide or cisapride, is commonly reported.[7,10,11] The efficacy of prokinetic drugs in rabbit is unclear,[19] and obstruction should be ruled out before starting a prokinetic treatment.

It is important to consider that GIS is typically secondary to another condition and specific treatment of the identified cause for GIS should be implemented, especially if the GIS is not responsive to medical therapy. For instance, omental torsion has been reported as a cause for GIS, and surgical removal of the necrotic omentum was necessary.[20] Three-month duration intermittent GIS, which was only partially responsive to medical treatment was reported in a rabbit who was subsequently diagnosed with mesenteric root torsion on necropsy, which is a condition requiring surgery in other species.[21] Other GI conditions have been reported to cause GIS, including enteric duplication cyst,[22] ileal pseudodiverticulum,[23] intestinal mycobacteriosis,[24] or intestinal lymphoma.[25] LLT is also commonly seen as a cause of GIS in rabbits and is discussed later in this article.

Rabbits diagnosed early and euthermic upon initial presentation[9] will typically respond well to subcutaneous or oral fluids with analgesia and syringe feeding. This allows for treatment on an outpatient basis, reducing the potential stress of being hospitalized, which could aggravate the GIS. If a rabbit is treated as an in-patient, all efforts should be made to keep the rabbit in a quiet area to reduce stress. If the rabbit remains stressed, a low dose of midazolam (0.2–0.5 mg/kg IM) could be used as an anxiolytic.[10,11]

GASTROINTESTINAL OBSTRUCTIVE DISORDERS

GI obstruction, also referred to as intestinal obstruction, gastric dilatation, or gastric bloat, is an acute and potentially fatal condition in pet rabbits. A mechanical obstruction causes buildup of fluids and gas proximal to the obstruction site. Rabbits are unable to vomit, so the fluid and gas accumulation eventually affects the stomach (even in case of distal obstruction) and causes gastric dilatation. The distended stomach compresses intra-abdominal vessels, thus reducing venous return and perfusion, and puts pressure on the diaphragm, reducing lung volume. The relocation of fluid from the intravascular space into the lumen of the GI tract, proximal to the obstruction also causes fluid loss and rapid hypovolemia, leading to shock.[7,10,26,27] Shock and hypovolemia can lead to death within a few hours, especially in rabbits with a proximal obstruction.

The most commonly reported cause of obstruction is a pellet of compressed hair.[7,10,16,26,27] Other causes such as foreign bodies (eg, carpet, cloth, plastic), neoplasia, adhesions, strictures, or other extraluminal compressions (eg, extraluminal mass) have been less frequently reported.[7,10,16,26,27]

Because of the life-threatening nature of GI obstructions, rapid and accurate diagnosis is essential for successful management. Initial presentation may resemble GIS, with commonly reported complaints being decreased appetite and fecal output, lethargy, and hunched posture. Thorough history and physical examination should always be performed, as some findings can be suggestive of a more severe condition. In case of an obstruction, the stomach typically feels distended, large and fluid-filled to tympanic gas-filled stomach (also known as meteorism or tympanites).[7,10] One study reported that rabbits that had not defecated in the 12 hours before admission, regardless of the cause, had twice the odds of dying compared to other rabbits.[28] This study assessed the prognosis value of rectal temperature at hospital admission and found hypothermia (rectal temperature < 38°C [<100.4°F]) upon admission to be associated with a three-time higher mortality risk compared to normothermic rabbits.[28] Other studies focused on gastric dilatation or obstruction in rabbits reported that 66%[29] to 81.2%[27] of rabbits were hypothermic on presentation, and hypothermia was not correlated with decreased survival in these studies. Another study reported temperatures on admission between 36 to 37°C (96.8–98.6°F) in obstructed rabbits.[30] Although hypothermia is not specific of GI obstruction in rabbits and may not always be associated with survival, it definitely appears to be a common physical examination finding.

Performing bloodwork is a common practice and can help assess the overall prognosis of the patient. A blood glucose (BG) performed with a point-of-care glucometer and more than 20 mmol/L (360 mg/dL) has been associated with more severe conditions or more critical illnesses in a study.[15] A prospective study conducted in 55 rabbits suffering from gastric dilatation found that 37% of them presented with hyperglycemia, and the mortality rate of rabbits with gastric dilatation and a BG more than 25 mmol/L (450 mg/dL) was 70%.[29] A retrospective study conducted on 141 rabbits with intestinal obstruction showed that 88.9% were hyperglycemic, 52.4% of which had a BG more than 20 mmol/L (360 mg/dL).[27] This study did not find a correlation between BG and survival, but another retrospective study found a higher mean BG in rabbits considered to be suffering from a life-threatening condition compared with unobstructed rabbits.[26] Azotemia has also been found to be a prognosis indicator in rabbits. A retrospective study showed that elevated blood urea nitrogen (BUN) was associated with decreased survival in rabbits, regardless of the cause for this elevation.[31] In rabbits suffering from gastric dilatation, a retrospective study showed that 72% of rabbits had elevated BUN, which was not correlated with survival in that study.[27] A prospective study showed that elevated creatinine was the most frequently observed biochemical change (51% of rabbits), and was associated with significantly higher mortality.[29] Among other changes reported in the bloodwork of rabbits suffering from GI obstruction, increased aspartate transferase activity was noticed in 44% of rabbits in 1 study, which also found hyponatremia in 43% of rabbits.[29] These findings were not associated with survival. Elevated plasma osmolarity and tonicity was found in 60.4% and 45.8% of rabbits in 1 study, and these findings were not correlated with survival.[27] Finally, a prospective study conducted in 30 rabbits suffering from either GIS or GI obstruction showed that 57% of the rabbits had acidosis (83% of which was metabolic), and the P_{CO_2}, HCO_3 and base excess were significantly lower in animals presented later in the course of the disease (12 hours after onset, compared to 6 hours after onset).[18]

Abdominal radiographs are the most used imaging modality to diagnose GI obstructions in rabbits. The most common features include a gastric content consisting of mostly liquid with a gas cap, the caudal aspect of the stomach extending past the second lumbar vertebral body, and direct contact between the gastric wall and the ventral abdomen.[16] Measurement of the gastric length and width can also be acquired on a lateral radiographs, and the sum of these 2 measurements should not exceed the length from the cranial end of the first lumbar vertebral body to the coxo-femoral joint.[16] Although not specific for obstruction as it was detected in a small number of nonobstruction cases, the sum of gastric length and gastric width being greater than or equal to the length from the first lumbar vertebra to the coxo-femoral joint should raise a suspicion of obstruction.[16]

Another study described a vertebral stomach score based on similar measurements expressed in lumbar vertebral units (LVU).[29] The gastric height and length are measured at a 90° angle from each other and transposed on the vertebral column starting at the first lumbar vertebra. A cut-off value of 9.3 LVU was determined, in which rabbits with gastric dilatation were 3.99 more likely to die if their vertebral stomach score was over 9.3 LVU.[29] The caudal extension of the stomach was also recorded in that study, which found that rabbits with gastric dilatation had a stomach extending significantly more caudally compared to nonobstructed rabbits, and that a stomach extending past the second lumbar vertebral body on a lateral radiograph was associated with significantly increased mortality.[29] A large amount of gas in the stomach (more than 50% of the content), and a ventral or central location of the gas on a lateral radiographs was also associated with significantly higher mortality in that study.[29] The use of iodinated contrast medium to determine whether or not an obstruction was present and moving through has been reported in rabbits.[18] Abdominal ultrasound could also be used to diagnose a GI obstruction in rabbits and be repeated to determine whether the obstruction is moving, and computed tomography (CT) scan can also be used for this purpose, as it is in other species.

Treatment of GI obstruction depends on the cause, and this article will focus on the treatment for compressed hair pellets obstructions as they are the most common. Initial stabilization with fluid resuscitation, analgesia, and supportive care should be implemented. The type and rate of fluids should be selected based on diagnosed acid-base and electrolyte disorders and should aim at correcting dehydration and possible shock. Recognition of hypovolemic shock is important as this is the main cause of mortality in obstructed rabbits. Bradycardia (below 180 beats per minute), hypothermia (below 36.1°C or 97°F), and hypotension (below 90 mm Hg systolic) are indicative of hypovolemic shock, and these patients require more aggressive fluid therapy.[13,30,32] Hypothermia if present should be managed by gradual warming.

Information regarding analgesia can be found in another article in this issue. Evidence of efficacy of prokinetic drugs and other supportive medications is lacking in rabbits; however, metoclopramide has been used successfully as part of a medical treatment protocol in rabbits with obstructions.[17,18,26,29] Ranitidine and various antibiotics have also been used as part of the supportive care protocol.[18,26,27] Support feeding has also been part of medical management protocols.[17]

A retrospective study conducted in rabbits with GI obstruction described orogastric tubing as a beneficial procedure in case of a life-threatening condition. These rabbits had a severely tympanic stomach with signs of hypovolemic shock and were sedated or anesthetized for stomach decompression. None of the rabbits in this study underwent surgery, making medical management alone a potentially viable option.[26] Other studies report successful medical management of GI obstructions in rabbits, various treatment protocols being described.[17,30] Decision for surgery is made on a case-by-case basis, and is typically based on various factors, including duration of clinical signs before presentation, poor clinical status, lack of response to medical treatment, or deterioration of clinical condition despite medical treatment, and willingness of the client to pursue surgery.[27] Depending on the location of the obstruction, gastrotomy and enterotomy have been described and can be performed, and if the gastric or intestinal wall appears devitalized, partial gastrectomy or enterectomy may be indicated.[7,10,33–35] It is generally recommended to avoid enterotomy whenever possible and milk the obstructing material either into the stomach to then perform a gastrotomy, or into the cecum instead, in which the obstructing material will be left.[10,27,34] Postoperative care should include intravenous fluids, analgesia, antibiotics, and support feeding.[27]

Other reported causes of GI obstructions include postovariohysterectomy colonic obstruction (4 days to 5 months postoperatively), caused by either adhesions, or a suture penetrating the colon.[36] None of these 3 rabbits survived, while a rabbit with colonic obstruction and jejunal adhesions recovered after colonic resection and anastomosis.[37]

APPENDICITIS

Although detailed descriptions of spontaneous appendicitis and its clinical features in pet rabbits are quite recent, early reports in laboratory rabbits were published in 1977 and 1987.[38,39] In addition, appendicitis can be induced by occlusion of the appendix in rabbit models.[40]

The primary etiology of appendicitis in rabbits is not yet elucidated. In humans, appendicitis seems to be associated with anaerobic bacteria. In pet rabbits, various aerobic and anaerobic bacteria have been cultured in diseased appendices: *E.coli, Yersinia pseudotuberculosis, Pseudomonas aeruginosa, Klebsiella variicola,* and *Bacteroides spp.*[40,41] Their significance is uncertain as many organisms have also been isolated from the appendices of presumed healthy farm rabbits, and a case report described mixed bacterial growth with no predominant organisms.[42] In farm rabbits, cases of fungal appendicitis have also been reported.[43]

The disease seems to affect rabbits of various ages, with a median age at presentation of 2 years in a retrospective study but ranging from 4 months to 7 years.[40] Cases were predominantly observed in the summer and fall seasons in that same study.

Clinical signs are mostly unspecific and consistent with GIS; some rabbits have no clinical signs or intermittent ones. Most rabbits have clinical signs for less than 48h at the time of presentation. Elevated rectal temperature, discomfort on abdominal palpation, and palpable tubular mass in the abdomen are noted in some rabbits and should prompt investigations for appendicitis.[40–42] Restlessness has also been reported in several rabbits with appendicitis.[40,41]

Radiographs and bloodwork show unspecific changes, such as signs of GIS or changes secondary to inflammation (leukocytosis, monocytosis,and anemia). Ultrasound seems to be the best option to assess the appendix[40–42] and normal appearance of the vermiform appendix in rabbits has been described.[44] However, GI content may hinder visualization of the appendix on ultrasound, so CT scan can be considered as an alternative, although only 50% of CT scans were suggestive of appendicitis in a study.[40,41,44] Typically, the appendix appears dilated with its wall thickened and loss of the typical multilayered structure of the wall. Sacculitis can accompany appendicitis, characterized by a thickening of the sacculus rotundus wall.[42] Based on the imaging findings, the main differential for appendicitis in rabbits is lymphoma. Definitive diagnosis relies on histopathology. In retrospective study, about a third of cases were diagnosed at necropsy, and the condition was not suspected before death or euthanasia.[40]

The treatment of choice is considered to be appendectomy. In rabbits, a retrospective study found a 62.5% survival rate postoperatively, with 50% surviving over 300 days.[40] However, data is still lacking regarding medical management as histopathology is necessary to confirm the diagnosis, making medical treatment difficult to study. The current recommended approach for surgery is via ventral midline approach. Cauterization and excision of the ileocecal fold is a crucial step before removal of the appendix as significant bleeding can occur. Then circumferential ligation of the appendix at its point of origin in the cecum is performed. The appendix can then be excised, leaving a residual appendiceal stump of maximum 3 mm long.[40] The removed appendix should be submitted for histopathology, and culture swabs should be taken for aerobic and anaerobic bacterial and fungal culture. Postoperative care should include broad-spectrum antibiotics (covering for Gram-positive and Gram-negative bacteria which should be modified as needed once bacterial culture results are available), analgesia, and supportive care. If surgery is not possible, medical management with antimicrobials and GIS management can be considered. All aerobic isolates were resistant to at least one antibiotic in a retrospective study, making empirical therapeutic choice difficult.[40]

DISEASES OF THE RECTUM
Rectal Prolapse

Rectal prolapse is typically observed in young rabbits, most often secondary to infectious diseases causing diarrhea. Cases in adults have been recently reported. Those rabbits had rectal prolapses secondary to masses, an inflammatory polyp in an 8-year-old neutered male and a leiomyosarcoma in a 4-year-old spayed female. Both had complete resolution and no relapse after surgical removal of the mass.[45]

LIVER DISEASES
Rabbit Hemorrhagic Disease

Rabbit hemorrhagic disease (RHD) is caused by a Calicivirus of the species *Lagovirus europaeus*.[46] Lagoviruses were initially thought to be host-specific as the classic variant (Rabbit Hemorrhagic Disease Virus 1, or RHDV1 or RHDV GI.1) only affects European rabbits (*Oryctolagus cuniculus*), and viruses from the GII genogroup (European brown hare syndrome virus and related nonpathogenic hare caliciviruses) only affect hares.[46] However, the genotype GI.2 that was first identified in 2010 in France, was then found to infect various species (lagomorphs including *Lepus* spp., *Sylvilagus* spp., *Brachylagus idahoensis*, *Pronolagus* spp., and non-lagomorphs such as the alpine musk deer [*Moschus sifanicus*] or the Eurasian badger [*Meles meles*]).[46–48] This feature, associated with slightly longer incubation period, variable apparent mortality (10%–90%), and possibly higher proportion of subacute or chronic forms, allowed this variant to spread rapidly and worldwide, especially in areas in which rabbit populations were abundant.[46] As GI.2 has become more common than GI.1 and has a worldwide distribution, the disease description, diagnosis, and management will focus on this variant.

Contrary to the *classic* variant (GI.1), GI.2 has been found to affect rabbits of all ages. In a retrospective study, the age of rabbits with characteristic histopathological lesions of RHD ranged from 4 weeks to 7 years.[49] Studies show variable incubation, disease course and mortalities, but overall GI.2 is considered to have a longer disease course (mortalities starting from 18h to up to 9 days after infection) and incubation period (3–5 days), as well as a variable mortality (10%–90%).[46,50,51] Surviving rabbits may excrete the virus for up to 2 months, and the subclinical carriers may shed for months without symptoms.[50] In an experimental study, the presence of infective viruses was assessed in the feces of rabbits inoculated with RHDV2. All surviving rabbits were found to have viral RNA in their feces, with irregular and variable detection timing. However, only 1 rabbit was found to excrete infective virus and was the only one who did not exhibit clear seroconversion after the infection.[52]

Clinical presentation ranges from a peracute form, where sudden death occurs with no or minimal premonitory signs, to subacute and chronic forms. Acute disease is typically characterized by unspecific signs (eg, depression, anorexia, GIS) that can be accompanied by hyperthermia or hypothermia, signs of circulatory shock, neurologic signs (eg, ataxia, opisthotonos, excitement, seizures), respiratory signs, subcutaneous and/or cutaneous hemorrhages, poor blood clotting, or jaundice.[10,46,49,50,53–55] Subacute to chronic forms seem to be more common with the GI.2 variant and manifest by protracted clinical disease including lethargy, anorexia, weight loss, and jaundice, with possible GI dilation, cardiac arrhythmia and murmurs, and neurologic abnormalities.[50] In a 2-year-old pet rabbit, chronic RHD was suspected to cause clinical signs for 4 months before the death of the animal.[53] In all cases, death and progression of the disease are generally attributed to liver failure and disseminated intravascular coagulation.[46,50]

Definitive diagnosis relies on viral detection, which is most often performed postmortem, but presumptive diagnosis is based on the combination of clinical signs, infection pattern in a population and clinical pathology and imaging findings. Radiographic findings are usually nonspecific and can sometimes show changes consistent with hepatomegaly or peritoneal effusion.[53,56] Ultrasonography can reveal signs of hepatitis or peritoneal effusion.[53,54,56] Complete blood count findings can include leukopenia, lymphopenia, heteropenia, thrombocytopenia and anemia.[49,50,53,54,56] Plasma biochemistry changes include elevated liver enzymes activities (although found to be markedly decreased in 2 cases), elevated bilirubin and bile acids, hypoglycemia and other changes consistent with liver failure.[46,49,53–56] Urinalysis can reveal aciduria, bilirubinuria, proteinuria, elevated urinary gamma-glutamyltransferase (GGT), and glucosuria.[54] Coagulation assessment typically shows prolonged prothrombin time and partial thromboplastin time.[50,53,54,56]

If RHD is suspected, molecular testing is necessary to confirm the diagnosis. Reverse transcription polymerase chain reaction (RT-PCR) is most commonly used.[50] Samples in which the virus RNA can be detected include tissues (liver, spleen), blood, effusion fluid, urine, feces, and swabs.[50,56,57] Most cases are confirmed postmortem, based on suggestive lesions (eg, hepatic necrosis, disseminated intravascular coagulation, splenic congestion, pulmonary hemorrhage or edema, cardiomyocyte necrosis) combined with virus identification (eg, RT-PCR on fresh or fixed tissues, electron microscopy, immunostaining).[50,54,58-61] However, 42% of pet rabbits with characteristic histopathological features of RHD did not exhibit any gross abnormalities in a retrospective study.[49] In addition, 8% of rabbits with positive RT-PCR lacked histologic changes postmortem in another study,[62] so RHD should not be ruled out even in the absence of suggestive lesions and RHDV molecular testing should be considered for every suspicious case.

There is no direct treatment, and so management mostly relies on supportive care.[50] Fresh plasma transfusion from a healthy vaccinated donor was associated with complete recovery in a rabbit with positive GI.2 blood RT-PCR and suggestive clinical and diagnostic findings.[56] Suspect or confirmed rabbits should be isolated and nonsymptomatic rabbits should be vaccinated.[50]

Given the limits of treatment options, prevention should be considered paramount. Biosecurity, rapid diagnosis, and vaccination are the main elements of prevention.[50] Caliciviruses are nonencapsulated viruses, which makes them resistant in the environment. Adequate cleaning and disinfection methods include incineration of infected material and animals or inactivation of the virus with sodium hypochlorite, formalin, or chloramine (at appropriate concentrations).[50]

Several vaccines are available depending on the countries, and recommendations vary with the epidemiologic situation. In endemic countries, such as European countries or Australia, vaccination against both variants is generally advised—GI.2 is the dominant variant in most places-; however, GI.1 was still found circulating in some countries in recent studies.[50,63] Vaccination against GI.2 is also advised in areas where outbreaks and/or endemic circulation of the virus have been reported. Available vaccines are either inactivated vaccines (from liver extracts) or recombinant vaccines (vectored or subunits) (**Table 1**). Most vaccines only require a yearly injection for appropriate seroconversion. Although vaccinal protection is satisfying, the main antigen (capsid protein VP60) varies between strains, and cases have been identified in vaccinated rabbits.[59,60,64]

PARASITIC DISEASES

Hepatic coccidiosis is caused by *Eimeria stiedae* and typically affects juvenile rabbits around weaning.[7,10] Clinical signs include diarrhea (with fecal material often staining

Table 1
Commercially available rabbit vaccines against RHDV GI.2 genotype

Vaccine	Type of Vaccine	Dosage
Eravac® (Hipra, Spain)	Inactivated, monovalent GI.2	SC, annually
Filavac K C + V® (Filavie, France)	Inactivated, bivalent GI.1 and GI.2	SC, annually
YURVAC® RHD (Hipra, Spain)	Recombinant RHD virus capsid protein (VP60)	SC, annually
Medgene® (Medgene, USA)	Recombinant subunit vaccine (VP60 protein of US strains of RHDV2)	SC, initially 2 doses 21 d apart then annually
Nobivac® Myxo-RHD Plus (MSD Animal Health, UK)	Recombinant vectored live myxoma RHD virus strains (capsid protein gene of GI.1 and GI.2)	SC, annually

Type of vaccine and dosage are extracted from manufacturers data sheets.

the perineum), anorexia, emaciation, rough hair coat, dulled appearance, distended abdomen, and pale mucous membranes. Plasma biochemistry can reveal elevated hepatic enzymes (alanine transaminase, alkaline phosphatase, GGT), hyperglobulinemia, hypoalbuminemia, and low BUN. Complete blood count can be suggestive of hemoconcentration due to dehydration associated with diarrhea, or changes consistent with inflammation such as anemia, lymphopenia, monocytosis, and eosinophilia. Thrombocytopenia was also associated with infection in a case study.[65] On ultrasound, nodules of varying shapes and diameters can be found, usually hyperechoic or with a target-like appearance (hypoechoic center and hyperechoic rim). In most cases, the parenchyma between the nodules has a normal appearance. The liver may appear enlarged with rounded edges. The gallbladder can be thickened or hyperechoic, and bile duct and hepatic blood vessels can appear dilated.[65,66] Treatment relies on anticoccidial medication, typically sulfamides and toltrazuril. However, prognosis is guarded, especially if rabbits are presented later in the disease course.

Cysticercosis due to *Taenia pisiformis* has been described in a rabbit, causing verminous hepatitis. Clinical signs were unspecific and consistent with GIS. On radiographs, hepatomegaly was observed. As the rabbit did not have access to outdoors, exposure was hypothesized to be via hay contaminated with dog or fox feces.[67]

Systemic toxoplasmosis has been associated with necrotizing hepatitis and other visceral lesions (splenitis, interstitial pneumonia, pancreatitis, peripancreatic steatitis, and lymphadenitis) in 2 young adult rabbits. Clinical signs were signs of GIS associated with pyrexia and a caudal abdominal mass in 1 case. Diagnostic was obtained postmortem and necessitated immunohistochemistry and polymerase chain reaction to confirm the etiology. As the rabbits were not exposed to cat feces, fomites or food were considered the most likely sources.[68]

LIVER LOBE TORSION

LLT prevalence was estimated at 0.7% in a recent retrospective study in rabbits.[69] The etiology of LLT is uncertain. Anatomic predisposition is suspected, but other factors such as abdominal organomegaly, trauma, or concurrent hepatopathy are also considered.[70] The torsion causes occlusion of the veins in the affected lobe, leading to passive congestion, increased hydrostatic pressure, and venous thrombosis. Ultimately, lobar necrosis and/or lobar capsular rupture and hemoperitoneum may occur. Pain and hypovolemic shock typically ensue, with possible systemic inflammatory reaction syndrome (SIRS), disseminated intravascular coagulation, and death as complications.[70]

Affected rabbits are typically older than 2 years.[70] The median age at diagnosis ranges from 2.15 and 4 year old depending on the study, but age can range from 6 months to 10 years.[69–73] Males are overrepresented in all retrospective studies, representing 56% to 83% of cases.[69–73] There is no clear breed predisposition although several studies observed a majority of lop-eared rabbits.[69,70,72]

Clinical signs are relatively unspecific and resemble GIS—reduced appetite, lethargy, reduced or absent defecation, and abnormal behavior. Most patients are presented within 1 to 2 days after clinical signs onset. On physical examination, the stomach and/or intestines may feel distended, with pain elicited upon palpation (mostly in the cranial abdomen). A mass may be palpable in the cranial abdomen, and mucous membranes may be pale. Signs suggestive of shock can often be noticed—dull mentation, hypothermia, tachycardia, and/or tachypnea.[69,70,72]

Plasma biochemistry and complete blood count can show suggestive changes. On plasma biochemistry, ALT is the most commonly increased liver enzyme.[69–73] AST and ALP are also commonly elevated, but up to 86% of patients had an ALP within normal ranges,[71] and up to 56% had normal AST[72] in various retrospective studies. Although rare, some patients may have no elevation of any of hepatic enzymes—5% of cases in 1 retrospective study.[69] Other common changes include azotemia, hyperglycemia, and hypoproteinemia.[69,70,72] On CBC, anemia is the most common finding with 59.5% to 83% of rabbits with LLT exhibiting some degree of anemia.[69–73] Thrombocytopenia and abnormal red blood cell morphology is reported in about half of the patients.[69,72]

Survey radiographs findings are not specific, most commonly consistent with GIS. Ultrasonography or CT is usually diagnostic. Ultrasonography was found diagnostic in all cases in 2 retrospective studies. Findings included hepatomegaly or abnormally large liver lobe, rounded lobar margins, mixed parenchymal echogenicity, peritoneal and/or pleural effusion, hyperechoic perihepatic mesentery, and hepatic or portal vein thrombosis,[69,72] but the most suggestive abnormality is the absence of blood flow on Doppler color flow mode.[69,72] As the flow Doppler is prone to motion artifact, findings can be inconclusive in some cases and the use of contrast-enhanced ultrasonography may confirm the absence of blood flow in the affected liver lobe.[74] CT is diagnostic in most cases, especially if intravenous contrast enhancement is used. The affected lobe can appear enlarged, rounded, hypoattenuating, and variably heterogeneous. Noncontrast to minimal contrast enhancement is observed. Mean Hounsfield units (HU) were found to be lower in affected lobes than in normal lobes, both precontrast and postcontrast.[70] Other findings on CT include free abdominal and/or pleural effusion, duodenal extraluminal compression adjacent to torsed lobe (when caudate lobe affected) and focal dilation, and stenosis of the caudal vena cava and/or portal system.[70,73]

The caudate lobe is the most commonly affected lobe, representing 63% to 95% of cases. The right lobe is the second most common (2.5%–31% cases), followed by the left lateral lobe (2.5%–13%). A case of left medial LLT was also described.[75] In some cases, 2 lobes can be involved.[69,70,72] The torsed lobe can be positioned either cranially or caudally to the pylorus.[70]

LLT can be managed either medically or surgically. Liver lobectomy is typically considered the best therapeutic option, with 77.2% to 100% survival rates.[69–72] However, life-threatening complications can occur in the perioperative and postoperative period: massive hemorrhage, anesthetic mortality, or postoperative multiorgan failure attributed to SIRS.[69–72] Perianesthetic mortality was as high as 17% in a retrospective study.[69] The paracostal approach described by Leonard and colleagues (2022)[71] may be preferred to the ventral midline approach when the caudate lobe is involved as the authors observed no complications and a quicker return of appetite with that technique. Postoperatively, histology and bacterial culture should be submitted to investigate underlying conditions and confirm the diagnosis. Bacteriology was rarely performed in the available literature and yielded no bacterial growth in most cases except for 1 occurrence where *Streptococcus epidermidis* was isolated.[69,70,72] Biopsies of unaffected liver lobes can also be considered as hepatocellular degeneration or necrosis; hepatitis or serositis were observed in other liver lobes in several rabbits in a retrospective study.[69]

Medical management involves fluid therapy, pain management, antimicrobials, syringe feeding, and supportive care. Depending on studies, survival rate with medical treatment only varied from 43% to 80%. In 1 study, recurrent episodes of GIS for 1 to 2 months after hospital stay was reported for patients treated medically.[72] Although no significant difference in survival rates between medical and surgical treatments was noted in the literature, a study observed that the median survival time was significantly shorter with medical treatment compared with surgery; medically managed rabbits had a median survival time of 530 days versus 1452 days with surgery.[69,70]

Overall, the reported survival rate is 61% to 75%.[69,70] Poorer outcomes were found associated with the degree of anemia. Rabbits were found to be significantly less likely to survive at 7 days when they had moderate to severe anemia (packed cell volume [PCV] < 26%) in 1 study,[69] and a 12% increase in odds of poor outcome was associated with each single percent decrease in PCV in another.[70] Decreased odds of survival were also associated with each additional day without defecating, with each additional mmol/L increase in BUN and with higher heart rates.[69,70] Caudate LLT had a significantly better prognosis than right LLT.[69]

HEPATOBILIARY NEOPLASIA

Biliary neoplasms have been described as case reports and as part of retrospective studies. Biliary cystadenomas seem to be most commonly reported. A bile duct adenoma and a biliary hamartoma with cholelithiasis were also reported.[76–80] In a retrospective of neoplastic and nonneoplastic lesions in rabbits, biliary neoplasms were described as comparatively common in rabbits from 4 to 8 year old.[79] Biliary cystadenomas have been described as case reports and were causing signs of GIS. They were both successfully removed surgically.[77,80]

Primary hepatic neoplasms are also reported, including cholangiocellular adenocarcinomas, soft tissue sarcomas, hepatic lymphoma, and cholangiosarcoma.[78,79] The liver is also a common site of metastasis.[78]

DISEASES OF THE PANCREAS

Pancreatic disorders are very scantly reported in the literature. Pancreatitis associated with systemic infections has been described such as with systemic toxoplasmosis.[68] Neoplasms of the pancreas seem rare. Histopathological retrospective studies mention few cases, and prevalence was less than 0.1% in a study.[78] Reported neoplasms include pancreatic acinar adenocarcinoma,[79] pancreatic adenocarcinoma with metastasis to the peritoneum, liver, gall bladder and kidneys,[78] and insulinoma.[15,81] Pancreatic nodular hyperplasia was also found postmortem in a rabbit.[78] As most cases have been reported as part of retrospective studies of histopathological results, there is very limited data regarding clinical signs, except for the insulinoma case. This rabbit was diagnosed at 9 years of age and was presenting GIS signs and intermittent neurologic signs (frantic movements, running into walls, slipping and falling over, and temporary weakness). Persistent hypoglycemia and concomitantly elevated insulin were considered diagnostic and treatment with prednisolone allowed for clinical remission for 1.5 years. Diagnosis was confirmed upon necropsy.[81]

SUMMARY

Digestive disorders are common in rabbits and can be either primary or secondary to a variety of causes. GIS is not a diagnosis but rather a syndrome that must be differentiated from GI obstruction, and the underlying cause for GIS must be investigated. More published data has become available in the last decade about other diseases affecting the GI tract of rabbits, including liver lobe torsion, RHDV, or appendicitis. Clinical signs for GI diseases in rabbits are often nonspecific, and diagnostic imaging and blood work are often warranted to achieve a diagnosis and determine a specific treatment plan.

CLINICS CARE POINTS

- Gastrointestinal disorders are a common cause of emergency presentation in rabbits.
- Gastrointestinal stasis (GIS) syndrome frequently occurs secondary to other diseases in rabbits and attempts should be made at identifying the underlying cause.
- GIS syndrome and gastrointestinal obstructions can initially present similarly and should be differentiated using a combination of clinical indicators, blood indicators, and radiographs. Additional imaging modalities, such as ultrasound or computed tomography scan, can also be used.
- Infectious diseases are overall less common than noninfectious diseases, but rabbit hemorrhagic disease has become worldwide and requires consideration given the risk for outbreaks.
- Clinicians should be aware of specific conditions such as liver lobe torsion or appendicitis when assessing a rabbit with GIS syndrome.

DISCLOSURE

The authors have nothing to disclose.

REFERENCES

1. Tokashiki EY, Rahal SC, Melchert A, et al. Retrospective study of conditions grouped by body systems in pet rabbits. J Exot Pet Med 2019;29:207–11.
2. O'Neill DG, Craven HC, Brodbelt DC, et al. Morbidity and mortality of domestic rabbits (Oryctolagus cuniculus) under primary veterinary care in England. Vet Rec 2020;186(14):451.
3. Robinson NJ, Lyons E, Grindlay D, et al. Veterinarian nominated common conditions of rabbits and Guinea pigs compared with published literature. Vet Sci 2017;4(4). https://doi.org/10.3390/vetsci4040058.
4. Smith SM. 13 - gastrointestinal physiology and nutrition of rabbits. In: Quesenberry KE, Orcutt CJ, Mans C, et al, editors. Ferrets, rabbits, and rodents. 4th edition. Louisville (MO): W.B. Saunders; 2020. p. 162–73.
5. Kohles M. Gastrointestinal anatomy and physiology of select exotic companion mammals. Vet Clin North Am Exot Anim Pract 2014;17(2):165–78.
6. Reusch B. Rabbit gastroenterology. Vet Clin North Am Exot Anim Pract 2005;8(2):351–75.
7. Varga Smith M. 5 - digestive disorders. In: Varga Smith M, editor. Textbook of rabbit medicine. 3rd edition. Elsevier; 2023. p. 156–91.
8. Huynh M, Vilmouth S, Gonzalez MS, et al. Retrospective cohort study of gastrointestinal stasis in pet rabbits. Vet Rec 2014;175(9):225.
9. Oparil KM, Gladden JN, Babyak JM, et al. Clinical characteristics and short-term outcomes for rabbits with signs of gastrointestinal tract dysfunction: 117 Cases (2014-2016). J Am Vet Med Assoc 2019;255(7):837–45.
10. Oglesbee BL, Lord B. 14 - gastrointestinal diseases of rabbits. In: Quesenberry KE, Orcutt CJ, Mans C, et al, editors. Ferrets, rabbits, and rodents. 4th edition. Louisville (MO): W.B. Saunders; 2020. p. 174–87.
11. DeCubellis J, Graham J. Gastrointestinal disease in Guinea pigs and rabbits. Vet Clin North Am Exot Anim Pract 2013;16(2):421–35.
12. Hasse K, Romano J, Emerson S, et al. Colocolic intussusception in a domestic rabbit (Oryctolagus cuniculus). J Exot Pet Med 2019;30:69–71.

13. Huynh M, Pignon C. Gastrointestinal disease in exotic small mammals. J Exot Pet Med 2013;22(2):118–31.
14. Ritzman TK. Diagnosis and clinical management of gastrointestinal conditions in exotic companion mammals (Rabbits, Guinea pigs, and Chinchillas). Vet Clin North Am Exot Anim Pract 2014;17(2):179–94.
15. Harcourt-Brown FM, Harcourt-Brown SF. Clinical value of blood glucose measurement in pet rabbits. Vet Rec 2012;170(26):674.
16. Debenham JJ, Brinchmann T, Sheen J, et al. Radiographic diagnosis of small intestinal obstruction in pet rabbits (*Oryctolagus cuniculus*): 63 cases. J Small Anim Pract 2019;60(11):691–6.
17. Schuhmann B, Cope I. Medical treatment of 145 cases of gastric dilatation in rabbits. Vet Rec 2014;175(19):484.
18. Brezina T, Fehr M, Neumüller M, et al. Acid-base-balance status and blood gas analysis in rabbits with gastric stasis and gastric dilation. J Exot Pet Med 2020;32:18–26.
19. Feldman ER, Singh B, Mishkin NG, et al. Effects of cisapride, buprenorphine, and their combination on gastrointestinal transit in New Zealand white rabbits. J Am Assoc Lab Anim Sci 2021;60(2):221–8.
20. Di Giuseppe M, Faraci L, Luparello M, et al. Omental torsion in a rabbit (Oryctolagus cuniculus). J Exot Pet Med 2016;25(2):163–7.
21. Gleeson M, Chen S, Fabiani M, et al. Mesenteric root and cecal torsion in a domestic rabbit (*Oryctolagus cuniculus*). J Exot Pet Med 2019;28:76–81.
22. McCready J, Gardhouse S, Barboza T, et al. Surgical resection of an enteric duplication cyst in a domestic rabbit (*Oryctolagus cuniculus*). J Exot Pet Med 2020;35:34–7.
23. Bertram CA, Müller K, Halter L, et al. Pseudodiverticula of the small intestine associated with idiopathic smooth muscle hypertrophy in domestic rabbits (*Oryctolagus cuniculus*). Vet Pathol 2019;56(1):152–6.
24. Bertram CA, Barth SA, Glockner B, et al. Intestinal *Mycobacterium avium* infection in pet dwarf Rabbits (*Oryctolagus cuniculus*). J Comp Pathol 2020;180:73–8.
25. Magnotti J, Bland D, Garner MM, et al. Primary intestinal lymphoma in rabbits. J Comp Pathol 2022;195:28–33.
26. Steinagel AC, Oglesbee BL. Clinicopathological and radiographic indicators for orogastric decompression in rabbits presenting with intestinal obstruction at a referral hospital (2015-2018). Vet Rec 2023;192(5):e2481.
27. Sheen JC, Sladakovic I, Finch S. Prognostic indicators for survival in surgically managed small intestinal obstruction in pet pabbits: 141 presentations (2011-2021). J Am Vet Med Assoc 2023;261(12):1–10.
28. Di Girolamo N. Prognostic value of rectal temperature at hospital admission in client-owned rabbits. J Am Vet Med Assoc 2016;248(3):288–97.
29. Böttcher A, Muller K. Radiological and laboratory prognostic parameters for gastric dilation in rabbits (*Oryctolagus cuniculus*). Vet Rec 2024;194(5):e3827.
30. Huckins GL, Tournade C, Patson C, et al. Lidocaine constant rate infusion improves the probability of survival in rabbits with gastrointestinal obstructions: 64 cases (2012-2021). J Am Vet Med Assoc 2024;262(1):61–7.
31. Zoller G, Di Girolamo N, Huynh M. Evaluation of blood urea nitrogen concentration and anorexia as predictors of nonsurvival in client-owned rabbits evaluated at a veterinary referral center. J Am Vet Med Assoc 2019;255(2):200–4.
32. Huynh M, Boyeaux A, Pignon C. Assessment and care of the critically ill rabbit. Vet Clin North Am Exot Anim Pract 2016;19(2):379–409.

33. Pignon C. 17 - rabbit basic surgery. In: Varga Smith M, editor. Textbook of rabbit medicine. 3rd edition. Elsevier; 2023. p. 401–10.

34. Bennett RA. Rabbit soft tissue surgery. Surgery of Exotic Animals 2021;240–76.

35. Szabo Z, Bradley K, Cahalane AK. Rabbit soft tissue surgery. Vet Clin North Am Exot Anim Pract 2016;19(1):159–88.

36. Guzman DS-M, Graham JE, Keller K, et al. Colonic obstruction following ovario-hysterectomy in rabbits: 3 cases. J Exot Pet Med 2015;24(1):112–9.

37. Lamb S. Large bowel resection and anastomosis in a domestic rabbit following obstruction. J Exot Pet Med 2017;26(3):224–9.

38. Fujiwara H, Uchida K, Takahashi M. Occurrence of granulomatous appendicitis in rabbits. Jikken Dobutsu 1987;36(3):277–80.

39. Mullink JW, Nikkels RJ. Mycotic appendicitis in rabbit mucoid enteropathy. Short communication. Z Versuchstierkd 1977;19(1–2):52–4.

40. Di Girolamo N, Petrini D, Szabo Z, et al. Clinical, surgical, and pathological findings in client-owned rabbits with histologically confirmed appendicitis: 19 cases (2015–2019). J Am Vet Med Assoc 2022;260(1):82–93.

41. Jekl V, Piskovska A, Drnkova I, et al. Case report: spontaneous appendicitis with suspected involvement of *Klebsiella variicola* in two pet rabbits. Front Vet Sci 2021;8:779517.

42. Longo M, Thierry F, Eatwell K, et al. Ultrasound and computed tomography of sacculitis and appendicitis in a rabbit. Vet Radiol Ultrasound 2018;59(5): E56–e60.

43. De Zan G, Bano L, Vascellari M, et al. Zygomycotic appendicitis in commercial fattening rabbits. J Comp Path 2014;150(1):95.

44. Nicoletti A, Di Girolamo N, Zeyen U, et al. Ultrasound morphology of cecal appendix in pet rabbits. J Ultrasound 2018;21(4):287–91.

45. Flenghi L, Bernhard C, Levrier C, et al. Rectal prolapse in two rabbits (*Oryctolagus cuniculi*) with rectal neoplasia. J Exot Pet Med 2021;39:64–7.

46. Asin J, Calvete C, Uzal FA, et al. Rabbit hemorrhagic disease virus 2, 2010–2023: a review of global detections and affected species. J Vet Diagn Invest 2024; 36(5):617–37.

47. Abade dos Santos FA, Pinto A, Burgoyne T, et al. Spillover events of rabbit haemorrhagic disease virus 2 (recombinant GI.4P-GI.2) from Lagomorpha to Eurasian badger. Transboundary and Emerging Diseases 2022;69(3):1030–45.

48. Bao S, An K, Liu C, et al. Rabbit hemorrhagic disease virus isolated from diseased alpine musk deer (Moschus sifanicus). Viruses 2020;12(8):897.

49. Harcourt-Brown N, Silkstone M, Whitbread TJ, et al. RHDV2 epidemic in UK pet rabbits. Part 1: clinical features, gross post mortem and histopathological findings. J Small Anim Pract 2020;61(7):419–27.

50. Gleeson M, Petritz OA. Emerging infectious diseases of rabbits. Veterinary Clinics 2020;23(2):249–61.

51. Williams LBA, Edmonds SE, Kerr SR, et al. Clinical and pathologic findings in an outbreak in rabbits of natural infection by rabbit hemorrhagic disease virus 2 in the northwestern United States. J Vet Diagn Invest 2021;33(4):732–5.

52. Calvete C, Sarto MP, Iguacel L, et al. Infectivity of rabbit haemorrhagic disease virus excreted in rabbit faecal pellets. Vet Microbiol 2021;257:109079.

53. Abade dos Santos FA, Magro C, Carvalho CL, et al. A potential atypical case of rabbit haemorrhagic disease in a dwarf rabbit. Animals 2021;11(1):40.

54. Bonvehí C, Ardiaca M, Montesinos A, et al. Clinicopathologic findings of naturally occurring Rabbit Hemorrhagic Disease Virus 2 infection in pet rabbits. Vet Clin Pathol 2019;48(1):89–95.

55. Pinto FF, Abrantes J, Ferreira PG, et al. Case series: four fatal rabbit hemorrhagic disease virus infections in urban pet rabbits. Front Vet Sci 2023;10:1144227.

56. Phouratsamay A, Barbarino A, Marolles G, et al. Successful medical management of a rabbit haemorrhagic disease virus 2 infection in a pet rabbit (*Oryctolagus cuniculus*). J Exot Pet Med 2024. https://doi.org/10.1053/j.jepm.2024.09.003.

57. Marschang RE, Weider K, Erhard H, et al. Rabbit hemorrhagic disease viruses detected in pet rabbits in a commercial laboratory in Europe. J Exot Pet Med 2018;27(4):27–30.

58. Albini S, Hetzel U, Cavadini P, et al. Inconspicuous post-mortem findings in rabbits from Switzerland naturally -infected with Rabbit Haemorrhagic -Disease Virus 2. Schweiz Arch Tierheilkd 2022;164(5):375–83.

59. Hänske GG, König P, Schuhmann B, et al. Death in four RHDV2-vaccinated pet rabbits due to rabbit haemorrhagic disease virus 2 (RHDV2). J Small Anim Pract 2021;62(8):700–3.

60. Harcourt-Brown FM, Harcourt-Brown N, Joudou LM. RHDV2 epidemic in UK pet rabbits. Part 2: PCR results and correlation with vaccination status. J Small Anim Pract 2020;61(8):487–93.

61. Katayama A, Miyazaki A, Okazaki N, et al. An outbreak of rabbit hemorrhagic disease (RHD) caused by Lagovirus europaeus GI.2/rabbit hemorrhagic disease virus 2 (RHDV2) in Ehime, Japan. J Vet Med Sci 2021;83(6):931–4.

62. Scarin G, Daly JM, Morey-Matamalas A, et al. Rabbit haemorrhagic disease virus type 2: how is the disease evolving in the UK? J Comp Pathol 2023;203:88.

63. Hrynkiewicz R, Bębnowska D, Kauppinen A, et al. Occurrence of lagovirus europaeus (rabbit hemorrhagic disease virus) in domestic rabbits in Southwestern Poland in 2019: case Report. Microbiol Spectr 2022;10(6). 022988-e2322.

64. Carvalho CL, Duarte EL, Monteiro M, et al. Challenges in the rabbit haemorrhagic disease 2 (RHDV2) molecular diagnosis of vaccinated rabbits. Vet Microbiol 2017;198:43–50.

65. Mlakar Hrženjak N, Zadravec M, Švara T, et al. Hepatic coccidiosis in two pet rabbits. J Exot Pet Med 2021;36:53–6.

66. Huismans M, Hermans K, Stock E. Ultrasonographic diagnosis of hepatic coccidiosis in rabbits. Vlaams Diergen Tijds 2022;91(2):55–61.

67. Graham-Brown J, Gilmore P, Harcourt-Brown F, et al. Lethal cysticercosis in a pet rabbit. Vet Rec Case Rep 2018;6(3):e000634.

68. Teo XH, Garrett KB, Akingbade G, et al. Systemic toxoplasmosis in 2 domestic rabbits in Georgia, United States. J Vet Diagn Invest 2024;10406-387241251834. https://doi.org/10.1177/10406387241251834.

69. Ozawa SM, Graham JE, Guzman DS, et al. Clinicopathological findings in and prognostic factors for domestic rabbits with liver lobe torsion: 82 cases (2010-2020). J Am Vet Med Assoc 2022;260(11):1334–42.

70. Sheen JC, Vella D, Hung L. Retrospective analysis of liver lobe torsion in pet rabbits: 40 cases (2016-2021). Vet Rec 2022;191(7):e1971.

71. Leonard KC, Zhao Q, Taber RH, et al. Paracostal versus ventral midline approach for caudate liver lobectomy in the rabbit. Vet Surg 2022;51(6):920–8.

72. Graham JE, Orcutt CJ, Casale SA, et al. Liver lobe torsion in rabbits: 16 Cases (2007 to 2012). J Exot Pet Med 2014;23(3):258–65.

73. Daggett A, Loeber S, Le Roux AB, et al. Computed tomography with hounsfield unit assessment is useful in the diagnosis of liver lobe torsion in pet rabbits (*Oryctolagus cuniculus*). Vet Radiol Ultrasound 2021;62(2):210–7.

74. Stock E, Vanderperren K, Moeremans I, et al. Use of contrast-enhanced ultrasonography in the diagnosis of a liver lobe torsion in a rabbit (*Oryctolagus cuniculus*). Vet Radiol Ultrasound 2020;61(4):31–5.

75. Chapple AR, Mikoni NA, Dutton CJ, et al. Left medial liver lobe torsion and post-operative acute gastric rupture in a 2.5-year-old male-castrated flemish giant rabbit (*Oryctolagus cuniculus*). Vet Radiol Ultrasound 2024;65(1):14–8.

76. Starost MF. Solitary biliary hamartoma with cholelithiasis in a domestic rabbit (*Oryctolagus cuniculus*). Vet Pathol 2007;44(1):92–5.

77. DeCubellis J, Kruse AM, McCarthy RJ, et al. Biliary cystadenoma in a rabbit (*Oryctolagus cuniculus*). J Exot Pet Med 2010;19(2):177–82.

78. Bertram CA, Bertram B, Bartel A, et al. Neoplasia and tumor-like lesions in pet rabbits (*Oryctolagus cuniculus*): a retrospective analysis of cases between 1995 and 2019. Vet Pathol 2021;58(5):901–11.

79. Baum B. Not just uterine adenocarcinoma-neoplastic and non-neoplastic masses in domestic pet rabbits (*Oryctolagus cuniculus*): a review. Vet Pathol 2021;58(5): 890–900.

80. Sabater M, Mancinelli E, Stidworthy MF. Biliary cystadenoma in a male domestic Dutch rabbit (*Oryctolagus cuniculus*). Vet Rec Case Rep 2014;2(1):e000037.

81. Foxx J, Mans C, Strunk A, et al. Long-term medical management of insulinoma in a rabbit. J Exot Pet Med 2022;42:47–9.

Ferret Gastroenterology

Mette L. Halck, DVM, Danish specialist (Small Mammal)[a,b,*],
Yvonne R.A. van Zeeland, DVM, MVR, PhD, Dip ECZM (Avian, Small Mammal)[c], Nico J. Schoemaker, DVM, PhD, Dip ECZM (Small Mammal, Avian)[c]

KEYWORDS

- Zoonosis • Foreign body • Gastritis • Reflux • Regurgitation • Vomitus • Diarrhea
- Melena

KEY POINTS

- Clinical signs of gastrointestinal disease in ferrets are often nonspecific and may include lethargy, anorexia, vomiting, and diarrhea. A systematic history-taking and work-up is required to make a diagnosis.
- Ferrets are notorious for ingesting foreign bodies. While gastric and esophageal foreign bodies often can be removed with flexible endoscopy, exploratory surgery is often indicated for intestinal foreign bodies.
- Enteritis in adult ferrets is often bacterial in origin and caused by feeding raw, uncooked diets.
- Hypoglycemia, hypovolemia, hypothermia, and anemia are not uncommon findings in ferrets presenting with gastrointestinal disease, and fast and adequate correction of these is vital.

INTRODUCTION

Spontaneous gastrointestinal (GI) tract diseases are common in ferrets (*Mustela putorius furo*), and as a result, ferrets have been used extensively as animal models for human GI tract diseases like reflux, ulcers, and neoplasia.[1] Despite the large variation in etiology, GI disease can be difficult to differentiate on initial presentation. Hence, a thorough history, physical examination, and systematic diagnostic approach are the key to obtaining a correct diagnosis. This review discusses the general work-up for ferret GI disease, including history taking, physical examination, and diagnostic tests. Furthermore, specific GI tract pathologies are described in oral to aboral direction, including their diagnosis and therapy. Additionally, the review will provide a short

[a] Department of Veterinary Clinical Sciences, University of Copenhagen, Frederiksberg, Denmark; [b] University Hospital for Companion Animals, Dyrlægevej 16, Frederiksberg C, Denmark; [c] Division of Zoological Medicine, Department of Clinical Sciences, Faculty of Veterinary Medicine, Utrecht University, Yalelaan 1, 3584 CL Utrecht, The Netherlands
* Corresponding author. Dyrlægevej 16, 1870 Frederiksberg, Denmark.
E-mail address: mettehalck@sund.ku.dk

Vet Clin Exot Anim 28 (2025) 227–261
https://doi.org/10.1016/j.cvex.2024.11.002
1094-9194/25/© 2024 Elsevier Inc. All rights reserved, including those for text and data mining, AI training, and similar technologies.
vetexotic.theclinics.com

Abbreviations	
ALT	alanine aminotransferase
AP	alkaline phosphatase
AST	aspartate aminotransferase
CDV	canine distemper virus
CT	computed tomography
ECE	epizoonotic catarrhal enteritis
ELISA	enzyme-linked immunosorbent assay
FECV	ferret enteric coronavirus
GI	gastroinstestinal
IBD	inflammatory bowel disease
PCR	polymerase chain reaction
SARS-CoV-2	severe acute respiratory syndrome coronavirus 2

overview of the anatomy and physiology of the digestive tract and its key features, as these are instrumental for the correct interpretation of clinical and diagnostic findings.

FERRET GASTROINTESTINAL ANATOMY AND PHYSIOLOGY

Ferrets are obligate carnivores with a short, simple digestive tract. A rapid GI transit time (1–8 hours, average 3–4 hours) combined with a small body weight, make ferrets prone to hypoglycemia with prolonged feeding regimens or vomitus.[2,3] GI tract motility is affected by vagal tone, which becomes clinically important when manipulation during tracheal intubation inadvertently stimulates the vagal nerve and decreases GI motility.[4]

Adult ferrets have a typical carnivore dentition with 34 brachydont teeth; 2(3/3, 1/1, 3/3, 1/2; **Fig. 1**).[5,6] Well-developed masticatory muscles provide the ferret with a powerful bite, grasping the prey tightly. The tongue is long, free, and mobile, and with a predilection site for penetrating grass awns in working ferrets. Five pairs of major salivary glands open into the oral cavity—parotid, submandibular, sublingual, molar, and zygomatic.[7] Fights between hobs can cause mucoceles, when bite wounds damage the salivary gland or ducts. The stomach is simple but has considerable storage capacity (~50 mL/kg). Unlike many other small mammals, the ferret lower esophageal sphincter allows for reflux and emesis. The small intestinal lumen is narrow, increasing the risk of foreign body entrapment. The remaining small intestine cannot be distinguished and passes directly into the ascending colon since neither an ileocolic junction or cecum is present.[8] The colon is approximately 7 cm in total, and divided into an ascending, transverse, and descending part.[9,10] The rectum and anus are 2 and 1 cm long, respectively. An internal sphincter of smooth muscle is followed by an external voluntary sphincter of striated muscle that covers the anal sac ducts, which open at approximately 4 and 8 o'clock positions with the ferret in dorsal recumbency.[11]

DIAGNOSING GASTROINTESTINAL DISEASE
History, Physical Examination, and Clinical Signs

Clinical signs of GI disease are often unspecific and may include anorexia, weight loss, lethargy, dehydration, and nausea (see also **Table 1**). Other clinical signs that are more specific, although not pathognomonic, to GI disease are regurgitation, vomiting, diarrhea, and melena.[12] A detailed clinical history should be obtained, with emphasis on the duration and progression of clinical signs, appetite, stool appearance and defecation, vomitus/regurgitation, housing, nutrition, contact with other ferrets, and possible

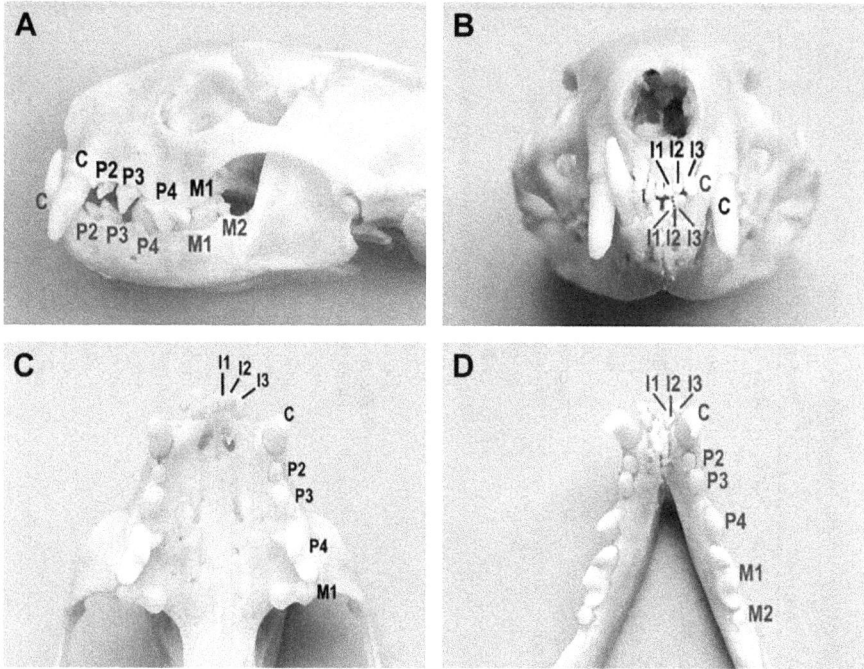

Fig. 1. Dentition of the ferret. Incisives (I), canines (C), premolars (P), molars (M) and their respective numbers are labeled. Note a number of dental abnormalities in this specimen, including malalignment of the incisors and blunting of the maxillary canine teeth. (*A*) Close-up of the dental arcades, lateral view. (*B*) Close-up of the dental arcades, rostral view. (*C*) Close-up of the maxillary arcades. Note the large carnassial tooth (fourth premolar or CT3) and the buccolingual direction of the molar tooth. (*D*) Close-up of the mandibular arcades. Note the large carnassial tooth (first molar or CT4) and that the second mandibular incisors are set back from the others. (*Courtesy of* Vittorio Capello, DVM. Previously published in "Johnson-Delaney CA. Diagnosis and treatment of dental disease in ferrets. J Exot Pet Med 2008;17(2):132-7".)

ingestion of toxins, drugs, or foreign bodies, which will greatly aid in the planning of any further workup and establishing a (differential) diagnosis. Asking the client to bring images or videos of excreted fluids and vomiting process can provide valuable information on color, consistency, and possible admixtures (eg, blood) in stool and/or vomit, as well as aid in differentiating regurgitation from vomiting, which can be challenging for clients as they may confuse reflux with gagging or coughing. Additionally, owners may not recognize pawing at the mouth as a sign of nausea.[13]

Due to their small body size, anorexic ferrets quickly become hypoglycemic, dehydrated, and hypothermic, especially if combined with fluid loss. Additionally, (prolonged) anorexia, vomiting, and/or diarrhea can lead to weight loss, muscle wasting, and depletion of fat reserves as a result of a negative energy balance. To discern whether aforementioned complicating sequela are present, a thorough physical examination, including at minimum an evaluation of mentation and alertness, body condition, posture, hydration status (skin turgor), pulse (frequency [200–400 bpm] quality), mucus membranes (color, moistness), capillary refill time, and body temperature (reference 37.8°–40°C [100–104°F]) will be needed.[14] Additionally, the physical examination should include a detailed examination of the digestive tract, including an

Table 1
Differential diagnosis, diagnostic work-up, and treatment options for common gastrointestinal disease presentations in ferrets

Clinical Sign	Differential Diagnoses	Diagnostic Work-Up Options	Treatment Options
Acute vomiting	GI foreign body Intoxication (food-related or other) Gastritis/gastroenteritis (eg, viral—coronavirus; bacterial—*Salmonella, E. coli*) Gastrointestinal (GI) obstruction/ileus Acute pancreatitis Acute renal failure Acute hepatitis Increased intracranial pressure (eg, head injury, meningitis) Motion sickness/vertigo Diabetic ketoacidosis (rare in ferrets) Sepsis, septic peritonitis	History (r/o toxicity, injury) Hematology and biochemistry (lipase, amylase, liver enzymes, bile acids, glucose, ketones, blood urea nitrogen [BUN], Ca, P, Na, K) Testing for specific pathogens Whole body radiographs Ultrasound Computed tomography Endoscopy (incl biopsy collection)	Anti-emetics: metoclopramide (Do not use in case of ileus/obstruction), maropitant Activated charcoal (in case of recent toxin ingestion) Laxatives (eg, lactulose) in case of trichobezoar Gastric protectants (eg, sucralfate) Antacids (eg, omeprazole, ranitidine) Antimicrobial therapy, for example, amoxicillin–clavulanic acid + metronidazole Nonsteroidal antiinflammatory drugs (meloxicam; CAVE: do not use in dehydrated patients or those with [suspected] gastrointestinal ulcers!) Assisted feeding Fluid therapy (if dehydrated, or diuresis is warranted eg, suspected intoxication or renal failure) Explorative laparotomy Endoscopic foreign body retrieval
Chronic vomiting	GI foreign body Gastric ulceration *Helicobacter mustelae* gastritis Gastritis/gastroenteritis Gastroparesis/delayed gastric emptying (eg, pyloric obstruction) GI neoplasia Azotemia (chronic renal insufficiency,	History Hematology and biochemistry (BUN, Ca, P, Ht, WBC, glucose, liver enzymes, bile acids, amylase, lipase, total protein, albumin, globulins, Na, K) (Contrast) radiography Fluoroscopy Ultrasound	Anti-emetics/prokinetics: metoclopramide, maropitant Antacids: omeprazole, ranitidine/cimetidine Gastric protectants, for example, sucralfate Antimicrobial therapy, for example, amoxicillin–clavulanic acid +

	Addisonian's disease) Hypoglycemia Chronic hepatitis/hepatopathy Hypercalcemia Drug-related Food allergy/hypersensitivity Pyometra Chronic pancreatitis Central nervous system disorders leading to increased intracranial pressure (eg, meningitis)	Computed Tomography Endoscopy PCR (gastric/duodenal biopsies, feces) Histopathology (silver stain) Elimination and challenge diet	metronidazole Nonsteroidal antiinflammatory drugs Iron supplements Assisted feeding Fluid therapy (forced diuresis) Endoscopic removal of foreign bodies Explorative laparotomy Chemotherapy
Regurgitation	Megaesophagus Hiatal herniation[a] Esophageal stricture[a] Myasthenia gravis Esophageal foreign body Esophageal neoplasia Gastric reflux	(Contrast) radiography Fluoroscopy Computed tomography Endoscopy Tensilon test Serology - Antibody titer for Myasthenia gravis (San Diego, California, USA)	Feed at higher position and maintain animal in vertical position for 10–15 min after a meal Prokinetics: metoclopramide Antacids: omeprazole, ranitidine/cimetidine Gastric protectants: sucralfate Endoscopic removal or surgical intervention
Diarrhea	Stress Foreign body ingestion (rubber, foam, plastic, other) Trichobezoar Bacterial infection (primary or secondary, eg, Salmonella spp E. coli, Clostridium spp, Campylobacter jejuni, Mycobacterium spp.) Proliferative bowel disease (Lawsonia, Desulfovibrio) Viral infection (eg, rotavirus, FECV, canine distemper) Parasitic disease: coccidiosis, giardiasis Neoplasia (lymphoma most common) Inflammatory bowel disease Food hypersensitivity/food intolerance	Signalment History Abdominal palpation Culture and sensitivity Fecal flotation, wet mount Cytology Elimination diet (Contrast) radiographs Ultrasound Endoscopy Histopathology of biopsies PCR testing (eg, Mycobacterium spp, FECV, rotavirus)	Modify living conditions Dietary adjustments, hypoallergenic diet Laxatives (eg, lactulose) Antimicrobial therapy, preferably based on culture and sensitivity results Antiparasitics: metronidazole, paromomycin, toltrazuril Antiinflammatories/immune suppressants (glucocorticoids) Assisted feeding (if anorectic) Fluid therapy (ORS, SC/IV/IO) Endoscopic retrieval of foreign objects Explorative laparotomy Chemotherapy

(continued on next page)

Table 1
(continued)

Clinical Sign	Differential Diagnoses	Diagnostic Work-Up Options	Treatment Options
Melena (confirm erythrocytes in the stool with a fecal occult blood test)	Gastritis Gastric or duodenal ulceration (eg, due to *Helicobacter mustelae*, renal azotemia) Gastric/intestinal neoplasia/polyp(s) Pancreatitis Parasitic infestation (eg, giardiasis, coccidiosis or cryptosporidiosis in young ferrets) Ulcerogenic medication Rodenticide poisoning Dysbiosis (eg, *Salmonella* spp) Sepsis	Complete history (drugs, known ingestion of toxins/foreign bodies) Fecal flotation, wet mount Hematology/biochemistry (coagulation profile) Whole body radiography Endoscopy Histopathology of biopsies	Discontinue medication Vitamin K (injections, oral) Antimicrobial therapy, preferably based on culture and sensitivity results; amoxicillin–clavulanic acid + metronidazole for *Helicobacter* Antiparasitics: metronidazole, paromomycin, toltrazuril Gastric protectants: sucralfate Antacids: omeprazole, ranitidine/cimetidine Antiinflammatories Iron supplements Fluid therapy Activated charcoal
Hematochezia (with formed or soft/diarrheic feces+/– mucus)	Constipation, too firm/dry feces Passage of foreign material Parasitic disease (giardiasis, coccidiosis, whip/hookworms) Bacterial colitis (eg, *Clostridium perfringens/difficile*, *Salmonella* spp, *Campylobacter jejuni*) Fungal colitis[a] Inflammatory bowel disease Perianal fistula Anal sac disease (infection or impaction) Coagulopathy (thrombocytopenia, thrombocytopathy, rodenticide intoxication) Rectal polyps, neoplasia, other rectal/anal growths Infiltrative neoplasia (primarily lymphoma)	Complete history (drugs, known ingestion of toxins/foreign bodies) Complete blood count (CBC), coagulation profile Fecal flotation, wet mount Culture and sensitivity FNA for cytology Radiographs Ultrasound Colonoscopy/proctoscopy Biopsy for histopathology	Dietary adjustments, hypoallergenic diet Laxatives (eg, lactulose) Cisapride (only if no physical obstruction present) Antimicrobial therapy (eg, metronidazole, sulfasalazine, tylosin), preferably based on culture and sensitivity results, where possible Antiparasitics (eg, fenbendazole, ronidazole, sulfonamides) Immunosuppressant drugs (eg, cyclosporin A, glucocorticoids) Chemotherapy Cryotherapy, laser therapy Surgical intervention

Dyschezia and tenesmus	Colonic disease (parasitism including coccidiosis, bacterial colitis, inflammatory bowel disease, stress colitis, food hypersensitivity, neoplasia, megacolon)	History	Laxatives (eg, lactulose)
		Fecal flotation, wet mount	Prokinetics (cisapride, only if no mechanical obstruction is present)
		Culture and sensitivity	
		CBC and biochemistry (frequently unremarkable)	Antiparasitics (eg, sulfonamides)
	Rectal/anal disease (eg, perianal fistula/hernia, rectal prolaps/stricture/polyp, proctitis, anal sacculitis, rectal/anal neoplasia)	FNA for cytology	Antimicrobial therapy, preferably based on culture and sensitivity
		Radiography	Antiinflammatory drugs (eg, sulfasalazine, prednisolone)
		Ultrasound	
	Prostatic disease (eg, related to hyperadrenocorticism)	Colonoscopy/proctoscopy	Immune modulatory drugs (cyclosporine A)
		Biopsy for histopathology	Chemotherapy
	Pelvic fracture, other trauma	Computed tomography	Cryotherapy, laser therapy
	Dysuria/stranguria		Surgical intervention
	Dystocia		

Abbreviations: BUN, blood urea nitrogen; Ca, calcium; FECV, ferret enteric coronavirus; FNA, fine needle aspiration; Ht, hematocrit; IO, intraosseus; IV, intravenous; K, potassium; Na, sodium; ORS, oral rehydration salts; P, phosphate; PCR, polymerase chain reaction; r/o, rule out; SC, subcutaneous; WBC, white blood cell count.
[a] Not previously diagnosed in ferrets.

evaluation of the oral cavity (including teeth, tongue), neck (esophageal or pharyngeal masses), abdomen (inspection, superficial and deep palpation, undulation), and perineal area. In case of suspected oropharyngeal pathology, a more thorough evaluation of these structures under sedation or anesthesia is warranted (**Fig. 2**).

Diagnostic Workup

The work-up for diagnosing GI disease in ferrets is mostly similar to that in dogs and cats, and may include a fecal examination, microbiological culture and sensitivity testing, hematology and biochemistry, whole body radiographs (with or without contrast), ultrasonography, computed tomography (CT), and/or endoscopy with biopsy collection for histopathology (see **Table 1**).

Fecal Examination: Screening for Pathogens, Parasitology, Culture and Sensitivity, and Fecal Occult Blood Test

A fecal examination is a relatively simple and inexpensive, yet a valuable tool that can be employed to identify the cause of gastrointestinal problems observed in a ferret. While parasitic diseases are relatively uncommon in ferrets, routine parasite testing should be performed in any ferret with diarrhea, hematochezia, or melena to exclude helminthiasis (eg, nematodiasis due to infestation with *Toxacara cati, Toxascaris leonina, Ancylostoma* spp, or cestodiasis due to infestation with *Mesocestoides* spp, *Dipylidium caninum*), or protozoal disease (eg, giardiasis, coccidiosis, cryptosporidiosis [particularly in young ferrets]). Such testing should include both a direct smear of fresh fecal material and flotation.

Microbiological culture and sensitivity of the stool can be useful to identify primary or secondary bacterial pathogens. For certain pathogens (eg, *Salmonella* spp.), the use of specific culture media or multiple-day testing (to increase the chance of detecting a pathogen that is shed intermittently) are recommended. Specific polymerase chain reaction (PCR) tests are also available to identify presence of ferret enteric coronavirus (FECV), canine distemper, rotavirus, *Helicobacter mustelae* (which is common in ferrets but difficult to culture), *Salmonella* spp, and *Mycobacterium* spp.

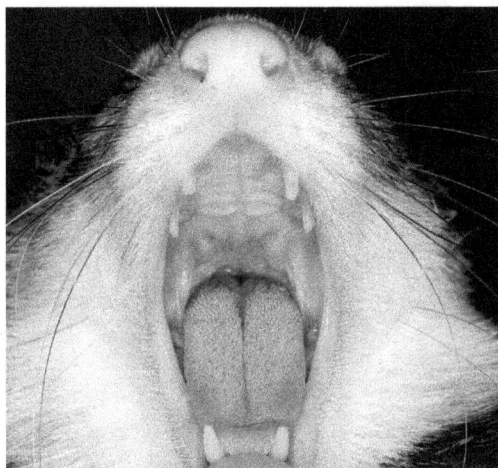

Fig. 2. Oral inspection in a ferret. Ferrets often open their mouths when being scruffed. If the oral cavity cannot be inspected sufficiently, sedation is needed for a more thorough inspection.

Some gastrointestinal diseases (eg, *Helicobacter*-related gastritis) can lead to hematochezia, but this may not be macroscopically visible. In such cases, fecal occult blood testing is helpful to confirm the presence of blood. It should be remembered that a single negative occult fecal blood test does not rule out gastrointestinal hemorrhage, as bleeding may be intermittent. Additionally, the ferret should be placed on a nonmeat diet (eg, Emeraid carnivore, Oxbow carnivore care) for at least 24 to 36 hours to avoid false-positive test results due to dietary heme.[12]

Hematology and Biochemistry

In many ferrets with GI disease, hematologic and biochemical changes will be reflective of dehydration, anorexia, and wasting that have occurred due to ongoing disease. Nevertheless, a complete blood count and chemistry panel can help to provide clues to diagnose and assess the overall clinical condition of the patient. If larger volumes are needed, the jugular vein or cranial vena cava can be used (sedation or anesthesia is recommended), while the cephalic or saphenous veins can be sampled in case smaller volumes are required or if clotting disorders are suspected. In healthy ferrets, approximately 10% of the total blood volume (4–6 mL) can be safely collected, but if anemia and/or hypovolemia are present or the animal is critically ill, it is safer to limit this volume to 5% (2–3 mL). With repeated samplings, the total blood volume sampled ideally is recorded to avoid iatrogenic anemia.

Anemia is commonly found in ferrets with severe GI bleeding or chronic inflammation. Evaluation of the reticulocyte count can help to differentiate regenerative (eg, in case of bleeding) from nonregenerative anemia (eg, in case of chronic inflammation). Similar to dogs and cats, the mean cell volume, mean cell hemoglobin, and mean cell hemoglobin concentration can be used to gain further insight into the size of the erythrocytes and their hemoglobin concentration, which can be helpful to discern between the various causes of anemia. Leukocyte counts can be decreased in case of acute infections, while moderate leukocytosis is often present with chronic infections Neutrophilia and/or monocytosis may also be observed.

In ferrets, alanine aminotransferase (ALT), aspartate aminotransferase (AST), alkaline phosphatase (AP), bilirubin, and bile acids can be used to assess liver function. Increases in AST and ALT can also be observed in animals with anorexia or primary intestinal disease. To evaluate kidney function, blood urea nitrogen, calcium, phosphate, potassium, and sodium can be evaluated. Creatinine has a very low sensitivity in ferrets and may remain normal in animals with severe kidney damage. Parameters used in many other species for diagnosing exocrine pancreatic insufficiency or pancreatitis are not properly established in ferrets. However, an increase in lipase (reference: 73–351 U/l) or amylase (reference: 19–62 U/l) can be associated with pancreatitis.[14] Glucose values <72 mg/dL (<4 mmol/L) in animals that have been fasted for 4 to 6 hours are highly suggestive of an insulinoma, although differentials may include severe septicemia, cachexia, or liver failure. Hypoproteinemia is frequently diagnosed in ferrets with GI disease and should ideally be corrected prior to anesthesia and surgical intervention (**Table 2**).[15] Elevated total protein can be seen in animals with acute or chronic inflammation, dehydration, liver disease, or lymphoma.

Diagnostic Imaging

Radiography can be useful in the diagnosis of GI disease. Survey radiographs can often reveal evidence of GI masses, thickened bowel loops, or abnormal gas patterns suggestive of foreign body obstruction or enteritis. Patency of the GI tract and transit time, megaesophagus, and obstructions are easily diagnosed with serial contrast

Table 2
Supportive care and medications commonly used in gastrointestinal disease in ferrets

	Product/Medication	Dose
Nutritional support (syringe-fed or via a nasogastric, esophageal or duodenojejunostomy tube)	Emeraid carnivore Oxbow critical care carnivore Royal Canine Recovery Liquid Trovet Recovery Liquid	Calculate a minimum daily intake of 400 kcal/kg BW, and divide into 4–6 feedings/day
Fluid therapy	Crystalloids, for example, lactated Ringer's	Replacement fluid volume (mL) with crystalloids = Estimated dehydration deficit (%) × body weight (kg) × 1000; maintenance = 70 mL/kg/day; PO/SC/IV/IO
	Colloids, for example, Hetastarch	3–5 mL/kg over 5 min IV/IO (for patients that are severely hypovolemic or hypoproteinemic)
	Glucose 5%, dextrose 2.5%–5%	0.25–2 mL IV (for hypoglycemia)
	Blood	6–12 mL/kg/h IV/IO (transfusion may be needed for anemic patients, PCV<25%); mix 1 mL of anticoagulant (citrate) with 6 mL of donor blood
Nutritional supplements	Cobalamin	25 µg/kg q7d SC × 6 wk, then q14 d SC × 6 wk (chronic diarrhea, with cobalamin malabsorption)
	Glutamine	0.5 g/kg q24 h PO (enterocyte supplementation with starvation)
	Iron dextran	10 mg/animal IM once (iron deficiency anemia)
	Pet-Tinic	0.2 mL/kg q24 h PO (iron deficiency anemia)
	Vitamin B12	½ capsule Cobalaplex q24 h PO
	Vitamin K	2.5–5 mg/kg q8–12 h SC/PO
Antacids/proton pump inhibitors	Cimetidine	5–10 mg/kg q6–8 h PO/SC/IM/IV
	Famotidine	0.25–2.5 mg/kg q24 h PO/SC/IV
	Omeprazole	1 mg/kg q12–24 h PO
	Ranitidine	2–5 mg/kg q12 h PO
Anti-diarrheal drugs	Loperamide	0.2 mg/kg q12 h PO

Category	Drug	Dosage
Antiemetics	Maropitant	1 mg/kg q24 h PO/IM
	Metoclopramide	0.2–1 mg/kg q6–12 h SC/PO/IV
	Ondansetron	0.5–1 mg/kg q12–24 h IM/IV/PO
Emetics	Apomorphine	0.04–0.2 mg/kg SC
	Ipecac (7%)	2.2–6.6 mL/animal PO
Gastrointestinal protectants	Bismuth subcitrate	6 mg/kg q12 h PO
	Bismuth subsalicylate	17.5 mg/kg q8 h PO
	Kaolin/pectin	1–2 mL/kg q2–6 h PO
	Sucralfate	25–125 mg/kg q6–12 h PO (give before meal, not simultaneous with other medication)
Laxatives	Feline hairball laxative	1–2 mL/animal q48 h PO
	Lactulose	0.15–0.75 mL/kg q12 h PO
Motility enhancers	Cisapride	0.5 mg/kg q8–12 h PO
	Metoclopramide	0.2–1 mg/kg q6–12 h SC/PO/IV
Antiparasitic drugs	Fenbendazole	20 mg/kg q24 h PO × 5 d (nematodiasis)
	Metronidazole	15–20 mg/kg q12 h PO × 5–14 d (gastrointestinal protozoa, eg, *Giardia*)
	Nitazoxanide	5 mg/kg q12 h PO (cryptosporidiosis)
	Paromomycin	165 mg/kg q12 h PO × 5 d (cryptosporidiosis)
	Piperazine citrate	50–100 mg/kg q14 d PO (nematodiasis)
	Ponazuril	30–50 mg/kg q24 h PO × 3–7 d (coccidiosis)
	Praziquantel	5–10 mg/kg PO/SC, repeat in 10 d (cestodiasis)
	Sulfamethoxine	25 mg/kg q24 h PO × 21 d (coccidiosis)
	Toltrazuril	20 mg/kg q24 h PO × 3–7 d (coccidiosis)
Antimicrobial agents	Amoxicillin + clavulanic acid	12.5–25 mg/kg q8–12 h PO
	Azithromycin	5 mg/kg q24 h PO
	Chloramphenicol	25–50 mg/kg q12 h PO/SC/IM/IV (14 d minimum for proliferative bowel disease)
	Clarithromycin	12.5 mg/kg q8–12 h PO
	Enrofloxacine	5–10 mg/kg q12 h PO/SC/IM
	Gentamycin	2–5 mg/kg q12–24 h PO/SC/IM/IV
	Metronidazole	15–20 mg/kg q12 h PO
	Trimethoprim/sulfa	15–30 mg/kg q12 h PO/SC
	Tylosin	5–10 mg/kg q12 h PO/SC/IM/IV

(continued on next page)

Table 2
(continued)

	Product/Medication	Dose
Analgesics	Buprenorphine	0.01–0.05 mg/kg q6–12h transmucosal/SC/IM/IV
	Butorphanol	0.05–0.5 mg/kg q8–12 h SC/IM (may cause sedation in higher dosages)
	Carprofen	1–5 mg/g q12–24 h PO (use with caution in dehydrated animals or those with gastritis/enteritis)
	Lidocaine	2 mg/kg q12–24 h topically
	Meloxicam	0.1–0.3 mg/kg q24 h PO/SC/IM (use with caution in dehydrated animals or those with gastritis/enteritis)
	Tramadol	5–10 mg/kg q12–24 h PO
Immune-modulating drugs	Azathioprine	0.9 mg/kg q24–7 2 h PO (chronic IBD, combine with prednisone)
	Cyclosporine	4–6 mg/kg q12 h PO
	Prednisone	0.5–2 mg/kg q12–24 h PO
	Sulfasalazine	62.5–125 mg/kg q8–12 h PO (colitis)
Miscellaneous	Activated charcoal	1–3 g/kg PO (adsorbent for gastrointestinal tract toxins/drug overdose)
	Cyproheptadine	0.5 mg/kg q12 h PO (appetite stimulant)
	Pyridostigmine	1 mg/kg q8–12 h PO (myasthenia gravis)

Abbreviations: IBD, inflammatory bowel disease; IM, intramuscular; IO, intraosseus; IV, intravenous; PCV, packed cell volume; PO, per os, orally; SC, subcutaneous.

radiographs (8–13 mL/kg, barium sulfate).[12] However, contrast should not be used in a sedated or anesthetized ferret without intubation as ferrets are likely to regurgitate and aspirate. Additionally, contrast agents such as barium can be damaging to the endoscopic equipment and should be avoided if endoscopy is planned.

Similar to dogs and cats, abdominal ultrasonography and CT can be extremely helpful for detailed visualization and evaluation of the size, shape, and density of the different parts of the GI tract and surrounding organs. Of the 2 techniques, ultrasound is cheaper and more readily available in clinical practice, but its sensitivity is highly operator dependent.[16] Additionally, newer technologies such as CT scans have become more affordable and available in private practices. Moreover, the disadvantage of the higher cost associated with CT scans is quickly outweighed by the fact that scans can be sent for external evaluation by a veterinary radiologist, if in doubt. Nevertheless, each technique has its merit for evaluating GI disease, as ultrasound is better at visualizing the individual intestinal layers, tissue blood flow, GI motility, and movement of chymus, while CT is superior at visualizing GI diameter, dilations, gastric trichobezoars, and foreign bodies.[15,17]

Endoscopy and Biopsy Collection for Histopathology

Despite their narrow diameter, the esophagus, stomach, duodenum, and upper jejunum are reachable by semiflexible or flexible endoscopy, allowing direct visualization of the intestinal lining and aiding in the diagnosis of, for example, gastric ulcers (**Fig. 3**). Similarly, colonoscopy is useful for visualization and obtaining biopsies during the diagnostic work up of chronic diarrhea, hematochezia on formed feces, or severe constipation. Because of the short large intestine, colonoscopy can be further advanced to a jejunoileoscopy. Flexible gastroscopy is commonly performed using a 100 cm long, 3 mm diameter bronchofiber flexible endoscope with a working channel of 1.2 mm, which is valuable for foreign body retrieval and biopsy sampling of the mucosa to help confirm the underlying cause of GI disease.[18] Alternatively, exploratory laparotomy can be considered for biopsy collection, especially in case of increased risk of intestinal wall perforation (eg, in case of intraluminal masses).

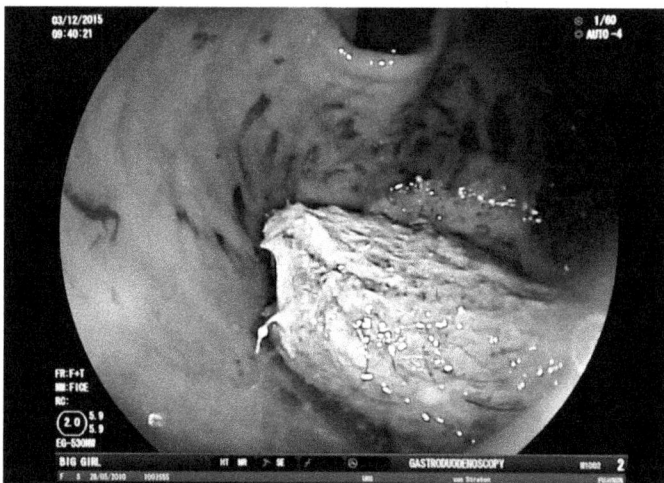

Fig. 3. Gastroscopic view of a hairball covered in sucralfate in a 5.5-year-old female chemically neutered ferret that was presented with chronic vomiting, anorexia, and weight loss.

Surgical biopsy also gives the added advantage of allowing visualization and targeting of grossly abnormal sections, and collection of full-thickness samples. Laparoscopy can be used for visualization and biopsy of the liver and/or pancreas via True-cut needle or simple clamshell or punch-style biopsy forceps.

For gastroduodenoscopy, a 4 to 6 hours fasting period will generally suffice, whereas colonoscopy can generally be accomplished following either a 12-hour fast or 8-hour provision of liquid carnivore diets (see **Table 2**) followed by a 4-hour fast. In fasted animals, sporadic monitoring of blood glucose may be considered to detect episodes of hypoglycemia, which should be treated prior to induction of anesthesia. During anesthesia, repeated boluses using a maximum of 20 mL/kg of warmed saline is introduced into the large intestine using a red rubber tube or large diameter urinary catheter, to empty remaining fecal content before commencing with the colonoscopy.[18]

SPECIFIC GASTROINTESTINAL DISEASE CONDITIONS
Dental Disease

Dental disease is common in ferrets, with a presentation, pathogenesis, and treatment similar to dental disease in dogs and cats.[19] Due to the high prevalence of acquired dental disease, a thorough inspection of the oral cavity is considered an important part of every physical examination, particularly in adult to older ferrets and patients that are hyporexic. Dental radiographs are helpful to exclude problems that are not readily visible during oral inspection.[20]

According to previous publications, common dental problems in ferrets include mild gingivitis (83.7%; **Fig. 4**), dental attrition (63%–72%), and fractures of the maxillary canines (30%–52%), while tooth resorption (21.9%) and severe periodontal disease (16.3%) are less commonly diagnosed.[20,21] Prevalence of malocclusion varies greatly among studies (24%–95%) with linguoversion of the secondary mandibular incisors being the most prevalent (93%).[20,21] Regardless of diet, dental calculus will gradually build up, leading to gingivitis, caries, periodontal disease, and eventually tooth root abscesses, if left untreated.[22] In rare instances, these abscesses may extend into the nasal cavity, leading to oronasal fistulas and unilateral nasal discharge.[23] To delay calculus build-up, daily tooth brushing is recommended, and often tolerated by ferrets if using meat flavored toothpaste.[24]

Oral Ulcerations and Neoplasia

Ferrets with oral ulcerations commonly present with pain, hypersalivation, nausea, anorexia, gagging, or pawing at the roof of the mouth. Such ulcerations can be

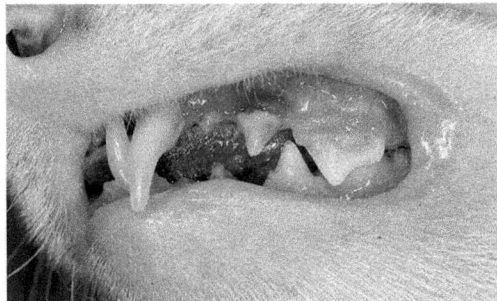

Fig. 4. Gingivitis and mild build-up of tartar seen around and on the maxillary teeth in a 6-year-old neutered female ferret that was presented for a routine check-up.

secondary to systemic or renal disease, gastric reflux, neoplasia, electrocution injuries, dental disease, or ingestion of caustic solutions. Ulcers can be directly visualized on the oral examination, and be present at any location.[6] Those associated with systemic disease are commonly found on the buccal mucosa, while those caused by ingestion of caustic substances are predominantly found on the rostral part of the tongue and mucosal lining.[25] A full work up including a detailed history, oral examination, bloodwork, urine analysis, and diagnostic imaging can aid in identifying the initiating cause.

Once the inciting cause is treated, ulcers will generally heal by themselves, but meanwhile alleviation of pain is recommended using analgesics such as tramadol, butorphanol, and/or nonsteroidal antiinflammatory drugs (NSAIDs). Additionally, oral liquid sucralfate can be provided, in addition to a soft to liquid diet to facilitate food intake.[26] For ferrets that are too painful and unwilling to eat by themselves, a nasogastric or esophageal tube can be placed to ensure adequate food intake while the oral lesions are allowed to heal. If left untreated, palatal ulcerations may erode through the hard palate to form oronasal fistulas. Healing of these is often complicated and will generally require surgical intervention.[27]

Mucosal lymphoma can occur in ferrets in association with oral ulcerations. Additionally, solid tumors of either benign or malignant origin have also been reported in ferrets. Cytology and/or histopathology of oral swellings is mandatory to differentiate neoplasia from abscesses and will help to determine the prognosis and course of treatment. While local resection of benign tumors like epulis can be achieved, more radical surgery should be considered in case of squamous cell carcinoma, osteoma, or multilobular tumors.[6] Hemimandibulectomies and adjunct radiation therapy may be considered in case of nonresectable tumors.[6,28]

Salivary Mucocele

Mucoceles have been reported in the zygomatic salivary glands in ferrets.[29,30] Obstruction of the salivary ducts can result from trauma, salivary microliths, oral neoplasia, or severe dental disease. The impaired drainage leads to progressive facial swelling with a build-up of mucous or seromucous fluids depending on which of the 5 types of salivary glands are affected.[7] Exophthalmos might be present.[29] Aside from the swelling, the ferret is usually unaffected.[11] Salivary mucoceles are diagnosed based on aspiration of the characteristic thick, viscous to mucinous, clear to light hemorrhagic fluid. CT is useful in identifying the affected gland and planning the surgical approach, which involves surgical drainage, marsupialization, or complete surgical resection to reduce the risk of reoccurrence.[6,29]

ESOPHAGEAL DISORDERS
Megaesophagus

Megaesophagus refers to dilation and lack of muscular motility of the esophagus. Thus far, megaesophagus has only been described in adult ferrets. The disease etiology is largely unknown.[31–33] Dilation of the esophagus can either be segmental or generalized, caused by neuromuscular dysfunction leading to a hypomotility and failure to transport the esophageal content to the stomach.[34] Intrathoracic, especially mediastinal, space-occupying lesions like thymomas and lymphomas compressing the esophagus can mimic the signs of megaesophagus, and should be excluded with diagnostic imaging.[35] Because of the hypomotility and delayed emptying, ferrets with megaesophagus often regurgitate after eating, and commonly display difficulties with swallowing. This results in coughing, choking, hyporexia, and weight loss.

Common complications include aspiration pneumonia, malnutrition, and hepatic lipidosis.[32] Affected ferrets often have concurrent gastritis and reflux, while a case reported myasthenia gravis as an underlying cause.[31] The dilated esophagus is best diagnosed on contrast radiographs using barium, while problems with motility can be assessed by fluoroscopy.[12,13] Treatment is often unrewarding, with survival times commonly being less than a week post diagnosis, except in 1 ferret with myasthenia gravis, that responded to pyridostigmine bromide (1 mg/kg, PO, q8h) treatment for a month.[31–33] Treatment consists of feeding liquid food at elevated locations, followed by restraining the ferret in an upright position for 10 minutes after the meal, medical prevention of (esophageal) ulcerations, and treatment of concurrent bronchopneumonia and GI-ulcerations, if present.[32]

Esophageal Foreign Bodies

The curious nature of young ferrets makes them prone to foreign body ingestion. Especially rubber and rubber-like materials, like ear plugs, seem to be highly preferred.[12] Foreign bodies can lodge throughout the GI tract, resulting in a variety of clinical signs, dependent on the size of the foreign body, the location, and the degree of luminal occlusion. Most often esophageal foreign bodies are identified on survey radiographs in ferrets with acute anorexia, vomiting, gagging, and lethargy, but some cases may require fluoroscopy, CT, or endoscopy to establish a diagnosis (**Fig. 5**).[36] Foreign body retrieval may be achieved endoscopically, whereby the object may be removed retrograde, or pushed into the stomach to allow natural passage or removal by gastrotomy.[13,36,37] Failure to dislodge the esophageal foreign body from the esophagus from both an oral and aboral (gastrotomy) direction complicates the removal and requires an esophagostomy through a thoracotomy. Temporary placement of a duodenojejunostomy tube can be used to allow for enteral nutrition during the healing and recovery.[38]

Esophagitis and Esophageal Strictures

Esophagitis is a common sequela to foreign bodies and other medical conditions, like megaesophagus and eosinophilic gastroenteritis. Gastric acid reflux during regurgitation or vomiting leads to erythema, inflammation, and erosion of the esophageal mucosal lining. Esophagoscopy can be used to assess the degree of esophagitis

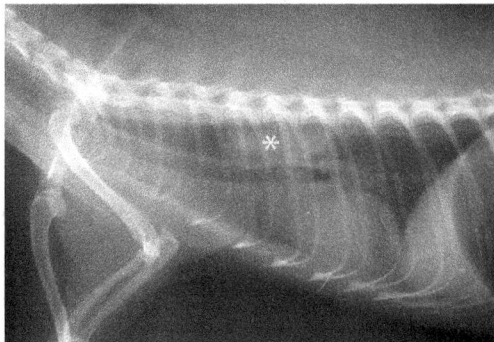

Fig. 5. Lateral projection of a radiograph of a 9-month-old intact male ferret that was presented with an acute onset of regurgitation directly after eating. A large foreign body can be seen craniodorsal to the heart (see *asterisk*). The foreign body proved to be a collapsed cat toy that could be removed endoscopically.

and presence of strictures.[18] Several reports on strictures exist, caused by chronic esophagitis, prolonged compression by a foreign body, or leakage of corrosive substances from such objects (eg, coin or button battery). Combined use of proton pump inhibitors, sucralfate, feeding of soft, liquefied foods, and surgical intervention with balloon dilation and stenting have shown moderate to good success in treating these conditions.[36,37,39,40]

DISORDERS OF THE STOMACH
Gastritis and Gastric Ulcerations

Signs associated with irritation of the gastric mucosa are generally mild and can include vomiting and hyporexia. A typical sign might be that the ferret shows interest in food, but once it starts to eat, it suddenly stops. If left untreated, gastritis may progress to gastric and duodenal ulceration or even perforation, with the ferret displaying hypersalivation, anorexia, weight loss, and teeth grinding as a result of abdominal pain, melena, anemia, and even death. Ferrets are sensitive to prolonged use of NSAIDs; hence, preventive use of gastroprotective drugs and/or antacids should be considered (see **Table 2**).[13] Renal azotemia and intoxications are other common causes, while neoplasia is rare. *H mustelae* is found in up to 100% of ferrets worldwide, and is commonly found in ferrets with gastritis, ulcerations, and even neoplasia (eg, gastric adenocarcinoma and mucosa-associated lymphoid tissue lymphoma).[41,42] However, many ferrets are subclinically infected, and disease seems mostly limited to individuals that are immunocompromised (eg, due to stress, crowding, other underlying disease). Hence, the relevance of the pathogen itself remains unclear. Radiographs are generally unremarkable, unless a gastric foreign body has caused gastric irritation or a pyloric perforation is present. Hematology may show varying levels of nonregenerative anemia, dependent on severity and chronicity of the bleeding. Gastroscopy is useful to assess the severity and distribution of gastric ulcerations (**Fig. 6**), and to obtain gastric and duodenal biopsies. *H mustelae* can be identified on histopathology using silver staining or following PCR analysis of biopsy specimens or fecal samples.[15] Blood serum immunoglobulin G enzyme-linked immunosorbent assay (ELISA) titers and a urea breath test can also be used to confirm *H mustelae*.[13] Nevertheless, due to the high prevalence of *H mustelae* in healthy ferrets, positive identification of the organism (without confirming its presence in lesions during histopathology) does not necessarily equal causation of clinical disease. Treatment is focused on gastroprotective drugs, antiemetics, supportive care, and antibiotics (see **Table 2**). In case of gastric neoplasia, due to the possible interaction with *H mustelae*, adjunct targeted antibiotic treatment is commonly advised in addition to chemotherapy.

Gastric Foreign Bodies and Gastric Distention

Ingested foreign bodies or trichobezoars are common in ferrets (see **Fig. 3**). Clinical signs are often nonspecific, with nausea, hypersalivation, hyporexia, and diarrhea. Vomiting is uncommon.[11,13] In rare cases, ferrets can present in lateral recumbency, and shock resulting from complete obstruction and associated gastric distention. Radiographs are diagnostic, and emergency treatment includes decompression of the stomach with an orogastric tube, treatment of hypovolemic shock, and stabilization of the patient prior to performing exploratory surgery.[13] Dependent on their nature, foreign bodies can easily be missed on initial survey radiographs, hence warranting 4 to 6 hours of fasting with follow-up radiographs in patients suspected of foreign body ingestion. Remaining gastric content at this point indicates delayed emptying

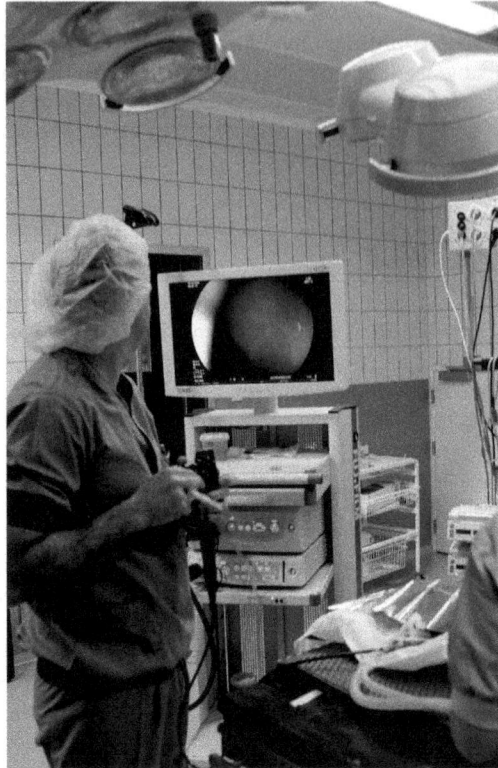

Fig. 6. Gastroscopy with a flexible endoscope in a 5.5-year-old female chemically neutered ferret that was presented with chronic vomiting, anorexia, and weight loss.

or entrapment of a foreign body. Additional techniques that can be used to assess gastric content include ultrasound and gastroscopy.[18] Endoscopic retrieval and/or surgical removal of a foreign body or trichobezoar may be attempted. Prevention is aimed at limiting exposure to rubber, foam, or plastic objects that the ferret can ingest. Additionally, frequent grooming and the use of cat laxatives are helpful to reduce the formation of trichobezoars.[43]

Neoplasia and Stenosis

Lymphoma is the most common gastric neoplasia in ferrets, while adenocarcinoma and neuroendocrine carcinomas are more rarely reported.[44] Both lymphoma and adenocarcinoma are suggested to coincide with *H mustelae* infection, as discussed previously.[41,42,45,46] Ferrets with gastric neoplasia commonly present with progressive lethargy, anorexia, vomiting, and weight loss (**Table 3**).[47,48] Radiographically, a cranial intraabdominal mass may be present, while ultrasonography may indicate thickening of the gastric mucosa or a nodular mass.[45,47] If the outflow of the pylorus is obstructed by a mass (or muscular hypertrophy), gastric distension may also be visible.[13,41,46–48] Gastric biopsies are required to obtain a definitive diagnosis. Samples can be obtained through endoscopy or laparotomy, and subsequently sent to a pathologist to help identify the tumor type and guide selection of the most appropriate chemotherapy protocol.[49] In case of confirmed pyloric neoplasia, euthanasia is generally

Table 3
Typical morphologic characteristics of diarrhea in ferrets caused by specific pathogens

Disease	Pathogen	Watery	Mucoid	Color	Hematochezia	Melena	Birdseed Like
Coccidiosis	Isospora spp, Eimeria spp				x	x	
Giardiasis	Giardia intestinalis, Giardia duodenalis						(x)
Cryptosporidiosis	Cryptosporidium parvum		x	Yellow			
Salmonellosis	Salmonella spp				x		
Campylobacteriosis	Campylobacter jejuni, Campylobacter coli	x	x	Green	x		
Proliferative bowel disease	Lawsonia intracellularis		x	Bright green	x		
Epizootic catarrhal enteritis	FECV		x	Bright green (acute stage)			x (chronic stage)
Parvo	Parvovirus					x	
Rotavirus diarrhea	Rotavirus		x	Green			
Canine distemper	Canine distemper virus					x	
Inflammatory bowel disease	N/A (immune mediated, possibly food intolerance/hypersensitivity)	x					x
Eosinophilic gastroenteritis	N/A	(x)	(x)	Green/dark	(x)		

Abbreviation: N/A, not applicable.
x, common clinical presentation, (x), can be present.

recommended, especially if the animal is in a poor condition. In case of muscular hypertrophy, reconstruction of the pylorus can be attempted.[12]

INTESTINAL DISORDERS
Intestinal Parasitism

While intestinal parasites are not a common cause of clinical disease, newly acquired, young, immunocompromised, stressed individuals, or ferrets housed in unsanitary conditions or high stocking densities are at greater risk of infection. Initial work-up includes a direct smear and serial fecal flotations. Since ferrets are often asymptomatic, routine testing of a newly acquired ferret should be considered, especially in multiferret households.

Coccidiosis

Clinical signs of coccidiosis range from a mild to severe diarrhea, dependent on degree and extent of atrophic enteritis (**Table 3**). If infection is severe, additional signs may include dehydration, hematochezia or melena, rectal prolapse, weight loss, and even death.[50,51] While ferrets of all ages are susceptible, young and immunocompromised individuals are most frequently affected.[51,52] In a study, oocysts were identified on fecal flotation in 4.7% of submitted fecal samples (n = 132/2805), with *Cystoisospora* (*Isospora*) *laidlawi* being twice as prevalent as *Eimeria furonis*. The same study also found a markedly higher prevalence of coccidiosis in European compared to Canadian samples (13% and 3.5%, respectively).[50] Since oocysts are shed intermittently, pooled or serial samples are recommended (**Fig. 7**).[51] If coccidiosis remains a viable diagnosis despite negative flotations, PCR and identification of the parasite on intestinal biopsies can be used to confirm the diagnosis.[50,51] Prognosis is grave in severe cases, though symptomatic treatment (assisted feeding, fluid therapy, blood transfusions, supplemental heat, etc.; see **Table 2**) can be attempted in combination with sulfamethoxine or sulfadimethoxine, ponazuril, or toltrazuril. Of these, ponazuril and toltrazuril are coccidiocidal and thereby the drugs of choice as sulfamethoxine is coccidiostatic.[51,53] Biliary coccidiosis due to *E furonis* has been reported in ferrets, resulting in hyperplasia of the biliary tree, cholecystitis, and cholangiohepatitis. Treatment was unsuccessful in both cases.[53,54]

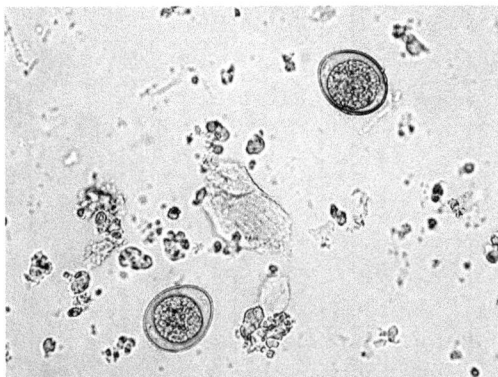

Fig. 7. Oocysts found after fecal flotation in a 4-month-old intact female ferret that was presented with persistent diarrhea.

Cryptosporidiosis

Similar to coccidia, cryptosporidia are single-celled protozoal organisms that can infest the gastrointestinal tract, predominantly the ileum, leading to chronic, watery to mucoid, yellow diarrhea (**Table 3**). In ferrets, cryptosporidiosis is most commonly associated with *Cryptosporidium parvum* which has zoonotic potential.[11] Ferrets of all ages can be affected, though the infection is usually subclinical in a large percentage of animals. Immunosuppression, caused by concurrent disease, suboptimal housing, or relocation, can escalate the diarrhea and result in anorexia, lethargy, and death occurring within 2 to 3 days after onset of clinical signs.[55,56] Affected animals excrete infective, sporulated oocysts in their feces, which can subsequently be identified in direct fresh fecal smears, following flotation, or using modified acid-fast staining or fluorescent antibodies. Alternative methods include the use of PCR, histopathology, or electron microscopy of intestinal biopsies.[55] A wide range of drugs (azithromycin, nitazoxanide, paromomycin) have been used to treat ferrets with cryptosporidiosis with variable success as continued autoinfection hinders successful eradication. In adult immunocompetent ferrets, the infection is usually self-limiting.

Giardiasis

Both *Giardia intestinalis* and *Giardia duodenalis* have been reported as a cause of giardiasis in ferrets.[57–59] *Giardia* spp infrequently cause anorexia and mild diarrhea in ferrets (**Table 3**), and may potentially be zoonotic, but rarely cause fatal disease in the absence of concurrent infections.[57–60] Fluorescent antibody coproscopy is considered the gold standard for diagnosing *Giardia,* but more commonly used methods include identification of motile flagellates or oocysts on fecal flotation (eg, Mini FLOTAC) with or without light microscopy or a positive *Giardia* coproantigen test.[61] In addition to symptomatic treatment, metronidazole can be used to eliminate infection (see **Table 2**).[55]

BACTERIAL GASTROENTERITIS

Feeding untreated or raw (whole) prey, eggs, and/or meat is the primary cause of bacterial gastroenteritis in ferrets.[13] As in other species, raw food products can be contaminated with *Campylobacter* spp, *Salmonella* spp, *Mycobacterium* spp, *Listeria* spp, and/or *Clostridium* spp. As these bacterial pathogens carry a potential zoonotic risk,[62] feeding raw food items to ferrets is discouraged at research facilities and in households with immunosuppressed family members.

Salmonellosis

Reports on *Salmonella* spp. causing enteritis in ferrets are rare, though infection may likely be underreported. *Salmonella* spp are readily transmitted by fecal-oral route,[63] with the serotype involved depending on the contaminated food source. Ferrets with clinical salmonellosis may demonstrate fever, lethargy, hemorrhagic diarrhea, anemia, balanitis, serous to seromucoid conjunctivitis, and pregnant jills might possibly abort (**Table 3**).[64] Mortality varies according to the strain involved. On necropsy, hyperemic small intestines with petechial hemorrhaging and bloody semi-solid contents may be observed. Histologically, the mucosal surface of the entire GI tract is inflamed with invasion of macrophages and lymphocytes, and missing intestinal tips on the villi. *Salmonella* is diagnosed on fecal cultures (repeated sampling is advised because of intermittent shedding), blood cultures (if septicemia is present), or culture of intestinal biopsies. Sensitivity testing is paramount to guide selection of antibiotic treatment. Sulfathalidine has been used with success in experimentally infected ferrets.[63] In addition to appropriate antibiosis, fluid therapy (including correction of electrolyte imbalances, if any), assisted feeding, reduction of environmental stressors, and treatment of concurrent diseases are advised (see **Table 2**).[13]

Campylobacteriosis

Campylobacteriosis in ferrets is common. Most often, infection is caused by *Campylobacter jejuni*, and—to a lesser extent—by *Campylobacter coli*. Ingestion of contaminated food and direct transmission at multiferret locations are the primary causes of infection.[65] Adult ferrets are usually asymptomatic carriers, while kits and immunodeficient individuals commonly develop diarrhea, usually within 24 hours following ingestion of the pathogen (**Table 3**).[66] *Campylobacter* colonizes the entire intestinal tract, leading to intermittent, mucoid, watery, green, or bloody diarrhea. Disease is often self-limiting, but infections can persist for more than 4 weeks.[41,46,50] *Campylobacter* can also cause placentitis and abortion in up to 100% of pregnant jills.[67] Infection can be confirmed by culturing the feces on selective media at 37°C and 42°C (98.6°F and 107.6°F) under microaerobic conditions for 48 to 72 hours.[11] PCR of intestinal biopsies or liver tissue can also be used to identify the pathogen. Treatment consists of supportive care and antibiotics based on antimicrobial sensitivity testing, as needed (see **Table 2**).[13]

Mycobacteriosis

Mycobacterial infections in ferrets are uncommon, except in New Zealand feral ferrets.[68,69] Infection typically involves *Mycobacterium bovis, M avium,* and *M triplex.* The primary cause of disease transmission is feeding of unheated raw meat products, but direct/indirect transmission from in-contact ferrets or wild animals also carries a risk.[70] Clinical signs of mycobacteriosis are often nonspecific and may include anorexia, diarrhea, weight loss, and lethargy (**Table 3**). In a study, mortality related to mycobacteriosis was reported to be 41% in ferrets with clinical disease.[71] Necropsy commonly reveals a granulomatous enteritis, enteric lymphadenitis, and hepatosplenomegaly with granulomas present in both organs.[69,72] Clinical diagnosis of mycobacteriosis can be difficult to achieve as many ferrets have subclinical disease, show nonspecific signs, and/or only have a single granuloma or no gross lesions on exploratory laparotomy or necropsy.[11] Old granulomas may calcify and be identified on radiographs. A delayed diagnosis increases the risk of zoonotic transmission or spread within the population and can therefore be problematic.[70] On cytology or histopathology (with or without immunohistochemistry), characteristic acid-fast staining rods can be identified in the granulomatous lesions. PCR testing and culture can be used to confirm the strain involved.[73] Reactions to tuberculin vary with the strain; hence, this test is considered unreliable in ferrets. Ferrets infected with mycobacterium tuberculosis complex (*M tuberculosis* or *M bovis*) should be euthanized for zoonotic reasons.[11] Be aware that strains of mycobacterium tuberculosis complex may be a notifiable disease depending on geographic regulations. In case of nontuberculous mycobacteria, rifampicin with/without enrofloxacin and azithromycin has been used. However, because of the granulomatous nature of the disease, clinical disease is likely to reoccur when antibiotic treatment is withdrawn.[71,73,74] Surgical removal of granulomas compressing or obstructing the GI-tract can be attempted to alleviate clinical signs, but chance of recurrence is high, hence making the overall prognosis guarded to poor.[72]

Proliferative Bowel Disease

Lawsonia intracellularis, formerly known as intracellular *Campylobacter*-like organism, is an uncommon cause of chronic, bright green, mucohemorrhagic diarrhea in very young or immunocompromised ferrets (**Table 3**).[13,75,76] *Lawsonia* invades the colonic intestinal wall, resulting in proliferation and infiltration of the intestinal wall with mixed inflammatory cells. This in turn leads to malabsorption. Upon clinical examination, thickened intestines may be palpable.[13] The ferret may cry in pain on defecation. Rectal prolapses may result from persisting chronic diarrhea and straining. Additionally, ferrets may show progressive anorexia, weight loss, and dehydration which can result in mortality if left untreated.[11,13,75] Coinfections with other pathogens like *Escherichia coli* may increase the risk of morbidity and mortality.[77] The thickened colonic wall can readily be diagnosed using abdominal ultrasound, while the organism can be diagnosed by PCR of feces or intestinal biopsies. Additionally, Warthin-Starry stain and immunohistochemistry can be used to identify the organism in the apical portion of the colonic enterocytes.[75,76,78] Treatment with oral chloramphenicol has been found effective.[79] Early treatment is vital to avoid chronic colonic malabsorption. Rectal prolapses, if present, usually do not require the use of purse-string sutures as these will generally not recur if the straining and diarrhea are resolved.

VIRAL GASTROENTERITIS
Epizootic Catarrhal Enteritis

Epizootic catarrhal enteritis (ECE) is a common cause of diarrhea caused by ferret enteric coronavirus.[80] Young ferrets are typically subclinical or only display very mild clinical signs, hence serving as an important reservoir for infecting adult ferrets. Adult ferrets, in contrast, develop smelly, bright green mucoid diarrhea within 2 to 3 days post infection, which lasts for weeks to even months (**Table 3**). As disease progresses, anorexia, vomiting, dehydration, weight loss, and lethargy may develop.[25] While mortality is low, morbidity may reach 100%.[11,13,81,82] Confirmation of infection can be achieved using PCR, identifying the coronavirus particles using transmission electron microscopy of fresh feces or intestinal biopsies or through detection of serum antibodies to ferret enteric virus using ELISA.[83] Histopathology of intestinal biopsies reveals atrophy and necrosis of intestinal villi and lymphocytic infiltration.[82] Ferrets with epizootic catarrhal enteritis must be isolated; supportive therapy, including prednisolone, is only necessary in anorexic or dehydrated ferrets. Nutritional support with an easily absorbed diet may improve the general clinical condition (see **Table 2**).[13] Chronic malabsorption, with feces typically containing undigested fat and starch and resembling birdseed (**Fig. 8**), is common in recovered ferrets. Due to the contagiousness of the disease, screening should be considered before introducing new individuals to multiferret households.

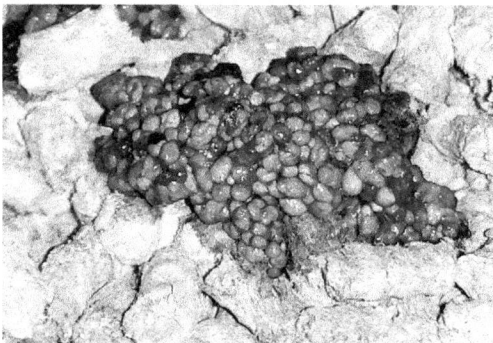

Fig. 8. Typical bird seed feces seen in a 4-year-old neutered male ferret that was presented with chronic poor appetite and irregular consistency of the feces.

Aside from causing ECE, it is speculated that ferret enteric coronavirus might mutate into a systemic form causing severe systemic disease, as known with feline coronavirus and feline infectious peritonitis.[25,84]

Rotavirus Diarrhea

Crowding and poor sanitary conditions are predisposing factors for rotavirus diarrhea. While adult ferrets usually display mild diarrhea or remain asymptomatic, morbidity and mortality can exceed 90% in 1 to 3 week old kits, especially in case of coinfections.[85] Transmission of the infection only requires ingestion of few fecal rotavirus particles, with kits developing a yellow to green mucoid diarrhea causing perineal soiling and erythema within 24 to 72 hours (**Table 3**).[13,86] Though clinical signs commonly only last for 3 to 4 days, the small size and undeveloped immune system of the kits predisposes them to severe dehydration, electrolyte imbalances, anorexia, and hypoglycemia.[87] Group A and C rotavirus infection can be demonstrated using electron microscopy, ELISA, or using reverse transcription PCR of fecal or tissue samples.[86,88,89] Gross postmortem examination of deceased kits will reveal an enlarged abdomen with gas-filled intestines, while histopathology confirms atrophic enteritis of the jejunum and ileum with blunted degenerated villous tips.[86,88] Treatment of affected kits generally requires intense supportive care (see **Table 2**). Rotavirus is almost impossible to eradicate in a population as virus particles are stable, especially in cooler climates. It is therefore important to maintain as sanitary conditions as possible, quarantine and screen new animals prior to introducing them into the population, and ensure ingestion of colostrum containing antibodies against rotavirus.[90]

Canine Distemper

Ferrets are highly susceptible to canine distemper virus (CDV), and readily develop disease following exposure to the virus if unvaccinated. Transmission occurs through direct contact or inhalation or ingestion of virus particles excreted in bodily fluids by other (unvaccinated) ferrets, as well as unvaccinated dogs, wild canines, mustelids, and procyonids.[89,91] Modified live virus vaccine-induced disease has also been documented.[92] After a 7 to 10-day incubation period, the ferret develops flu-like symptoms, and a pruritic rash which starts on the chin and progresses to the ventrum. GI signs including melena and diarrhea may be seen, though these are less common.[93,94] Progressing leukopenia results in secondary bacterial infections, including pneumonia. If the animal survives the initial stage, neurologic signs, including seizures, will develop prior to death.[13,89] In unvaccinated populations, mortality reaches up to 100%.[95] Infection with CDV can be confirmed by immunofluorescence test on blood or conjunctival scrapings, or by reverse transcriptase-PCR on peripheral blood.[96] Treatment consists of supportive care, symptomatic therapy, and treatment of secondary bacterial infections using antibiosis, but is rarely successful, and may only prolong the development of neurologic signs.[89] Euthanasia should therefore be considered as a realistic alternative to palliative treatment. Prevention is by serial vaccination, which may also help to reduce risk of spread and severity of disease after exposure.[95] Currently, PureVax Ferret Distemper Vaccine (Boehringer-Ingelheim) is the only licensed vaccine for ferrets. Unfortunately, this vaccine is unavailable in many countries. Canine vaccines, most notably Nobivac Puppy-DPv (Merck Animal Health), have successfully been used as an alternative. However, efficacy and safety studies for this and many other vaccines are lacking. With some of these vaccines inducing myofasciitis, caution is warranted when considering using a new vaccine.[97]

Influenza

Enteritis in ferrets with influenza can occur when viral particles invade the intestinal epithelium. However, ferrets infected with influenza virus more commonly present with respiratory signs, pyrexia, anorexia, and conjunctivitis.[13,62] Influenza is a zoonosis, but ferrets are also susceptible to transmission from humans.[98,99] Diagnosis is based on clinical signs, and spontaneous recovery occurs within 7 to 10 days. Nutritional support, cough suppressants, and NSAIDs can be used to alleviate symptoms.

In young kits, infection can be fatal because of secondary bacterial pneumonia.[89,100] A thorough history and PCR are important to differentiate influenza from canine distemper, because of the difference in prognosis.

Coronavirus Disease 2019

Acute gastroenteritis with lethargy, anorexia, vomiting, and profuse mucoid diarrhea has been observed in a ferret that became infected with severe acute respiratory syndrome coronavirus 2 (SARS-CoV-2) by a symptomatic human. The ferret recovered after symptomatic treatment, including amoxicillin and dexamethasone.[101] This report not only indicates that SARS-CoV-2 should be considered in the differential diagnosis for ferrets with GI disease, but also emphasizes the disease to be an anthropozoonosis. Hence, caution is warranted to prevent transmission to ferrets in the household in case of SARS-CoV-2-positive family members.

MISCELLANEOUS INTESTINAL DISORDERS
Inflammatory Bowel Disease

The cause of inflammatory bowel disease (IBD) in ferrets is unknown, but chronic inflammation of the GI tract caused by diet, atypical immune response, genetics, or hypersensitivity has been proposed.[13] IBD is common in young to middle-aged ferrets, with a study identifying GI inflammation in up to 92% of necropsied ferrets. Initially, clinical signs can be subtle and intermittent, including hyporexia, vomiting, and diarrhea; in the later stages of the disease, loose birdseed poop, anorexia, weight loss, and lethargy may be noted (**Table 3**).[11] If left untreated, IBD has been suggested to progress to intestinal lymphoma.[102]

Diagnostic workup is important to distinguish IBD from ferret coronavirus, lymphoma, eosinophilic gastroenteritis, and dietary indiscretion.[13] Initial history taking should include current diet, possible exposure to ferret corona virus, and response to a diet trial (if performed). Hematology and biochemistry are often unremarkable or nonspecific with increased liver enzymes, hyperglobulinemia, and lymphocytosis. A final diagnosis and differentiation from lymphoma and eosinophilic gastroenteritis can be made using full-thickness intestinal biopsies. Histology of jejunum shows villous atrophy, distended crypts, and an inflammation characterized by lymphocytes and plasma cells, and occasionally low numbers of eosinophils.[103,104] Immunohistochemistry (using CD3 and CD79a) is slightly superior in distinguishing IBD from lymphoma and should be considered.[102] Prednisone and/or azathioprine can be used to reduce intestinal inflammation, with both drugs being well tolerated by ferrets (see **Table 2**).[105] No hydrolyzed diets for ferrets are available; hence, the use of hypoallergenic diets for cats or a nutritionally balanced homemade diet using a novel protein source should be considered while keeping the general nutritional requirements for ferrets in mind.

Eosinophilic Gastroenteritis

Reports of confirmed eosinophilic gastroenteritis in ferrets are rare. Eosinophilic gastroenteritis is a noncontagious disease, characterized by eosinophilic infiltration of multiple tissues (GI tract, associated lymph nodes, liver, and lungs) and persistent eosinophilia in peripheral blood.[11,13,106] Clinical signs are related to the degree of GI infiltration and affected segments, and include vomiting, thickened intestines, lethargy, weight loss, and green mucoid diarrhea (**Table 3**).[106] The condition has only been reported in adult ferrets and is thought to be triggered by genetics or chronic intestinal irritation caused by commercial diets low in protein (<35%–55% of dry matter).[1] Biopsies of intestines and associated tissues are required to identify the diffuse eosinophilia of multiple tissues, which allows distinction between eosinophilic gastroenteritis, intestinal lymphoma, and IBD. Reports on treatment include the use of azathioprine, prednisone, ampicillin, cyclosporine, ivermectin, hypoallergenic diets, or combinations of these.[13,106,107] Treatment in other species indicates that immunosuppressive therapy in combination with hypoallergenic diets might be useful (see **Table 2**).[1] Unfortunately, current data are insufficient to recommend a specific treatment regimen in ferrets.

Food Hypersensitivity

Confirmed cases of food allergy have not been reported in ferrets, but GI signs with mild diarrhea that resolve following a diet change are not uncommon. Reports on the effect of elimination diets alone are currently not available, but a hydrolyzed hypoallergic diet (Hill's Prescription Diet z/d for cats) did not seem to decrease GI inflammation in a ferret with eosinophilic gastroenteritis.[107] A nutritionally balanced, novel protein home cooked diet might be superior to commercial hypoallergenic cat food, while also meeting the specific nutritional requirements of the ferret, but further research is required. Furthermore, care should be taken if using grain-free diets, as these have been associated with development of cystine urolithiasis.[108]

Intoxications

Accidental ingestion of toxic agents like household chemicals, plants, creams, soaps, paint, human food items, or medications are common in ferrets. Ferret-proofing the environment is therefore paramount.[109,110] Even small amounts of ingested toxins can cause significant morbidity and mortality, due to the small body weight of the ferret.[111] A thorough history should be obtained, and owners should be encouraged to bring packaging from ingested materials to aid in identifying potential toxic ingredients. Common toxicoses causing GI symptoms are theobromine, caffeine, and ibuprofen. Treatment depends on the type and amount of the toxin that is ingested and the clinical signs that are observed.[109,112] In case of a recent ingestion of a noncorrosive toxin, emesis can be induced with apomorphine. Activated charcoal (1-3 mg/kg orally) can be used to reduce GI absorption.[109,112]

Aside from household toxins, toxicity may also result from enterotoxins produced by bacteria. For example, severe yellow mucoid diarrhea may develop in neonatal kits following exposure to enterotoxins produced by *Staphylococcus delphini*. *E coli* is another enterotoxin-producing bacterium that leads to diarrhea; the type of diarrhea seen is strain dependent.[113,114] Enterotoxemia can quickly lead to severe dehydration, and—together with septicemia—to high mortality rates. Diagnosis is rarely made antemortem. If enterotoxemia is suspected, treatment using antibiotics, fluid therapy, and electrolytes should be initiated as soon as possible. Bacterial culture and PCR may be used to identify the strain and serotype involved.[114]

Intestinal Neoplastic Disease

Both benign and malignant intestinal neoplasias have been described in ferrets. Polyps are often asymptomatic and incidentally found on endoscopy.[110]

Intestinal lymphoma is the most common malignant intestinal tumor, and often diagnosed in older ferrets (mean age: 6.8 years).[44,115,116] Nodules can be present, but more commonly intestinal lymphoma results in diffuse intestinal thickening, with enlarged mesenteric lymph nodes.[115,117] Clinical signs can be subtle with slowly progressive weight loss, chronic diarrhea, and malabsorption. Lymphoma is readily misdiagnosed as IBD or eosinophile gastroenteritis,[22] requiring histopathology and immunohistochemistry of full-thickness intestinal biopsies to differentiate lymphoma from other causes of chronic diarrhea, and allowing the neoplasia to be immunophenotyped as either T-cell or B-cell lymphoma. IBD has been suggested as a precursor for lymphoma, making early stage disease especially difficult to distinguish.[102,115] T-cell lymphoma is more common than B-cell lymphoma (56% and 31%), with a slightly shorter median survival time (5 and 8.4 months, respectively).[118] Lymphoma can be staged, depending on the degree of organ involvement, with lower stages resembling less infiltration and better prognosis.[110,116] Several chemotherapeutic protocols have been utilized, but further research is required to define the treatment of choice, considering efficacy, safety, and quality of life during treatment.[117]

Intestinal adenocarcinoma and leiomyoma have also been described in ferrets but are rare. Generally, these neoplasms cause distinct nodular masses in the intestinal wall, with the ferrets developing progressive weight loss and nonresponsive diarrhea. If the tumor obstructs the intestinal lumen, vomiting and anorexia may be seen, thereby mimicking the clinical signs of intestinal foreign body entrapment.[44,110,119] The nodular mass may be identified using diagnostic imaging or be discovered as an incidental finding during abdominal palpation or exploratory laparotomy. Prior to starting chemotherapy, enterectomy with end-to-end anastomosis should be performed to remove the neoplasia and obstructed portion of the bowel. As regional and distant metastasis may already be present at the time of diagnosis, prognosis in case of adenocarcinomas is usually grave, and euthanasia should be considered.

Foreign Bodies

In addition to the stomach, the jejunum and duodenum are common sites where gastrointestinal foreign bodies get lodged.[110] Clinical signs include acute anorexia, apathy, diarrhea, profuse vomiting, bruxism, and ptyalism; time of onset is related to the time of luminal obstruction.[120,121] While some intestinal foreign bodies are readily palpable on abdominal palpation, abdominal radiographs with/without contrast or abdominal ultrasound are often used to confirm their presence.[121] As ferrets are notorious for ingesting rubber, foam, or plastic objects, it is not uncommon for them to have ingested multiple foreign bodies at once. Therefore, the entire GI tract should be thoroughly palpated, even if a foreign body has already been identified.[110,122] Linear foreign bodies are rare and can be more difficult to diagnose on radiographs, unless a curled-up intestine is identified on abdominal radiographs. As intestinal foreign bodies are unlikely to pass, enterotomy is indicated after initial stabilization (see **Table 2**). Postoperative care includes assisted feeding with liquid diets, analgesia, heat, and fluid therapy, as needed (see **Table 2**). In older ferrets, full-thickness intestinal biopsies for lymphoma/IBD screening as well as careful evaluation and palpation of the pancreas are recommended during exploratory surgery. In absence of perforations and (pre-) perforative peritonitis, the prognosis after foreign body removal is good.[120–122]

Stress-Related Diarrhea

Some ferrets are very sensible to environmental change. Traveling, altered routines, or a new human/animal family member can pose enough stress to the ferret, and subsequently lead to (Helicobacter-associated) gastritis and intermittent diarrhea. Generally, ferrets will show little, if any, other clinical signs and commonly have a good body condition, which enables distinction from other causes of diarrhea. Diagnosis is based on history and exclusion of other causes of diarrhea. Modifications of the living environment to reduce exposure to stressors will suffice to resolve the problem.

DISTAL ENTERIC DISEASE
Rectal Prolapse

Any disease causing straining or prolonged diarrhea (see **Table 1**) can result in rectal prolapse. In young ferrets, rectal prolapse is most commonly seen in animals with enteritis and profuse diarrhea. In older animals, in addition to primary GI disease, rectal prolapses are also commonly seen with other conditions, including urinary straining caused by prostatic disease, neoplasia, obstructive urolithiasis; dystocia; or sublumbar lymphadenopathy.[11,12,103] In countries where anal gland removal is not prohibited, poor surgical technique may also cause rectal prolapse.[110] Diagnosis and treatment are focused on identifying and alleviating the initiating cause, following which most prolapses will resolve by themselves. Irritation or discomfort from mild prolapse can be alleviated using hemorrhoid cream or lidocaine-containing gel/ointment. If the rectal prolapse is severe, placement of a purse-string suture can be considered to prevent recurrence and protect the mucosal lining. Sutures can be left in place for 2 up to 21 days while the underlying cause is being treated.[11,13,103,110] Necrotic tissue should be removed, if present.[110]

Rectal Masses and Fistulas

Mild intermittent hematochezia, straining, or rectal prolapse can be an indication of rectal masses. Typically, these masses protrude into the lumen or compress the rectum, as can be visualized during CT or proctoscopy. Rectal polyps are usually benign and can be biopsied and removed with proctoscopy.[13] Rectal neoplasia includes lymphoma and leiomyosarcoma, which require a more complex treatment using radical surgical debulking, possible rectoplasty, and chemotherapy with/without radiation, dependent on tumor type and initial staging.[119,123] Removal of the entire tumor is often not feasible because of its anatomic location, and the risk of regrowth with local invasion is high, resulting in a poor prognosis.[13]

Rectovaginal fistulas have been described in 2 ferrets with fecal incontinence through the vulva, causing chronic vaginitis. Contrast radiographs and CT were used to identify the fistula path, before attempting surgical closure. Refistulation is possible, and quality of life should be considered in case of reoccurrence.[124,125]

Anal Gland Disease

Reports of anal gland disease in ferrets are few, but likely underreported since anal glands are routinely surgically removed in many countries.[126] Anal sacs can become impacted or infected, resulting in unilateral/bilateral perianal swelling. Emptying should be performed under sedation in a well-ventilated room, for the sake of the veterinary personnel. Antibiotics are rarely required after emptying and flushing, but analgesics are recommended to prevent discomfort.[13,110] Anal gland neoplasia can easily be mistaken for anal gland impaction; hence, it is recommended to carefully palpate the anal sacs after emptying. Both anal gland squamous cell carcinoma and adenocarcinomas have been reported. Surgical removal in combination with radiotherapy and/or chemotherapy usually carries a good prognosis.[127–129] In case of malignancy, screening for metastases is important, as adenocarcinomas may metastasize to regional lymph nodes or distant organs, including liver, spleen, and lung.[127]

SUMMARY

Ferrets are commonly affected by GI diseases of both infectious and noninfectious origin, resulting in clinical signs that are often nonspecific such as lethargy, anorexia, vomiting, and diarrhea. Noninfectious disease is often related to ingestion of foreign objects, trichobezoars, gastric reflux, neoplasia, or dental disease. Amongst the infectious causes, viral and bacterial gastroenteritis are most commonly encountered, with the latter frequently being associated with consumption of raw food. Diagnostic workup and therapeutic principles largely follow similar guidelines as those established in other companion animals, while preventive measures include maintaining the ferret on a high-protein diet, ensuring vaccination against canine distemper, ferret proofing the house, and adequate quarantine and routine fecal parasite screening when new ferrets enter the household.

CLINICS CARE POINTS

- Histopathology and immunohistochemistry of full-thickness intestinal biopsies are required to differentiate IBD from intestinal lymphoma.
- In contrast to many other small mammals, ferrets are prone to gastric reflux, causing esophagitis and oral ulcerations. Gastritis is also common, and often suggested to be related to *H mustelae* infection.
- Screening for epizootic catarrhal enteritis through fecal PCR or serum antibodies should be considered before introducing new ferrets into multiferret households, as young kits serve as a reservoir, transmitting disease to other, adult ferrets.
- While the cause at current remains uncertain, eosinophilic gastroenteritis in ferrets might be triggered by long-term feeding of a diet low in protein (<35–55% of dry matter).
- In elderly ferrets, full-thickness intestinal biopsies for lymphoma/inflammatory bowel disease screening as well as careful evaluation and palpation of the pancreas are recommended during exploratory surgery.

DISCLOSURE

The authors have nothing to disclose.

REFERENCES

1. Kinoshita Y, Oouchi S, Fujisawa T. Eosinophilic gastrointestinal diseases - pathogenesis, diagnosis, and treatment. Allergol Int 2019;68(4):420–9.
2. Bell JA. Ensuring proper nutrition in ferrets. Vet Med 1996;91(12):1098–103.
3. Fodor K, Prohácik A, Andrásofszky E, et al. Determination of transit time in ferret and domestic cat. Magy Allatorv Lapja 2006;128(11):674–9.
4. Mackay TW, Andrews PL. A comparative study of the vagal innervation of the stomach in man and the ferret. J Anat 1983;136(Pt 3):449–81.
5. Johnson-Delaney CA. Diagnosis and treatment of dental disease in ferrets. J Exot Pet Med 2008;17(2):132–7.
6. Johnson-Delaney CA. Anatomy and disorders of the oral cavity of ferrets and other exotic companion carnivores. Vet Clin North Am Exot Anim Pract 2016; 19(3):901–28.
7. Poddar S, Jacob S. Gross and microscopic anatomy of the major salivary glands of the ferret. Acta Anat (Basel) 1977;98(4):434–43.

8. Poddar S, Murgatroyd L. Morphological and histological study of the gastro-intestinal tract of the ferret. Acta Anat 2008;96(3):321–34.
9. Evans H, An NQ. Anatomy of the ferret. In: Fox JG, Marini RP, editors. Biology and diseases of the ferret. 3rd edition. Newark, United States: John Wiley & Sons; 2014. p. 23–67. Incorporated.
10. Bueno L, Fioramonti J, More J. Is there a functional large intestine in the ferret? Experientia 1981;37(3):275–7.
11. Maurer KJ, Fox JG. Diseases of the gastrointestinal system. In: Fox JG, Marini RP, editors. Biology and diseases of the ferret. 3rd edition. Newark, United States: John Wiley & Sons; 2014. p. 363–75. Incorporated.
12. Lennox AM. Gastrointestinal diseases of the ferret. Vet Clin North Am Exot Anim Pract 2005;8(2):213–25.
13. Hoefer HL. 3 - gastrointestinal diseases of ferrets. In: Quesenberry KE, Orcutt CJ, Mans C, et al, editors. Ferrets, rabbits, and rodents. 4thEdition. Philadelphia: W.B. Saunders; 2020. p. 27–38.
14. Fox JG. Normal clinical and biological parameters. In: Fox JG, Marini RP, editors. Biology and diseases of the ferret. 3rd edition. Newark, United States: John Wiley & Sons; 2014. p. 157–85. Incorporated.
15. Devaux L, Huynh M, Hernandez J, et al. Upper gastrointestinal endoscopy in ferret and the histological assessment of the endoscopic biopsies. Vet Rec 2016;178(4):96.
16. van Randen A, Laméris W, van Es HW, et al. A comparison of the accuracy of ultrasound and computed tomography in common diagnoses causing acute abdominal pain. Eur Radiol 2011;21(7):1535–45.
17. Miniter BM, Gonçalves Arruda A, Zuckerman J, et al. Use of computed tomography (CT) for the diagnosis of mechanical gastrointestinal obstruction in canines and felines. PLoS One 2019;14(8):e0219748.
18. Pignon C, Huynh M, Husnik R, et al. Flexible gastrointestinal endoscopy in ferrets (Mustela putorius furo). Vet Clin North Am Exot Anim Pract 2015;18(3):369–400.
19. Verstraete FM. Advances in diagnosis and treatment of small exotic mammal dental disease. Seminars Avian Exot Pet Med 2003;12(1):37–48.
20. Nemec A, Zadravec M, Račnik J. Oral and dental diseases in a population of domestic ferrets (Mustela putorius furo). JSAP (J Small Anim Pract) 2016;57(10):553–60.
21. Eroshin VV, Reiter AM, Rosenthal K, et al. Oral examination results in rescued ferrets: clinical findings. J Vet Dent 2011;28(1):8–15.
22. Hoppes SM. The senior ferret (Mustela putorius furo). Vet Clin North Am Exot Anim Pract 2010;13(1):107–22.
23. Thas I, Cohen-Solal NA. Acquired oronasal fistula in a domestic ferret (Mustela putorius furo). J Exot Pet Med 2014;23(4):409–14.
24. Kling MA, Powers LV. Section two: ferrets, hedgehogs, sugar gliders, and small pet marsupials. 30th annual association of avian veterinarians conference & expo with the association of exotic mammal vetererinarians and the 16th annual association of reptilian and Amphibian veterinarians conference. Milwaukee, Wisconsin: AEMV; 2009.
25. Johnson-Delaney CA. Emerging ferret diseases. J Exot Pet Med 2010;19(3):207–15.
26. Williams BH. Therapeutics in ferrets. Vet Clin North Am Exot Anim Pract 2000;3(1):131–153, vi.

27. Fossum TW. Small animal surgery. 5th edition. Philadelphia, United States: Elsevier; 2018.

28. Blackwell RP, Lennox AM, Tobias J, et al. Successful treatment of a mandibular multilobular tumor of bone in a ferret (Mustela putorius furo). J Exot Pet Med 2024;49:9–11.

29. Fehr M, Thiele A, Gerdwilker A, et al. Salivary mucocele (Zygomatic gland) in a ferret (Mustela putorius furo). Kleintierpraxis 2006;51(4):210.

30. Miller PE, Pickett JP. Zygomatic salivary gland mucocele in a ferret. J Am Vet Med Assoc 1989;194(10):1437–8.

31. Couturier J, Huynh M, Boussarie D, et al. Autoimmune myasthenia gravis in a ferret. J Am Vet Med Assoc 2009;235(12):1462–6.

32. Blanco MC, Fox JG, Rosenthal K, et al. Megaesophagus in 9 ferrets. J Am Vet Med Assoc 1994;205(3):444–7.

33. Harms CA, Andrews GA. Megaesophagus in a domestic ferret. Lab Anim Sci 1993;43:506.

34. Gaschen L. Chapter 30 - canine and feline esophagus. In: Thrall DE, editor. Textbook of veterinary diagnostic radiology. 7th Edition. W.B. Saunders; 2018. p. 596–617.

35. Taylor TG, Carpenter JL. Thymoma in two ferrets. Lab Anim Sci 1995;45(4): 363–5.

36. Webb J, Graham J, Fordham M, et al. Diagnosis and treatment of esophageal foreign body or stricture in three ferrets (Mustela putorius furo). J Am Vet Med Assoc 2017;251(4):451–7.

37. Caligiuri R, Bellah JR, Collins BR, et al. Medical and surgical management of eosophagal foreign body in a ferret. J Am Vet Med Assoc 1989;195(7):969–71.

38. Adamovicz L, Applegate J, Harris J, et al. Use of a gastrostomy and jejunostomy tube for management of gastric distention following pyloric outflow obstruction in a ferret (Mustela putorius furo). J Exot Pet Med 2018;28. https://doi.org/10.1053/j.jepm.2018.02.040.

39. Preliminary evaluation of esophageal stenting for recurrent benign esophageal strictures in 1 ferret and 2 dogs. 26th annual forum of the American college of veterinary internal medicine; June 4–7, 2008; San Antonio, TX.

40. Diagnosis and management of esophageal strictures in a ferret (Mustela putorius furo). 12th annual conference of the association of exotic mammal veterinarians, September 14–19, 2013; Indianapolis, IN.

41. Fox J, Dangler C, Sager W, et al. Helicobacter mustelae-associated gastric adenocarcinoma in ferrets (Mustela putorius furo). Vet Pathol 1997;34(3):225–9.

42. Fox JG, Marini RP. Helicobacter mustelae infection in ferrets: pathogenesis, epizootiology, diagnosis, and treatment. Seminars Avian Exot Pet Med 2001; 10(1):36–44.

43. Vinke CM, Schoemaker NJ. The welfare of ferrets (Mustela putorius furo T): a review on the housing and management of pet ferrets. Appl Anim Behav Sci 2012; 139(3):155–68.

44. Avallone G, Forlani A, Tecilla M, et al. Neoplastic diseases in the domestic ferret (Mustela putorius furo) in Italy: classification and tissue distribution of 856 cases (2000-2010). BMC Vet Res 2016;12:8.

45. Bousquet T, Bravo-Araya M, Davies JL. Gastric neuroendocrine carcinoma (carcinoid) in a ferret (Mustela putorius furo). Can Vet J 2022;63(11):1109–13.

46. Nakanishi M, Kuwamura M, Yamate J, et al. Gastric adenocarcinoma with ossification in a ferret (Mustela putorius furo). J Vet Med Sci 2005;67(9):939–41.

47. Rice LE, Stahl SJ, McLeod CG. Pyloric adenocarcinoma in a ferret. J Am Vet Med Assoc 1992;200(8):1117–8.
48. Sleeman JM, Clyde VL, Jones MP, et al. 2 cases of pyloric adenocarcinoma in the ferret (Mustela putorius furo). Vet Rec 1995;137(11):272–3.
49. Antinoff N, Hahn K. Ferret oncology: diseases, diagnostics, and therapeutics. Vet Clin North Am Exot Anim Pract 2004;7(3):579–625, vi.
50. Pastor AR, Smith DA, Barta JR. Molecular characterization of enteric coccidia from domestic ferrets (Mustela putorius furo). Vet Parasitol Reg Stud Reports 2021;23:8.
51. Sledge DG, Bolin SR, Lim A, et al. Outbreaks of severe enteric disease associated with Eimeria furonis infection in ferrets (Mustela putorius furo) of 3 densely populated groups. J Am Vet Med Assoc 2011;239(12):1584–8.
52. Blankenshipparis TL, Chang JJ, Bagnell CR. Enteric coccidiosis in a ferret. Lab Anim Sci 1993;43(4):361–3.
53. Kaye SW, Ossiboff RJ, Noonan B, et al. Biliary coccidiosis associated with immunosuppressive treatment of pure red cell aplasia in an adult ferret (Mustela putorius furo). J Exot Pet Med 2015;24(2):215–22.
54. Williams BH, Chimes MJ, Gardiner CH. Biliary coccidiosis in a ferret (Mustela putorius furo). Vet Pathol 1996;33(4):437–9.
55. Bell JA. Parasites of domesticated pet ferrets. Compend Continuing Educ Pract Vet 1994;16(5):617–20.
56. Gómez-Villamandos JC, Carrasco L, Mozos E, et al. Fatal cryptosporidiosis in ferrets (Mustela putorius furo): a morphopathologic study. JZWM 1995;26(4): 539–44.
57. Pantchev N, Broglia A, Paoletti B, et al. Occurrence and molecular typing of Giardia isolates in pet rabbits, chinchillas, Guinea pigs and ferrets collected in Europe during 2006-2012. Vet Rec 2014;175(1):18.
58. Abe N, Tanoue T, Noguchi E, et al. Molecular characterization of Giardia duodenalis isolates from domestic ferrets. Parasitol Res 2010;106(3):733–6.
59. Abe N, Read C, Thompson RCA, et al. Zoonotic genotype of Giardia intestinalis detected in a ferret. J Parasitol 2005;91(1):179–82.
60. Kurnosova OP, Arisov MV, Odoyevskaya IM. Intestinal parasites of pets and other house-kept animals in Moscow. Helminthologia 2019;56(2):108–17.
61. Pantchev N, Gassmann D, Globokar-Vrhovec M. Increasing numbers of Giardia (but not coccidian) infections in ferrets, 2002 to 2010. Vet Rec 2011;168(19):1.
62. Fox JG, Broome R. Housing and management. In: Fox JG, Marini RP, editors. Biology and diseases of the ferret. 3rd edition. Newark, United States: John Wiley & Sons; 2014. p. 145–55. Incorporated.
63. Coburn DR, Morris JA. The treatment of Salmonella typhimurium infection in ferrets. Cornell Vet 1949;39(2):198–201.
64. Morris JA, Coburn DR. The isolation of Salmonella typhimurium from ferrets. J Bacteriol 1948;55(3):419–20.
65. Fox JG, Ackerman JI, Newcomer CE. Ferret as a potential reservoir for human campylobacteriosis. Am J Vet Res 1983;44(6):1049–52.
66. Bell JA, Manning DD. A domestic ferret model of immunity to Campylobacter jejuni induced enteric disease. Infect Immun 1990;58(6):1848–52.
67. Bell JA, Manning DD. Reproductive failure in mink and ferrets after intravenous or oral inoculation of Camylobacter jejuni. Can J Vet Res 1990;54(4):432–7.
68. de Lisle GW, Pamela Kawakami R, Yates GF, et al. Isolation of Mycobacterium bovis and other mycobacterial species from ferrets and stoats. Vet Microbiol 2008;132(3):402–7.

69. Pollock C. Mycobacterial infection in the ferret. Vet Clin Exot Anim Pract 2012; 15(1):121–9.
70. Qureshi T, Labes RE, Lambeth M, et al. Transmission of Mycobacterium bovis from experimentally infected ferrets to non-infected ferrets (Mustela furo). N Z Vet J 2000;48(4):99–104.
71. Mentré V, Bulliot C. A retrospective study of 17 cases of mycobacteriosis in domestic ferrets (Mustela putorius furo) between 2005 and 2013. J Exot Pet Med 2015;24(3):340–9.
72. Schultheiss PC, Dolginow SZ. Granulomatous enteritis caused by Mycobacterium avium in a ferret. J Am Vet Med Assoc 1994;204(8):1217–8.
73. Lucas J, Lucas A, Furber H, et al. Mycobacterium genavense infection in two aged ferrets with conjunctival lesions. Aust Vet J 2000;78(10):685–9.
74. Piseddu E, Trotta M, Tortoli E, et al. Detection and molecular characterization of Mycobacterium celatum as a cause of splenitis in a domestic ferret (Mustela putorius furo). J Comp Pathol 2011;144(2–3):214–8. https://doi.org/10.1016/j.jcpa.2010.08.004.
75. Fox JG, Murphy JC, Ackerman JI, et al. Proliferative colitis in ferrets. Am J Vet Res 1982;43(5):858–64.
76. Krogstad AP, Dixon LW. Gross pathology of small mammals. Seminars Avian Exot Pet Med 2003;12(2):106–22.
77. Schauer DB, McCathey SN, Daft BM, et al. Proliferative enterocolitis associated with dual infection with enteropathogenic Escherichia coli and awsonia intracellularis in rabbits. J Clin Microbiol 1998;36(6):1700–3.
78. Ohta T, Kimura K, Katsuda K, et al. Proliferative enteropathy caused by Lawsonia intracellularis in chickens. J Comp Pathol 2017;156(2–3):158–61.
79. Krueger KL, Murphy JC, Fox JG. Treatment of proliferative colitis in ferrets. J Am Vet Med Assoc 1989;194(10):1435–6.
80. Li TC, Yoshizaki S, Kataoka M, et al. Determination of ferret enteric coronavirus genome in laboratory ferrets. Emerg Infect Dis 2017;23(9):1568–70.
81. Wise AG, Kiupel M, Maes RK. Molecular characterization of a novel coronavirus associated with epizootic catarrhal enteritis (ECE) in ferrets. Virology 2006; 349(1):164–74.
82. Williams BH, Kiupel M, West KH, et al. Coronavirus-associated epizootic catarrhal enteritis in ferrets. J Am Vet Med Assoc 2000;217(4):526–30.
83. Minami S, Terada Y, Shimoda H, et al. Establishment of serological test to detect antibody against ferret coronavirus. J Vet Med Sci 2016;78(6):1013–7.
84. Shigemoto J, Muraoka Y, Wise AG, et al. Two cases of systemic coronavirus-associated disease resembling feline infectious peritonitis in domestic ferrets in Japan. J Exot Pet Med 2014;23(2):196–200.
85. Fox GJ, Bell JA, Broome R. Growth and reproduction. In: Fox JG, Marini RP, editors. Biology and diseases of the ferret. 3rd edition. Newark, USA: John Wiley & Sons; 2014. p. 187–210. Incorporated.
86. Torresmedina A. Isolation of atypical rotavirus causing diarrhea in neonatal ferrets. Lab Anim Sci 1987;37(2):167–71.
87. Grimprel E, Rodrigo C, Desselberger U. Rotavirus disease: impact of coinfections. Pediatr Infect 2008;27(1):S3–10.
88. Wise AG, Smedley RC, Kiupel M, et al. Detection of Group C rotavirus in juvenile ferrets (Mustela putorius furo) with diarrhea by reverse transcription polymerase chain reaction: sequencing and analysis of the complete coding region of the VP6 gene. Vet Pathol 2009;46(5):985–91.

89. Langlois I. Viral diseases of ferrets. Vet Clin North Am Exot Anim Pract 2005;8(1): 139–60.

90. Van de Perre P. Transfer of antibody via mother's milk. Vaccine 2003;21(24): 3374–6.

91. Shen DT, Gorham JR. Contact transmission of distemper virus in ferrets. Res Vet Sci 1978;24(1):118–9.

92. Gonzalez-Jassi HA, Fithian J, Doden G, et al. Vaccine-induced distemper in domestic ferrets (Mustela putorius furo): 5 cases (2022). J Exot Pet Med 2024; 51:20–6.

93. George AM, Wille M, Wang J, et al. A novel and highly divergent Canine Distemper Virus lineage causing distemper in ferrets in Australia. Virology 2022;576: 117–26.

94. Guercio A, Mira F, Di Bella S, et al. Biomolecular analysis of canine distemper virus strains in two domestic ferrets (Mustela putorius furo). Vet Sci 2023; 10(6):12.

95. Wyllie SE, Kelman M, Ward MP. Epidemiology and clinical presentation of canine distemper disease in dogs and ferrets in Australia, 2006-2014. Aust Vet J 2016;94(7):215–22.

96. Stephensen CB, Welter J, Thaker SR, et al. Canine distemper virus (CDV) infection of ferrets as a model for testing Morbillivirus vaccine strategies: NYVAC- and ALVAC-based CDV recombinants protect against symptomatic infection. J Virol 1997;71(2):1506–13.

97. Quesenberry KE, de Matos R. 2 - basic approach to veterinary care of ferrets. In: Quesenberry KE, Orcutt CJ, Mans C, et al, editors. Ferrets, rabbits, and rodents. 4th Edition. Philadelphia: W.B. Saunders; 2020. p. 13–26.

98. Smith W, Stuart-Harris CH. Influenza infection of man from the ferret. Lancet 1936;2:21.

99. H S, C S. Lessons for human influenza from pathogenicity studies in ferrets. Rev Infect Dis 1998;10:56–75.

100. A ferret model of synergism between influenza virus and Streptococcus pneumoniae. 5th international conference on options for the control of influenza; Oct 07–11, 2003; Okinawa, Japan. Elsevier Science Bv.

101. Račnik J, Kočevar A, Slavec B, et al. Transmission of SARS-CoV-2 from human to domestic ferret. Emerg Infect Dis 2021;27(9):2450–3.

102. Watson MK, Cazzini P, Mayer J, et al. Histology and immunohistochemistry of severe inflammatory bowel disease versus lymphoma in the ferret (Mustela putorius furo). J Vet Diagn Invest 2016;28(3):198–206.

103. Burgess ME. Ferret gastrointestinal and hepatic diseases. In: Lewington JH, editor. Ferret husbandry, medicine and surgery. 2nd edition. WB Saunders; 2007. p. 15.

104. Cazzini P, Watson MK, Gottdenker N, et al. Proposed grading scheme for inflammatory bowel disease in ferrets and correlation with clinical signs. J Vet Diagn Invest 2020;32(1):17–24.

105. Burgess M, Garner M. Clinical aspects of inflammatory bowel disease in ferrets. Exot Dvm 2002;4:29–34.

106. Fazakas S. Eosinophilic gastroenteritis in a domestic ferret. Can Vet J 2000; 41(9):707–9.

107. Carmel B. Eosinophilic gastroenteritis in three ferrets. Vet Clin North Am Exot Anim Pract 2006;9(3):707–12.

108. Lamglait B, Brieger A, Rainville EM, et al. Retrospective case control study of pet ferrets with cystine urolithiasis in Quebec, Canada: epidemiological and clinical features. J Vet Med Sci 2021;5.

109. Dunayer E. Toxicology of ferrets. Vet Clin North Am Exot Anim Pract 2008;11(2): 301–14.

110. Livingstone M. Dealing with gastrointestinal disease in ferrets. In Pract 2022; 44(3):169–79.

111. Richardson J, Balabuszko R. Managing ferret toxicoses. Exot Dvm 2000; 2(4):23–6.

112. Cathers TE, Isaza R, Oehme F. Acute ibuprofen toxicosis in a ferret. J Am Vet Med Assoc 2000;216(9):1426.

113. Gary JM, Langohr IM, Lim A, et al. Enteric colonization by Staphylococcus delphini in four ferret kits with diarrhoea. J Comp Pathol 2014;151(4):314–7.

114. Swennes AG, Fox GJ. Bacterial and mycoplasmal diseases. In: Fox JG, Marini RP, editors. Biology and diseases of the ferret. 3rd edition. Newark, United States: John Wiley & Sons; 2014. p. 519–52. Incorporated.

115. Onuma M, Kondo H, Ono S, et al. Cytomorphological and immunohistochemical features of lymphoma in ferrets. J Vet Med Sci 2008;70(9):893–8.

116. Mayer J, Burgess K. An update on ferret lymphoma: a proposal for a standardized classification of ferret lymphoma. J Exot Pet Med 2012;21(4):343–6.

117. Huynh M, Pignon C. Gastrointestinal disease in exotic small mammals. J Exot Pet Med 2013;22(2):118–31.

118. Ammersbach M, DeLay J, Caswell JL, et al. Laboratory findings, histopathology, and immunophenotype of lymphoma in domestic ferrets. Vet Pathol 2008;45(5): 663–73.

119. Li XT, Fox JG, Padrid PA. Neoplastic diseases in ferrets: 574 cases (1968-1997). J Am Vet Med Assoc 1998;212(9):1402.

120. Biétrix J. Upper intestinal occlusion by a foreign body in a ferret. Point Vet 2007; 38(276):67.

121. Mehler SJ. Surgery. In: Fox JG, Marini RP, editors. Biology and diseases of the ferret. 3rd edition. Newark, United States: John Wiley & Sons; 2014. p. 285–310. Incorporated.

122. Mullen HS, Scavelli TD, Quesenberry KE, et al. Gastrointestinal foreign body in ferrets - 25 cases (1986 to 1990). J Am Anim Hosp Assoc 1992;28(1):13–9.

123. Williams BH, Wyre NR. Neoplasia in ferrets. In: Quesenberry KE, Orcutt CJ, Mans C, et al, editors. Ferrets, rabbits, and rodents. 4thEdition. Philadelphia: W.B. Saunders; 2020. p. 92–108.

124. Schlax K, Quiévreux L, Mélin M, et al. A rectovaginal fistula in a ferret (Mustela putorius furo) with a normal anus: a case report. J Exot Pet Med 2020; 35(C):20–2.

125. Rectovaginal fistula with atresia ani in a ferret (Mustela putorius furo). ICARE 2024; 2024; Ghent, Belgium.

126. Reviron T, Haffar A. Routine operations on the ferret. Point Vet 1998; 29(188):51–5.

127. Vilalta L, Meléndez-Lazo A, Canturri A, et al. Anal sac adenocarcinoma with metastasis and hypercalcemia in a ferret (Mustela putorius furo). J Exot Pet Med 2017;26(2):143–9.

128. Nakata M, Miwa Y, Nakayama H, et al. Localised radiotherapy for a ferret with possible anal sac apocrine adenocarcinoma. JSAMP 2008;49(9):476–8.

129. Müller S, Puff C, Thöle M, et al. Squamous cell carcinoma of the anal sac in a ferret - a case report. Kleintierpraxis 2015;60(12):646–51.

Gastroenterology in Rodents

Vladimír Jekl, MVDr, PhD, Dip ECZM (Small Mammal Medicine and Surgery), EBVS
European Recognized Veterinary Specialist in zoological Medicine (Small Mammal Medicine
and Surgery)[a,b,*], David Modry, MVDr, PhD[c,d,e]

KEYWORDS

- Guinea pig • Chinchilla • Degu • Hamster • Rat • Gastrointestinal disease
- Gastric dilatation and volvulus • Enteritis

KEY POINTS

- Gastrointestinal diseases are very common in companion rodents. The gastrointestinal syndrom is commonly due to concurrent illness, stress, or pain.
- Gastric dilatation and volvulus in guinea pigs is life-threatening and must be treated as soon as possible.
- Chinchillas are commonly carriers of *Giardia intestinalis*. All rodents should be routinely examined for intestinal parasites.
- Degus suffer from gas accumulation in the stomach and intestines due to obstructive nasal disease.
- "Wet tail" in hamsters is just a syndrome whose primary cause needs to be identified.

INTRODUCTION

Gastrointestinal (GI) diseases are frequently diagnosed in pet rodents.[1–4] Clinical signs are usually nonspecific and include anorexia, weight loss, chronic wasting, abdominal discomfort, gas accumulation in the intestines and stomach, and diarrhea. The main goal of treatment is to address the primary disease and stabilize the patient, which includes fluid therapy, analgesia, assisted feeding, and other supportive measures. The prognosis of the patient with GI disease depends on the primary cause, the time of diagnosis, and the initiation of appropriate treatment. Disease prevention is based

[a] Department of Pharmacology and Pharmacy, Faculty of Veterinary Medicine, Veterinary University Brno, Brno, Czech Republic; [b] Jekl & Hauptman Veterinary Clinic – Focused on Exotic Companion Mammal Care, Brno, Czech Republic; [c] Deptartment of Veterinary Sciences and CINeZ, FAPPZ, Czech University of Life Sciences Prague, Kamýcká 129, 165 21 Praha 6 - Suchdol Prague, Czech Republic; [d] Deptartment of Botany and Zoology, Masaryk University, Brno, Czech Republic; [e] Parasitological Institute of CAS, Biology Center, České Budějovice, Czech Republic
* Corresponding author. Jezeruvky 525/1, Brno 62100, Czech Republic.
E-mail address: vladimirjekl@gmail.com

Vet Clin Exot Anim 28 (2025) 263–294
https://doi.org/10.1016/j.cvex.2024.12.002
vetexotic.theclinics.com

Abbreviations	
CSM	colonic separation mechanism
ELISA	enzyme-linked immunosorbent assay
GD	gastric dilatation
GDV	gastric dilatation and volvulus
GI	gastrointestinal
IDIRs	infectious diarrhea of infant rats
PCR	polymerase chain reaction

on appropriate housing and nutrition and avoidance of stress and pain. To prevent nutritional problems, which are one of the most common causes of GI diseases, it is important to consider the nutritional needs of each species and its microbial population. The choice of dietary components must be adapted accordingly: high-fiber, low-sugar, and low-starch diets for strict herbivores, with slightly more starch and less fiber allowed for granivores and omnivores.[5] Selected anatomic features of the GI tract can be found in **Table 1**.[6–20] One important characteristic of some small mammals is coprophagy. Guinea pigs, like chinchillas and degus, are hindgut fermenters and coprophagic. Although the belief is that coprophagy is an important function in these species, its contribution to nutritional needs has not been fully characterized. In some small mammal species, the colonic separation mechanism (CSM) is referred as the "mucous trap."[21] Guinea pigs, chinchillas, and degus have particular colonic anatomic features, the colonic grooves or furrows, that are essential for the functionality of the mucous trap CSM. In this groove, mucous and bacteria are trapped and transported in a retrograde direction through antiperistalsis back to the cecum. This feature allows for the rapid passage of less-digestible food particles while retaining microorganisms, fluids, and more digestible food particles in the cecum to allow adequate opportunity for fermentation.[22] At certain intervals, the separation mechanism ceases to function, and cecotrophs are formed. The nitrogen concentration in the contents of the large intestine fluctuates greatly within 24 hours, which is related to the production of 2 types of pellets, one rich in nitrogen (cecotrophs) and one poor in nitrogen (fecal pellets). The ratio of nitrogen concentration between these 2 types can be up to 3 times higher in the same animal.[21–23]

When evaluating the GI function of rodents, a thorough history is essential and should be structured in the same way as for other mammalian species, with particular attention to signalment, diet, and husbandry. This includes any recent changes in diet, group size, disease in other animals kept in the same household, previous contact with other animals (eg, pet shows), new additions, onset and duration of clinical signs, course of disease, and any previous treatments. Clinical examination can be challenging in smaller species, but a systematic approach will help to ensure that nothing is missed (**Fig. 1**). Clinical assessment can be complemented with a variety of diagnostic imaging modalities (**Table 2**) and other diagnostics (**Table 3**).

GUINEA PIGS

Guinea pigs are strictly herbivorous rodents, which belongs to the family Caviidae in the rodent suborder Hystricomorpha. They are crepuscular animals and are one of the most popular species of exotic pets due to their small size, docile nature, and relatively easy care.[24,25] GI tract disease is a common clinical disorder in guinea pigs. Minarikova and colleagues[26] recorded a GI disease prevalence of 13.1% (131 out of 1000 animals). GI tract disorders are mainly secondary; however, life-threatening acute

Table 1
Selected information on gastrointestinal tract anatomy of the guinea pig, chinchilla, degu, hamster, and a rat[12,21–25,58–62,90,117,118]

	Stomach	Cecum and Colon—Anatomy	Miscellaneous
Guinea pig	• Simple • Completely glandular • Gastric emptying time is approximately 2 h	• Cecum: up to 65% volume of the entire GI tract • *Taenia coli* running in 3 thin bands along its entire length, causing protrusions or haustra in the intervening wall	• The perineal sac of the male opens as longitudinal slit between scrotal pouches • The smaller and shallower perineal sac of the female opens transversely between the vagina and anus • Cecotrophy takes place during the day and night
Chinchilla	• Simple • Completely glandular	• Cecum: up to 22% volume of the entire GI tract • There are sacculations in the proximal portion of the cecum • The second portion is more tubular and includes fewer but larger haustra • Colon has numerous haustra	• Cecotrophy only takes place during the day and only releases their fecal pellets at night • The chinchilla produces approximately the same amount of cecotrophs as fecal pellets within 24 h • 10 most common abundant microbiota bacterial genera/families in the gastrointestinal tract of chinchillas are *Lactobacillus*, Muribaculaceae, Sarcina and *Streptococcus*, Erysipelotrichaceae, *Ruminococcus*, Clostridia_UCG-014, Atopobiaceae, and Lachnospiraceae
Degu	• Simple • Completely glandular	• The cecum has *Taenia* separated by haustra • Colon lacks the haustra	

Hamster	• Compound
	  ○ Larger blind forestomach
	  ○ Small glandular stomach
		• Large helical structure	• The mucous membrane of cecum and colon is pale and smooth, and free of villi

Rat	• Compound
	  ○ Nonglandular part is used to store the food
	  ○ Glandular part contains gastric glands
		• The comma-shaped cecum	

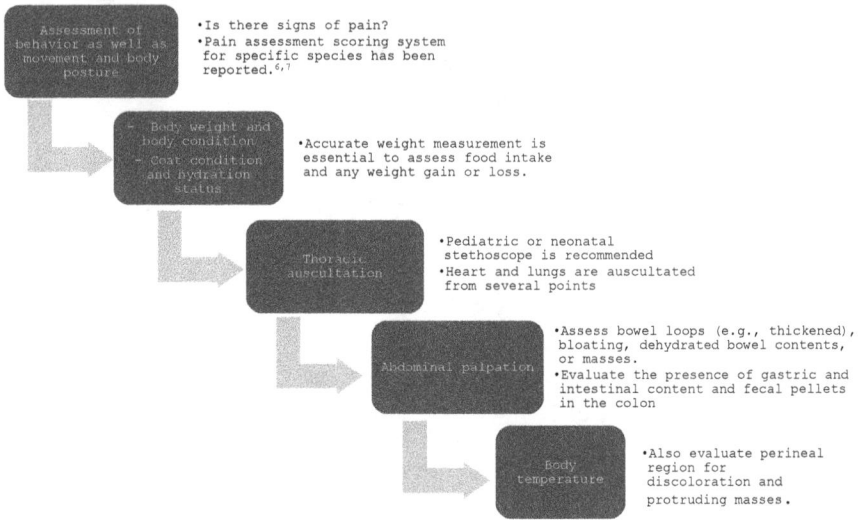

Fig. 1. Flow chart 1: Systematic and standard approach of the clinical examination will help to ensure that nothing is missed.

gastric dilation and torsion can be also seen (**Fig. 2**A–D).[2,26,27] In a retrospective study with 1000 guinea pigs, changes in the consistency of the fecal pellets were mainly observed in connection with dental diseases or in animals that were obese and/or were predominantly fed a commercial muesli-like diet.[26]

Viral and Bacterial Diseases

Primary infectious diseases of the GI tract are rarely seen in guinea pigs. A suspected coronavirus enteritis has been reported in 3 to 4 week old laboratory guinea pigs, characterized by diarrhea, anorexia, weight loss, and death associated with enteritis. The disease has low morbidity and low mortality rates.[28] Bacterial diarrhea occurs mainly in weaned animals, pregnant females and immunocompromised or chronically stressed animals.[2] *Escherichia coli*, *Salmonella typhimurium*, *Salmonella enteritidis*, *Salmonella ochiogu*, *Lawsonia intracellularis*, *Yersinia pseudotuberculosis*, *Clostridium piliforme* (Tyzzer's disease), *Clostridium perfringens*, *Pseudomonas aeruginosa*, *Listeria monocytogenes*, and *Citrobacter freundii* are among bacterial pathogens causing enteritis.[1,29] Diagnosis is based on clinical signs and bacterial culture. Treatment consists of fluid therapy, supportive care, assisted feeding, and antibiotics.

Parasitic Infections

The digestive tract of guinea pigs is colonized by a relatively small number of parasitic protists and helminths, only some of which are present in captive animals and are potentially pathogenic. While some of the parasites are considered commensals under normal circumstances (eg, *Trichomonas*, *Balantioides coli*, and *Entamoeba caviae*), others can occasionally cause GI disorders. As all these parasites have a direct life cycle and oral infection, environmental conditions, breeding group composition, diet and general husbandry play a crucial role in infection intensity and consequences.[30] In a survey of endoparasites in 60 pet guinea pigs in Italy, only *Paraspidodera uncinata* eggs, *Nippostrongylus*-like eggs, and *Eimeria caviae* were detected. None of the samples was positive for *Cryptosporidium* or *Giardia* sp.[17]

Table 2
Diagnostic imaging modalities used for the rodent gastrointestinal tract examination

Imaging Modality	Recommended Images and Other Applications	Limitations	Notes
Abdominal radiographs	• Ventrodorsal (Fig. 2) • Lateral views	• Moderate loss of definition of the serosal surfaces, which makes visualization of the margins of the abdominal organs difficult • Overlap of gases in the GI tract (mainly the cecum)	• Entire abdomen, ventral, dorsal, and lateral soft tissue margins, including the gluteal muscles and perianal region, should be visible on the radiograph[8]
Abdominal ultrasound	• Dorsal • And/or lateral recumbency to assess the entire GI tract	• A large amount of gas in the digestive tract impacts the visualization of the abdominal organs[9]	• Can be used to assess the abdominal organs and to detect ascites or hemabdomen • Provides real-time information • Ultrasound data for rats and guinea pigs has been published[9-11]
Computed tomography	• Whole body view • Abdominal-only view	• It may not always be available	• Reference data for CT of the liver and other abdominal organs in chinchillas has been published[12]
Flexible endoscopy	• Gastroscopy • Colonoscopy	• Insufflation can lead to gastric and intestinal distention and pain	• Rodents cannot vomit and are very sensitive to dysbiosis • Endoscopy should always be performed with caution • All gas must be removed when the examination is completed

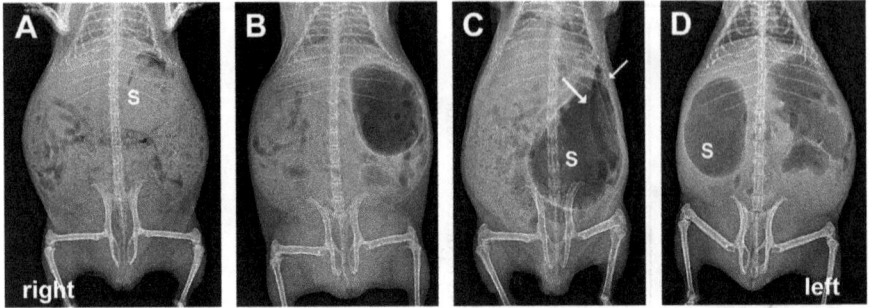

Fig. 2. Ventrodorsal radiographs of the abdomen of various guinea pigs. (A) Healthy guinea pig with stomach (S) and the entire gastrointestinal tract filled with food ingesta. There is a just small amount of gas located in the right cranial region of the stomach. (B) Guinea pig with distended stomach (S) with air swallowed during anesthesia. The stomach is mainly located on the left side of the abdomen. (C) Gastric dilatation and torsion of the stomach. The duodenum is displaced and located on the left side of the abdominal cavity (*arrows*). The small intestines are located cranially to the stomach. (D) A guinea pig with gastric dilatation (S) and omental torsion with gas in the cecum. The stomach is filled with air and fluid, and it is located on the right side. The loss of organ detail indicates the presence of ascites. (*Courtesy of* Vladimir Jekl, DVM.)

Eimeria caviae

E caviae is the only species of *Eimeria* that infects guinea pigs (**Fig. 3**A).[3] This organism is species-specific. Endogenous development takes place in the large intestine. Massive infection can lead to severe destruction of the mucosa, followed by colitis. Infection is usually more severe in young animals; nonsterile immunity develops after infection. Infection is easily detected by the presence of

Table 3
Other diagnostics used in pet rodents with gastrointestinal tract disorders

Diagnostic Method	Notes
Hematology and biochemistry results	• Often nonspecific • Can show inflammatory response, anemia, and azotemia (commonly due to dehydration) • Can show hypoproteinemia and hypoalbuminemia (commonly associated with anorexia or malabsorption (endoparasites, enteritis)[16]
Fecal parasitology (qualitative [eg, wet preparation and simple flotation] and quantitative coprologic methods [eg, McMaster, quantitative diagnostic techniques sufficiently accurate to estimate the number of parasites in fecal samples [FLOTAC] or others])	• Used to identify and quantify the parasite load • Some endoparasites do not shed regularly; therefore, collection of feces should be done over multiple days • If pinworms are suspected, a "tape test" from the perianal region should be performed[1] • PCR and immunoassays may also be available (eg, *Giardia* and *Cryptosporidium*)[17]
Microbial culture and sensitivity	• May allow the identification of specific organisms/pathogens • Aim therapy of bacterial infections

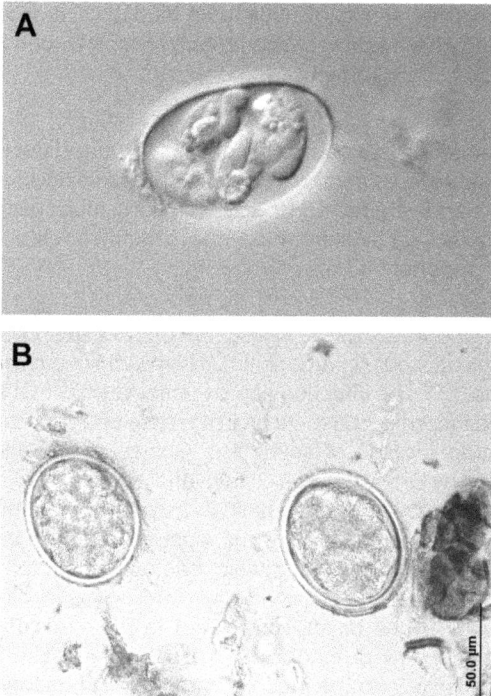

Fig. 3. Endoparasites of guinea pigs. (*A*) *E caviae*, a moderately pathogenic coccidium, is usually clinically manifested by lethargy, anorexia, and pasty stool diarrhea in weanlings; (*B*) *P uncinata* is a common helminth of guinea pigs, which inhabits the cecum and large intestine mucosa. (*Courtesy of* David Modry, DVM.)

unsporulated oocysts on coproscopic examination using the flotation technique. As with other rodent species, toltrazuril/diclazuril or ponazuril is the drug of choice against coccidia.

Cryptosporidium sp

Infections with *Cryptosporidium wrairi* and *Cryptosporidium homai* are known to occur occasionally in captive guinea pigs. Developmental stages are found in the microvilli of the intestinal mucosa and tiny oocysts are excreted in the feces. Infections are usually asymptomatic, but the parasite is potentially zoonotic.[31,32] In young animals, weanlings, or immunocompromised animals, the disease can be clinically associated with anorexia, weight loss, diarrhea, and death. Morbidity and mortality can be up to 50%. Immunocompetent guinea pigs recover from the infection within 4 weeks and become resistant to reinfection.[1] At necropsy, watery content is found in the intestines. Diagnosis is based on fecal examination, phase microscopy, and electron microscopy. There is no curative treatment, but sulfonamides can suppress outbreaks.

Paraspidodera uncinata

Known as guinea pig pinworm, *P uncinata* is a medium-sized heteracid nematode that inhabits the large intestine and cecum (**Fig. 3**B). The eggs survive in moist bedding and the intensity of infection depends on hygiene measures. Mild infections are usually subclinical, severe infections lead to anorexia, diarrhea, and weight loss.

Benzimidazoles such as fenbendazole (20 mg/kg for 5 days) or febantel (10 mg/kg for 3 days), both repeated after 14 days are commonly recommended anthelmintics; ivermectin (0.3 mg/kg s.c.) can also be used.

Trichuris sp

A rarely occurring nematode that causes infection of the large intestine. Mild infections are usually subclinical, severe infections can lead to chronic colitis. Diagnosis by fecal flotation with typical barrel-shaped eggs. Eggs survive in moist bedding and the intensity of infection depends on hygiene measures. Treatment as above, resistance to ivermectin has been reported in Peru.[33]

Enterotoxemia

Enterotoxemia can be caused by pathogenic *Clostridium spiroforme*, *Clostridium difficile*, or *C perfringens*.[34,35] The infection can be associated with a fecal–oral infection with *C spiroforme* via the fecal–oral route or, in the case of *C difficile* and *C perfringens*, secondary to inappropriate use of antibiotics. Guinea pigs, chinchillas, and degus possess a predominantly Gram-positive GI flora and are exquisitely sensitive to antibiotics targeting those bacteria. Oral drugs such as penicillin, ampicillin, clindamycin, erythromycin, and lincomycin will destroy the most susceptible Gram-positive organisms, permitting overgrowth of pathogenic bacteria such as *C difficile* and *C perfringens*.[36]

The pathophysiology of the disease is related to the exotoxins of the clostridia, which are either enterotoxins or cytotoxins. These toxins cause fluid secretion into the intestinal lumen, damage to the mucosa, and an inflammatory reaction. The disease is usually peracute. Clinical symptoms include anorexia, dehydration, hypothermia, abdominal distension, diarrhea (**Fig. 4**), abdominal pain, and, in severe cases, acute death. Diagnosis is based on the history, clinical examination and results of fecal cytology and microbiology. At postmortem examination, the intestinal loops are distended with serosal hemorrhages, hepatomegaly, and splenomegaly. The prognosis is very guarded to poor. Treatment includes fluid therapy, thermal and nutritional support, cholestyramine, and the administration of metronidazole or chloramphenicol. Use probiotics alone (eg, *Lactobacillus* sp) is not recommend as its administration was not shown to be effective.[37] In addition to clostridial infections secondary to enterotoxemia, staphylococcal enterocolitis has also been reported as a complication of antibiotic therapy.[38]

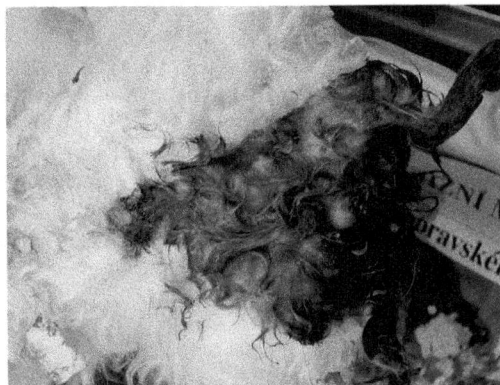

Fig. 4. A guinea pig with severe watery diarrhea associated with oral beta-lactam antibiotic administration. (*Courtesy of* Vladimir Jekl, DVM.)

Gastrointestinal Stasis/Gastrointestinal Syndrome

The most common disorder of the GI tract in herbivorous exotic companion rodents is GI stasis.[1-3] In rabbits, the term GI syndrome or rabbit GI syndrome is used to better define a complex of clinical signs, symptoms, and concurrent pathologic conditions affecting the rabbit's digestive system.[39] The following pathologic conditions may be included and often occur in combination: gastric obstruction, gastric gas accumulation, intestinal obstruction, intestinal gas accumulation, intestinal obstruction, primary gastroenteritis, adhesions, neoplasia, pancreatitis, and liver disease. The pathophysiology of primary GI stasis and secondary diseases is, in fact, even more complex in exotic domestic mammals. Therefore, the term "GI syndrome" can also be used in herbivorous pet rodents. GI syndrome is defined as disruption of the normal motor activity of the GI tract by nonmechanical mechanisms (synonyms: paralytic ileus and functional ileus) or by pylorus/bowel obstruction (synonyms: mechanical ileus and mechanical obstruction). The cause of the obstruction can be outside the intestine (extramural), inside the intestinal wall, or due to a luminal defect/foreign body that prevents the passage of GI contents (intraluminal). The intestinal obstruction may be partial or complete. The most common cause of bowel obstruction in exotic companion rodents is the presence of an intraluminal foreign body (eg, trichobezoar) or gastric dilatation and volvulus (GDV).

GI stasis in guinea pigs, chinchillas, and degus is commonly associated with an inappropriate diet (low-fiber, high digestible carbohydrates). However, GI stasis can be associated with any stressful situation or condition that stimulates the sympathetic nervous system, including pain (eg, dental disease), systemic illness, or surgery.

As GI motility decreases, the digesta retention is prolonged and the normal, balanced ecosystem in the gut (especially in the cecum) is disrupted. The pH value in the cecum is altered and allows the overgrowth of potentially pathogenic bacteria (Clostridium sp and E coli). The bacterial overload/dysbiosis described earlier may lead to either clinical enteritis/typhlitis or enterotoxemia. In case of prolonged digesta retention in the stomach for a longer period, there is a risk of developing a gastric ulcer, which leads to an additional source of pain. GI hypomotility leads to gas formation in the intestines and cecum or in the stomach. The GI tract gas distension is painful, stimulates the sympathetic nervous system and aggravates the situation. Secondary impaction can result from excessive accumulation of normal GI contents due to alterations in gastric and intestinal motility or desiccation of normal contents due to dehydration. Metabolic acidosis is a common consequence of negative energy balance due to anorexia and malabsorption.

The diagnosis of GI syndrome includes a complete medical history, physical examination, fecal examination, and radiographic examination. Palpation of the abdomen reveals gas and fluid in the bowel and cecum with minimal contents of the colon. In the case of colonic or cecal impaction, the dehydrated contents will be palpated as a hard mass. Gentle palpation is recommended as excessive pressure can lead to damage to the colonic or cecal wall. Radiographs may confirm the clinical findings. An ultrasound examination can also be carried out, although flatulence in the bowel makes it difficult to perform an ultrasound examination. Hematology and blood biochemistry may be helpful in detecting electrolyte imbalance and/or organ failure.

GI syndrome management is based on the treatment of the underlying condition. The goal is to restore appetite and reverse the negative energy balance. If no obstruction is present, correction of the hydration status, body temperature, and analgesia is of paramount importance. Continuous rate infusions of analgesics are also recommended (eg, lidocaine, fentanyl, and ketamine). There are several drugs used for the stimulation of peristalsis used in herbivorous rodents with GI stasis/postoperative ileus.[40–42] Supportive feeding with commercial recovery foods (Emeraid Herbivore [Emeraid Intensive Care Herbivore, EmerAid, USA], Supreme Science Selective Recovery Plus [Supreme Petfoods, UK], Oxbow Critical Care [Oxbow Animal Health, USA], etc.) is recommended. Syringe feeding is essential as the aim is to create a positive energy balance. Digestible fiber (small fibers) is important to provide nutrients for the cecal bacteria (eg, Emeraid). Indigestible fibers (eg, Supreme Recovery, Oxbow Critical Care Herbivore) are necessary to promote motility of the digestive tract, even if they are difficult to administer by syringe due to the long fibers. Feeding prebiotics and probiotics may help prevent dysbiosis. For analgesia, a combination of opioids and nonsteroidal anti-inflammatory drugs is the best choice in well-hydrated animals. Among prokinetics, ranitidine, metoclopramide, itopride, or cisapride can be used (**Table 4**). Prokinetics are contraindicated in cecal/colonic impaction and may be less effective in cases where the primary cause is not adequately treated. Other medications that may be used include probiotics (*Saccharomyces cerevisiae* and *Enterococcus* sp), and prebiotics; however, there is still lack of clinical studies in the literature to prove the positive effect on a rodent GI tract. Studies on probiotic supplementation in guinea pigs have produced inconsistent results. Most studies aim to increase productive performance.[43,44] In a recent study, bacteria with possible probiotic potential were identified by molecular analysis: *Leuconostoc citreum* (cepa MG5373 and cepa BGL7), *Enterococcus gallinarum*, *Exiguobacterium* sp, and *Lactococcus lactis*.[45]

Gastric Dilatation and Volvulus

Gastric dilatation (GD) or GDV are life-threatening emergencies that must be treated immediately.[1–3] GDV is typically observed in 1.5 to 3 year old guinea pigs.[2,27] In cases of GDV, the stomach rotates on its axis, creating a functional obstruction. Fluid and gas are trapped in the lumen and bacterial fermentation in the stomach leads to further distension of the stomach and thus to increased pressure in the abdominal cavity. This reduces venous flow in the caudal vena cava and portal vein, leading to portal hypertension, systemic hypotension, venous stasis, and cardiac dysfunction. This, in turn, can lead to cardiogenic shock. The venous stasis itself causes death of the gastric mucosa and bacterial dislocation. The pressure of the distended stomach on the diaphragm impacts inspiration.

GDV is a well-recognized and highly prevalent condition in guinea pigs older than 2 years.[2,26,27,46–49] In a retrospective study of 1000 pet guinea pigs, GD was found in 1% (10 out of 1000) and GDV in 3.4% (34 out of 1000) of animals.[26] Another publication described 6 breeding animals with GDV in a colony of 253 animals within a period of 18 months.[49]

Table 4
Prokinetic effect of selected drugs on guinea pig and rat colon[40–42]

Drug	Oral Dose (mg/kg)	Effect on Guinea Pig Colon	Effect on Rat Colon
Itopride	10	Prokinetic effect	Prokinetic effect
Cisapride	10	No prokinetic effect	No prokinetic effect
Mosapride	10	No prokinetic effect	Prokinetic effect
Prucalopride	5–10	Prokinetic effect	Not known

The factors predisposing guinea pigs to GDV are still unknown; however, the presence of trichobezoar, bloat, dysbiosis, delayed gastric emptying, poor nutrition, pain, and dental disease can lead to GI stasis, and gas formation with subsequent GDV.[1,48] Once distended, the stomach could rotate with certain movements of the animal (eg, repositioning during anesthesia).[50] Clinicians should be aware of this possibility and avoid excessive repositioning of guinea pigs with GD when performing radiographs[48] or when the animal is under anesthesia.

The most common type of torsion in dogs is a 180° clockwise torsion; however, 90° clockwise torsion as well as 360° and 540° clockwise volvulus have also been documented in the literature.[27] Similar findings (180° and 360° clockwise volvulus) were observed by the author (VJ) in guinea pigs. The pylorus and proximal duodenum move ventrally then cranial to the body of the stomach.

Clinical manifestations of GD or GDV include apathy, reluctance to move, shallow breathing, cyanosis of the mucous membranes, tachycardia, tachypnea, abdominal distention, and absence of normal borborygmi. In severe cases, affected animals can be found dead with no prior clinical signs of disease. The cause of death in guinea pigs with GDV appears to be respiratory compromise due to compression of the diaphragm by the gas-distended stomach, hypothermia, hypovolemic shock, and cardiovascular failure associated with extramural compression of the caudal vena cava.[49,50]

The diagnosis is based on clinical signs and abdominal radiographic findings (**Figs. 2** and **5**). Abdominal radiographs confirm marked GD with bloating and displacement of the stomach to the right side of the abdominal cavity with intestinal loops cranial to the stomach, which are pathognomonic findings for GDV. The stomach may appear septated and gas may also be present in the small intestine and cecum. In a mesenteric root torsion/volvulus, the stomach can be also located either on the right side of the body or caudal to the small bowel loops.[51] Based on the author experience (VJ), many guinea pigs are in metabolic acidosis, so acid–base balance disorders need to be addressed too.

Treatment is very challenging, and the prognosis in most cases is guarded to poor. Treatment of GDV includes aggressive intravenous fluid therapy, thermal support, and pain management. Placement of an orogastric tube is recommended to achieve gastric decompression prior to gastric repositioning; however, occlusion of the distal esophagus in GDV can make passage of the tube into the stomach difficult, so

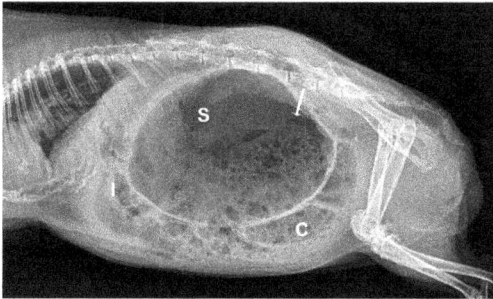

Fig. 5. Lateral abdominal radiograph of a 5 year old intact male guinea pig presented with acute onset of lethargy. The stomach (S) is markedly distended with gas and displaced caudodorsally. The small intestine (I) is displaced cranially to the stomach. The cecum (C) is located caudoventrally. A small amount of gas is also present in the large intestine (*arrow*), no feces are visible. These radiograph findings were consistent with gastric dilatation-volvulus. (*Courtesy of* Vladimir Jekl, DVM.)

extreme caution is required when passing the tube. The stomach content is usually semisolid, so it can be difficult to aspirate them. The stomach should be palpated carefully to determine when the pressure has eased. Percutaneous decompression of the stomach with a needle, as can be performed in dogs,[52] is not recommended due to the potential leakage of gastric contents unless performed during surgery. Surgical attempts have been made to correct GDV in guinea pigs, but there are few cases that have successfully recovered. During midline laparotomy, the abdominal organs are carefully revised, the stomach is decompressed, and then returned to a physiologic position. Gastropexy is one of the options during surgery to prevent further movement of the stomach, whereby the stomach is sutured to the abdominal wall. However, due to the small survival rate and small number of reported cases, it is not possible to say whether this technique is helpful or not.[49]

Gastric Trichobezoars

Gastric bezoars are a mixture of indigestible material, which may or may not be organic, in the GI tract. In guinea pigs, bezoars are thought to be the result of excessive ingestion of hair, particularly in Peruvian-type breeds.[53] Excessive grooming during shedding, licking of local dermatologic medications and chewing of fur due to lack of fiber or boredom may contribute to increased ingestion of fur. Reduced GI motility due to stress factors (eg, malnutrition, stress, and lack of exercise) is thought to lead to anorexia, dehydration, and accumulation of hair and food debris in the stomach and intestines. As a result, the stomach contents accumulate, preventing adequate gastric emptying.

Bezoar is considered a rare finding in guinea pigs. Trichobezoars can be diagnosed by palpation of the abdomen as hard objects of varying size, usually located in the gastric lumen, but often the physical examination remains inconclusive. In the author's (VJ) experience, repeated palpation in sedated animals or animals under general anesthesia during other procedures (blood sampling, intravenous catheter placement, and so forth) significantly increases the diagnostic results of abdominal palpation. Radiographic and ultrasound examinations can help to confirm the presence of a foreign body in the GI tract.[54]

There is some information on medical/conservative and surgical treatment options.[53–55] Treatment consists primarily of stabilization of the patient (fluid therapy, pain management and other supportive measures, oral hydration, and administration of convalescent diet) and gastrotomy.

Several measures should be taken to prevent recurrence of gastric trichobezoar: a high-fiber diet with ad libitum access to grass hay, optimal hair care, reduction of environmental stressors and diagnosis of possible complicating disease conditions (eg, dental pathology).[53] High-fiber pellet diet alone without hay supply did not reduce hair loss in a feeding experiment and, therefore, may not prevent trichobezoars.[53]

Anal Sac/Rectal Impactions

In older guinea pigs (especially boars) or guinea pigs that have lost weight for various reasons, fecal impaction in the anus may occur (**Fig. 6**). Loss of muscle tone and inability to perform coprophagy are possible etiologic factors. The clinical signs are related to abnormal fecal excretion and a foul-smelling accumulation of feces in the anus. Diagnosis is based on clinical examination, but the primary cause must be identified. Treatment consists of gentle manual removal of the impacted material and disinfection of the anus.

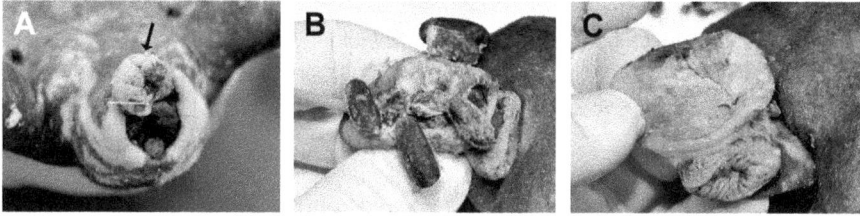

Fig. 6. The male guinea pigs (5-year-old (*A*), and 3-year-old (*B*, *C*) was presented with constipation and a foul-smelling anal area. On clinical examination, anal sac/rectal impaction was diagnosed, the colon, cecum, and intestine were normal on palpation, and no constipation was noted. In both cases, prepucium was also slightly enlarged (*arrow*, *A*). Treatment included gentle removal of accumulated feces, anal gland secretions, and other debris (*B*, *C*). (*Courtesy of* Vladimir Jekl, DVM)

Neoplasia

Spontaneous tumors of the GI tract of guinea pigs are rare. Reported cases include gastric leiomyoma, gastric leiomyosarcoma, GI stromal tumor of the cecum, lymphoma, and lymphosarcoma.[56,57]

CHINCHILLAS

Chinchillas are social rodents living in extreme climates at high altitudes in South American mountains. Chinchillas are grazing herbivores and hind-gut fermenters with a unique gastrointestinal digestive system (see **Table 1**).[21,58–62] GI disorders, apart from dental disease and giardiasis, are not as common in chinchillas as these are in guinea pigs or rabbits. Disorders of the GI tract of noninfectious origin are more common and mostly related to inappropriate diet.

Infectious Diseases

Bacterial infections are rare in pet chinchillas and are mainly seen in young animals or breeding females.[1] Predisposing factors include suboptimal husbandry conditions, dietary change, low-fiber diet, high-energy diet, and stress, overcrowding included. As a cause of gastroenteritis, *Yersinia enterocolitica*, *E coli*, *Staphylococcus* spp, *Pasteurella* spp, *Proteus mirabilis*, and *Klebsiella pneumoniae* were described.[1] Reavill[63] suggested that *K pneumoniae* remains a common cause of enteritis and systemic infections in young chinchillas; however, it is rarely seen by authors. Also, some bacteria causing septicemia (eg, *P aeruginosa*, *L monocytogenes*, and *Listeria ivanovii*) may be associated with enteritis. *Y enterocolitica* has also been associated with sporadic outbreaks of death in chinchilla colonies. The lesions were of granulomatous hepatitis, splenitis, and fibrinous enterocolitis, closely resembling the classic lesions of *Y pseudotuberculosis*.[63]

Clinically affected chinchillas are anorectic, apathetic, dehydrated, and suffering from diarrhea or constipation. Excessive accumulation of mucus in the intestinal lumen is a commonly reported finding.[63,64] Other clinical signs may be associated with systemic bacterial infection/septicemia and may be seen as dyspnea (eg, *P aeruginosa*), ataxia, or seizures (eg, *L monocytogenes*). Peracute cases may die within 2 to 3 days of the onset of clinical signs. Diagnosis is based on the clinical signs and isolation of the pathogen from the feces (colonic swab). The disease may be associated with leukocytosis, leukopenia, anemia, and azotemia. Treatment is based on supportive care, fluid therapy, and antibiotic administration.

Enterotoxemia and gastrointestinal stasis

These conditions in chinchillas are similar to guinea pigs. For more information, see "Enterotoxemia" and "Gastrointestinal Stasis/Gastrointestinal Syndrome" sections.

Parasitic infections

In captive animals, *Giardia duodenalis* is broadly distributed, and chinchillas are sensitive to occasional infection by parasites acquired from other rodents, such as *Trichuris* sp, *Eimeria* spp, and *Cryptosporidium* spp.[65,66]

Giardia duodenalis

Captive chinchillas are known for the high prevalence of various genotypes of *Giardia*.[67–69] Detected genotypes involve both zoonotic and nonzoonotic lineages (assemblages). Infections are commonly asymptomatic. The zoonotic risk should always be considered, especially in immunocompromised owners. The life cycle of *G duodenalis* consists of 2 stages: trophozoite and cyst. The trophozoite is the vegetative form and replicates in the small intestine of the host. The 8 flagella provide motility, and the ventral disk provides attachment to the intestinal wall, where it gains its nutrients. More distally, in the small intestine and even extending to the large intestine, the trophozoite transforms into a cyst that is environmentally stable and can be transmitted to the next host through the fecal–oral route.[70] The main predisposing factors are poor husbandry, stress, or concurrent disease. Clinical signs and symptoms include apathy, anorexia, weight loss, poor coat condition, and diarrhea. In cases of dehydration, constipation may be also present. Diagnosis is mainly based on findings and microscopic identification of cysts or adult giardia in stool samples, but immunological-based assay and molecular methods are available. Orally administered metronidazole (20 mg/kg) can be used to treat giardia; however, metronidazole administration commonly results in a temporary reduction of food intake.[71,72]

Cestodiasis. Chinchillas may serve as intermediate hosts for the cestodes *Taenia serialis*, *Taenia pisiformis*, *Taenia crassiceps*, *Echinococcus granulosus*, and *Hymenolepis (Rodentolepis) nana*.[1]

Oxyurids. There is only one case report describing a pinworm infection in a pet chinchilla, which is presented with perianal swelling.[73] The chinchilla was treated with oral fenbendazole (20 mg/kg, once a day for 5 days), with uneventful recovery.[73]

Noninfectious Diseases

GI stasis/tympany

Gastrointestinal stasis and/or tympany may be associated with the feeding of an inappropriate diet rich in carbohydrates and low in fiber.

Rectal prolapse

Rectal prolapse may be seen in chinchillas more commonly than in other species. It occurs secondary to diarrhea, partition, mesenteric torsion, or constipation (**Fig. 7**). The main diagnostic purpose is to determine the primary cause and to find out if the prolapsed tissue is only the distal colon or not. If the prolapse is only minor, cleaning of the prolapsed tissue and repositioning using cotton tips is indicated; a purse-string suture may be applied to the anal opening. In more severe cases, the combination of manual reduction and laparotomy is needed; however, prognosis and treatment are mostly unsuccessful.

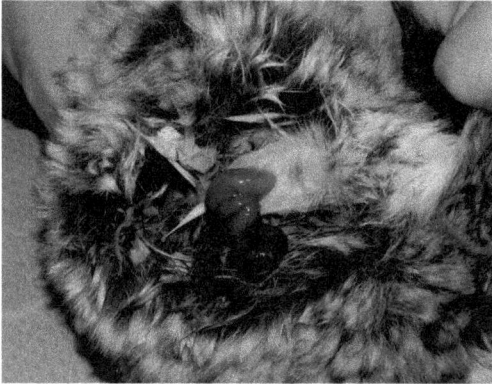

Fig. 7. Rectal prolapse in a chinchilla associated with severe straining simultaneous infection of *E coli* and *Giardia intestinalis*. (*Courtesy of* Vladimir Jekl, DVM.)

DEGUS

Degus are members of the Octodontidae family. Degus are social, diurnal rodents that are native to the western slopes of the Andes in northern and central Chile and feed exclusively on plants. In the wild, they are among the smallest South American hystricomorph rodents and live in areas of medium altitude, that is, up to 1200 m.[74,75] Anatomic features of the GI tract are given in **Table 1**.[76–79] In a retrospective study of 300 pet degus, gastrointestinal disease occurred in 10% of the animals (30 out of 300; some with more than one disorder), including GD (25 cases), diarrhea (10 cases), liver failure (4 cases), pancreatitis (6 cases), and cecal or colonic impaction (7 cases).[76]

Bacterial Diseases

Infectious diseases of the GI tract are extremely rare in pet degus, and no primary GI tract infectious disease was recorded in 300 degus.[76] In a study of 39 degus by Nagy and colleagues,[80] *E coli* was isolated from 2 cases and was seen together with the accumulation of mucoid material in intestines. One case of typhlitis was also recorded; however, no treatment was described.[80]

Parasitic Infections

Degus are broadly distributed in South America and free-ranging populations host a broad-spectrum of endoparasites, including anoplocephalid tapeworms, *Trichuris bradleyi* (zoonotic), and *Graphidioides taglei*, *Longistriata degusi*, and *Physaloptera* spp (zoonotic), and strongyloid nematodes.[71,81] Intestinal parasites are very rare in captive degus.[1,76]

Sporadic *Giardia* infections are reported from captive animals, usually as asymptomatic cases.[82] Najecki and Tate[83] described fatal diarrhea associated with *Giardia* spp in adult and pup degus. Diagnosis is based on coprological testing (flotation, wet mount cytology, and cytology) and/or fecal enzyme-linked immunosorbent assay (ELISA). Treatment includes oral administration of fenbendazole (25mg/kg q24 h for 5 consecutive days).

Noninfectious Disease

Gastrointestinal syndrome

GI syndrome etiology and pathophysiology is similar to listed earlier.[84] Abnormalities in physiologic peristalsis lead to an imbalance in the bacterial GI microflora, followed by an increased fermentation process and gas production, leading to bloating of the stomach and/or intestine, which exacerbates the abnormalities of GI motility. Gas can also accumulate in the stomach in obstructive upper airway diseases, which are often associated with apical elongation of the maxillary molars and the formation of elodontomas (**Fig. 8**) or due to the presence of other intranasal tumors.[85–87] The presence of gas in the stomach and GD are also observed due to gasping and aerophagia and immediately after isoflurane anesthesia. When GI syndrome occurs, the animal rapidly develops hepatic lipidosis, which can be fatal. Clinical signs and symptoms include those associated with the underlying disease, such as anorexia, apathy, dehydration (skin tenting), immobility, and abdominal distension. For additional information on diagnostics and therapy, see "Gastrointestinal Stasis/Gastrointestinal Syndrome" section.

Enterotoxemia
Similar to previous descriptions. For more information, see "Enterotoxemia" section.

HAMSTERS

Hamsters are members of the order Rodentia, suborder Myomorpha, superfamily Muroidea and in family Cricetidae. Species kept as pet animals mostly include the Syrian or golden (*Mesocricetus auratus*), the Chinese or striped-back (*Cricetulus griseus*), the Russian dwarf (*Phodopus campbelli*), Djungarian or Siberian dwarf (*Phodopus sungorus*), and the Roborovski hamster (*Phodopus roborovskii*).

Bacterial Diseases

GI diseases are a significant cause of morbidity and mortality, especially in Syrian hamsters, often due to bacterial diseases caused by *L intracellularis*, *C piliforme*, *S typhimurium*, *S enteritidis*, *Campylobacter jejuni*, and *E coli*.[88,89] Diarrhea is also one of the most frequent emergency complaints.[89]

Clinical signs are associated with weight loss, low activity, hunched posture, liquid feces, and perineal fecal staining. The term "wet-tail" was commonly used in the case of infection with *L intracellularis*; however, "wet-tail" (perineal fecal staining) is just a clinical symptom and can be associated with any GI tract disorder resulting in diarrhea (**Fig. 9**). The demographic study of clinical disorders in hamsters in United Kingdom showed that enteropathy was the second most common disorder group reported across all species, affecting 11.26% of hamsters, and was the most common disorder

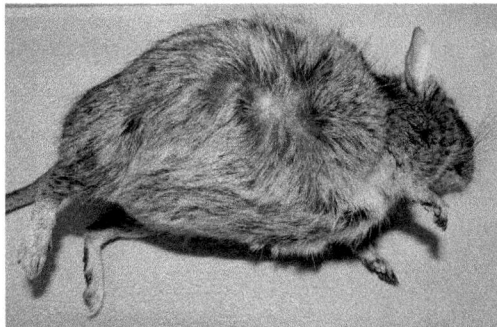

Fig. 8. A degu with severe abdominal distension due to gastrointestinal bloating associated with air swallowing due to nasal cavity obstruction with elodontoma. (*Courtesy of* Vladimir Jekl, DVM.)

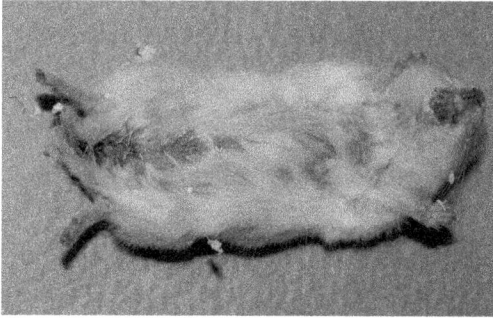

Fig. 9. A hamster with severe perineal fecal staining (wet tail). The term "wet tail" was commonly used in the case of infection with *L intracellularis*. However, the "wet tail" is a clinical symptom and can be associated with any gastrointestinal disease leading to diarrhea. (*Courtesy of* Vladimir Jekl, DVM.)

group reported in Syrian hamsters. "Wet-tail" was seen in 7.33% of animals.[88] The term "wet tail" is a symptom and should not be used as a sole disease entity, as it covers all the numerous conditions that may cause diarrhea in hamsters, and it is even sometimes extended to describe any perineal soiling by urinary tract or reproductive tract discharges.

Proliferative ileitis

Proliferative ileitis (PE) is a unique intestinal disease that is grossly characterized by segmental mucosal hypertrophy. The causative agent of PE is *L intracellularis*, a Gram-negative, non–spore-forming, slightly curved rod (1.25–1.75 × 0.25–0.43 μm), which also causes the disease in other species such as pigs, ferrets, horses, deer, and rabbits.[90,91] This obligate intracellular bacterium infects mitotically active enterocytes and prevents these cells from differentiating into mature enterocytes, resulting in enterocyte proliferation.[92] In hamsters, the bacterium enters the immature epithelial cell via an entry vacuole, which then breaks down and releases bacteria to freely multiply uncontained in the cell cytoplasm. These infected crypt epithelial cells continue to undergo mitosis and transmit the organisms to daughter cells. Eventually, the bacteria are released from cytoplasmic extrusions on the epithelial cells, which are located at the villous apices or between crypts.[93] Infection may spread to the entire ileum, distal jejunum, cecum, and colon. The histologic lesions of PE are equally distinctive and consist of crypt hyperplasia with large numbers of small, curved, intracellular bacteria in the apical cytoplasm of proliferating enterocytes. The results of Vannucci and colleagues[94] showed that a lower intestinal absorption as an important mechanism of diarrhea in hamsters experimentally infected with *L intracellularis*. Therefore, malabsorption should be considered as the main mechanism involved in the pathophysiology of the diarrhea in *L intracellularis*-infected animals.

Hamsters are usually resistant to experimental diseases by 10 to 12 weeks of age[91]; however, spontaneous disease is seen commonly in weaning hamsters (4–8 weeks old), but also older animals can be infected. Predisposing factors include diet changes, transportation, overcrowding, litter from primiparous females, and experimental treatments. There is no sex predilection. The disease's morbidity and mortality rate can reach up to 90%.[95] In early outbreaks, the infection is epizootic, but after several months, the disease becomes enzootic with only sporadic cases identified.[96]

Proliferative ileitis has been divided into different stages, based on clinical manifestation. In the acute stage, which typically occurs 7 to 10 days after infection, hamsters exhibit profuse hemorrhagic diarrhea. The subacute presentation is characterized by retarded growth, diarrhea, and palpable abdominal masses, usually begins between 21 and 30 days after infection. The chronic disease syndrome is characterized by an absence of clinical signs, normal growth rates or occasional deaths, palpable abdominal masses due to thickening of the ileum, abscesses, and enlarged lymph nodes.[96]

Typically, hamsters die within 24 to 48 hours after exhibiting clinical symptoms. Early in the course of the disease, symptoms include agitation, ruffled hair coat, lethargy, anorexia, and rapid weight loss. Soon after, the peritoneum, tail, and ventral abdomen develop wet, matted hair and a foul, watery diarrhea, which leads to dehydration, lethargy, and a hunched posture suggestive of pain. Before the death, the patient is hypothermic, has its abdomen distended, and has convulsions. Animals that survive the initial infection will show signs of emaciation and cachexia. Some hamsters may present with a bloody, intestinal intussusception, or prolapsed colon.[96]

Diagnosis of PE is based on clinical signs and finding the typical histopathological changes. The L intracellularis cannot be cultivated using conventional microbiologic techniques but can be grown in tissue culture. Although experimentally infected animals develop high serologic titers, these titers are not of clinical use in hamsters. Warthin–Starry silver stain will reveal brown haze numerous organisms, in the apical cytoplasm of mucosal and crypt epithelial cells. A fecal DNA-polymerase chain reaction (PCR) assay is also currently available.[97]

Trimethoprim/sulfonamide (30 mg/kg orally every 12 hours for 5–7 days), tetracyclines (400 mg/L of drinking water for 10 days or 10 mg/kg orally every 12 hours for 5–7 days), and enrofloxacin (10 mg/kg orally every 12 hours for 5–7 days) are all appropriate empirical antibiotic options.[97] Chloramphenicol (50 mg/kg intramuscular route of administration [IM], subcutaneous route of administration [SC], or oral route of administration [PO] q12 h) can be used in hamsters as well. In addition to analgesics and antibiotics, and oral bismuth subsalicylate, treatment involves vigorous supportive care with fluid therapy, thermal, and nutritional support. The effectiveness of this approach varies.

Prognosis is very guarded to poor. Control strategies aim to eliminate the pathogen with strict hygiene, isolating afflicted individuals, and optimizing husbandry to reduce stress.

Clostridium difficile infections

C difficile is a Gram-positive, anaerobic, spore-forming bacterium that is frequently associated with diarrhea, typhlitis, and colitis. Among the animals commonly used for laboratory research, Syrian hamsters are the most susceptible to the naturally acquired disease.[98,99] Two protein toxins, A (enterotoxin) and B (cytotoxin), play a major role in the pathogenesis of C difficile infection/toxemia.[100] In addition to the direct pathogenic effect on the enterocytes, the triggering of an inflammatory cascade, which can lead to increased damage to the host tissue and exudation of fluid, is of particular importance. When the toxins are produced in vivo, they trigger a severe, often fatal hemorrhagic ileitis or typhlitis, with ulceration, formation of a pseudomembrane and watery and bloody diarrhea.[100] The cecum is often distended by fluid, with multiple petechial to ecchymotic hemorrhages on the cecal wall. Histopathological findings consistent with Clostridium-induced typhlitis include necrosis, epithelial denudation, vascular congestion, and hemorrhage. Signs of a more chronic disease process may include hyperplasia of the cecal mucosa and renal amyloidosis.[101]

Three forms of diarrhea can be observed.[102] The most common form is profuse and watery diarrhea. A chronic form presents with semiformed, thin feces that discolor the perianal region. The third form is hemorrhagic. Mortality is high in animals with acute watery or hemorrhagic diarrhea. Animals with semiformed soft stools are dehydrated, have a roughened hair-coat, and hunched posture. The diagnosis is based on clinical signs, microbiological culture, and histopathological findings. Even if the presence of the bacteria cannot be confirmed, the presence of *C difficile* toxin is diagnostic. PCR detection of *C difficile* is a highly sensitive method and can differentiate between toxigenic and nontoxigenic strains of the organism by detecting toxin-producing genes. Other diagnostic measures include isolation of the pathogen from fecal samples and the detection of *C difficile* toxins using ELISA.[3,103]

Clostridial enterotoxemia can be associated with the oral administration of penicillin, lincosamides, aminoglycosides, cephalosporins, and erythromycin, which leads to suppression of the normal intestinal microbial flora with an overgrowth of clostridia. In hamsters that develop diarrhea after starting antibiotic treatment, usually the administration of antibiotics is stopped immediately and supportive treatment is given.

Tyzzer's disease

Tyzzer's disease is caused by *C piliforme* and can be associated with a high mortality rate. The infection is usually considered opportunistic, because of severe stress such as overcrowding, poor hygiene, and inadequate nutrition. Clinical signs include acute pale-yellow watery diarrhea, lethargy, dehydration, and death. Postmortem findings show distension of the cecum and mesenteric lymphadenopathy. Histologically, necrotizing typhlitis and hepatitis are present. Typical lesions associated with Tyzzer's disease (ie, hepatomegaly with multiple pale foci of hepatic necrosis) may not be seen.[104] Warthin–Starry silver-stained tissue sections can reveal clusters of *C piliforme* within the cytoplasm of intestinal epithelial cells, smooth muscle cells, hepatocytes, and myocytes bordering foci of necrosis in the intestines, liver, and heart.[105] Tetracycline and oxytetracycline have been reported to control mortality.[104]

Zoonotic bacteria

Salmonellosis in hamsters caused by *S typhimurium* was described as peracute with unexpected death.[63] On gross examination, the small intestine and cecum are filled with fluid and gas. The infection is systemic, and the lungs also show a patchy, hemorrhagic, greyish appearance with small white foci in the liver. These lesions are caused by both bacteremia and thrombi, especially in the lungs.[63] *Helicobacter* spp and *Campylobacter* spp have been isolated from the intestinal tracts of hamsters with clinical signs of GI disease and in asymptomatic animals.[106] Both have potential zoonotic potential. Antibiotic therapy should be based on culture and sensitivity testing.

Parasitic Infections

The most common parasites of the Syrian hamster are pinworms and *H nana*. The digestive tract is colonized by a number of nonpathogenic flagellates, including *Trichomonas*, *Spironucleus*, and *Giardia* species.[107] Infections by *Trichuris* sp and *Eimeria* sp have been reported, but without detailed information.[108]

Spironucleus muris (syn. *Hexamita muris*) is a small, bilaterally symmetric, pear-shaped flagellate (7–9 × 2–3 μm) related to *Giardia*. The egg-shaped cysts with a size of 7.4 × 4.0 μm are excreted with the feces, where they can be detected by a flotation technique. The host specificity is unclear, *S muris* clones from mice were also able to infect Syrian hamsters.[109] This flagellate does not cause clinical disease in hamsters and treatment is not required.

Syrian hamsters as laboratory and pet animals are frequently infected with oxyurid nematodes of the genera *Syphacia, Aspiculuris,* and *Dentostomella. Syphacia mesocricetus* is probably the most typical species of Syrian hamsters. *Syphacia obvelata* has a direct life cycle, with an oro–fecal transmission, and the parasite eggs are found around the anus of the infected host. The eggs have a sticky outer layer and are resistant to rapid environmental degradation. In immunocompetent animals, infestation with *S obvelata* does not lead to obvious clinical disease. Clinical signs of disease attributed to the pinworm include rectal prolapse, poor hair coat, and cachexia. In the body, *S obvelata* are generally found in the cecum and to a lesser extent in the colon and may be associated with signs of mild enteritis.[3] The typical elongated eggs are detected by fecal flotation (*Aspiculuris* and *Dentostomella*) or by a perianal sticky strip test or smear (*Syphacia*). Pinworm infections are generally nonpathogenic and rarely require medical treatment. As the eggs are resistant to desiccation, thorough decontamination of the environment is necessary. Pinworm eggs are susceptible to high ambient temperatures. The recommended treatment for hamster pinworms is fenbendazole 20 to 50 mg/kg once daily orally for 5 days or ivermectin 2 mg/kg once topically.[110]

H nana and *Hymenolepis diminuta* are common small tapeworms in rodents. Both species parasitize the small intestine. The life cycle involves insects as intermediate hosts; however, *H nana* is an exception due to its optional direct life cycle and endogenous autoinfection. Infections in hamsters are usually asymptomatic. Clinical signs of severe infestation include poor weight gain, distended abdomen, and diarrhea. A definitive diagnosis is made through fecal flotation. Both *H nana* and *H diminuta* are considered zoonotic, although experimental transmission between rats and humans has failed in some cases.[111] Praziquantel (5–15 mg/kg orally, twice 10 days apart) is recommended for treatment.

Noninfectious Diseases

Diarrhea can have various causes, but it is usually associated with a change in diet, a high number of vegetables and fruit or excessive feeding.[18,112] Intestinal intussusception has been reported in hamsters fed high levels of sucrose (65% of the diet).[113] Alteration of GI motility and reduction of mucus production in the large intestine, leading to the formation of fecal bolus or diarrhea as a result of water retention in the large intestine due to excess sucrose. Bile secretion is reduced, and the gallbladder becomes distended, which impairs fat digestion. As a result, the intestinal transit time is shortened and the fat content in the feces is increased. Clinical signs include lethargy, weight loss, diarrhea, distended gallbladder, steatorrhea, ileal–cecal hemorrhage, and cramps.[113] Improper housing may also be associated with chronic emaciation and diarrhea. Inappropriate bedding can lead to intestinal blockage and obstruction.

Neoplasia

The incidence of alimentary neoplasia is very low.[114] The most reported tumors are benign, such as gastric squamous papillomas, gastric adenocarcinoma, and intestinal adenomas, although cases of intestinal lymphosarcoma and lymphoma (**Fig. 10**) have also been reported.[1,115] Gastric or intestinal carcinomas and lymphomas of the small intestine are reported, and metastases may occur.[115,116] The clinical signs of alimentary neoplasia include decreased appetite, weight loss, and palpable abdominal masses. Solitary neoplasms can be surgically resected, and chemotherapy protocols have been anecdotally reported for diffuse disease.[116]

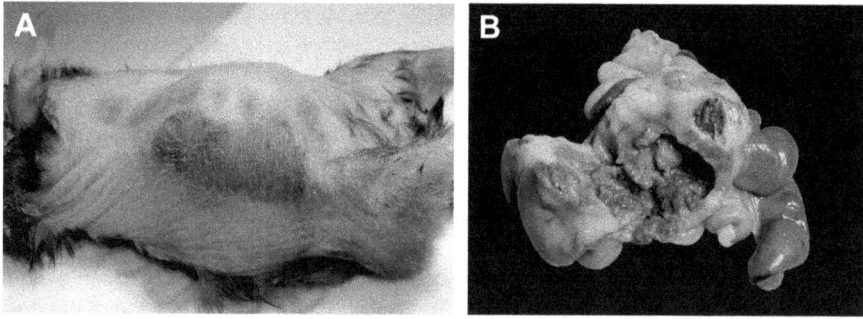

Fig. 10. A 2 year old Syrian hamster with a distended abdomen due to intestinal lymphoma, intestinal abscess, peritonitis, and abdominal wall necrosis. Note the obvious hyperemia and skin necrosis (A). The intestines had a dilated lumen and thickened walls (B). (*Courtesy of* Vladimir Jekl, DVM.)

RATS

The rat belongs to the order Rodentia and the family Muridae. Rats are very popular animals due to their calm nature. Rats are omnivorous animals. Selected anatomic features are given in **Table 1**.[117–119] Diseases of the digestive system are relatively rare in pet rats. In a retrospective study of 375 cases, only 10 animals had a disease of the gastrointestinal tract, 3 of which had an unspecified neoplasia of the gastrointestinal tract.[117]

Viral Infections

An epidemic of diarrhea in infant rats, known as infectious diarrhea of infant rats (IDIRs), has been attributed to a group B rotavirus. Transmission occurs via the fecal–oral route. The virus can be transmitted via fomites, dusts, and human contact. Suckling rats are infected. From 2 weeks of age, rats are naturally resistant to the disease. Clinical signs, which appear 24 to 48 hours after infection, are associated with growth retardation, diarrhea, and perianal dermatitis.[120] On gross necropsy, the stomach usually contains milk curds and watery contents in the small intestine. The ileum and large intestine are filled with yellow brown to greenish fluid and gas. Histopathological changes include intestinal villus attenuation, necrosis of the enterocytes, and pathognomonic epithelial syncytia in which eosinophilic intracytoplasmic inclusions are seen. Viral antigen could be detected in small intestinal enterocytes and rarely in the colonic epithelium, but only for 1 to 2 days. Viral precursor material and rotaviral particles can be visualized in cells by electron microscopy.[121] This virus is probably of human origin. Inoculation of infant rats with human isolates of group B rotavirus resulted in a diarrheal disease identical to IDIR. IDIR has not been reported since the first observation, but the potential for re-emergence remains as the agent is likely of human origin.

Bacterial Infections

Tyzzer's disease

Tyzzer's diseases lead in rats to pronounced dilatation of the ileum. Morbidity is generally low, but mortality is high. It is assumed that transmission occurs via the fecal–oral route. In utero transmission to the fetus has been demonstrated under experimental conditions.[1,3] Tyzzer's disease in weaned or stressed animals is an acute, enzootic condition characterized by lethargy, rough coat, and mortality within 48 to 72 hours. Chronically infected animals, in which the liver lesions are more pronounced, show weight loss, coarse fur, abdominal distension, and death. Diarrhea is not a common sign in rats.[1] Sparse to abundant gray, white or yellow foci 1 to 2 mm in diameter, either on the liver surface or on parenchyma, are the predominant lesion associated with C piliforme infection; the myocardium of rats may show analogous changes. In severe cases, edema, congestion, hemorrhage, and local ulcerations of the intestine may occur, particularly at the ileocecal–colonic junction. Segmental dilatation and inflammation of the ileum refer to the intestinal lesion as "megaloileitis." Nevertheless, ileal dilatation is not consistently observed. Intracellular organisms can be observed in the epithelium of the crypts and villi. Intracytoplasmic bacteria can be observed in hepatocytes at the periphery of the lesion, but in minimal amounts, making them difficult to detect. PCR of feces, intestinal tissue, or liver can detect the presence of the bacterium. Serologic tests and indirect fluorescent antibody tests can also be used. Although intradermal tests exist, their use is not widespread.

The acute (1–4 days) course of the disease and the intracellular location of the organism reduce the effectiveness of treatment. Oxytetracycline, administered at a concentration of 0.1 g/L in drinking water for 30 days, has suppressed an outbreak of the disease. Tetracycline, administered at a concentration of 10 mg/kg body weight for 5 days in an "on–off–on" regimen or at a concentration of 400 mg/L for 10 days, has also been used. Penicillin, streptomycin, and erythromycin can all effectively treat C piliforme infection.

Infectious spore-like bodies can survive for a year or more in bedding, soil, or contaminated feed. Routine cleaning of cages is likely to be ineffective in eradicating C piliforme spores. Exposure of the organism to 80°C for 30 minutes has been shown to be effective in inactivating them. Sodium hypochlorite (0.3%) and peracetic acid serve as effective disinfectants. The spores are resistant to ethanol and quaternary ammonium chemicals.

Salmonellosis

Rats are very susceptible to Salmonella infections and can carry subclinical infections for long periods. Salmonella species that infect rats include S enteritidis, S typhimurium, Salmonella dublin, and Salmonella meleagridis. S typhimurium and S enteritidis are the species most frequently isolated from laboratory animals. Infection in pet rats is extremely rare. Transmission occurs via the fecal–oral route through the ingestion of feces or feed or bedding contaminated with feces. Salmonellosis in rats is an intestinal and systemic infection that can be either enzootic or epizootic. Specific signs include anorexia, reduced activity, coarse hair coat, weight loss, pale, soft feces, ocular discharge and conjunctivitis, dyspnea, small litters, and abortions. Diagnosis is based on bacterial isolation using specific agars (eg, MacConkey's or brilliant green agar). One of the possible treatments is the oral administration of oxytetracycline added to the drinking water at a rate of 10 g/L for 10 days or 250 mg/kg body weight per day. Infected animals must be isolated. There are chronic carriers that make it difficult to eliminate the infection. To prevent the disease, new animals must be quarantined and contamination of feed by birds and wild rodents must be prevented. Due to the zoonotic nature of the disease, strict hygiene precautions must be taken and consultation with a human epidemiologist is essential. The main source of Salmonella in humans is not domestic animals but wild rats.[122,123]

Parasitic Infections

Due to their lifestyle, ecological plasticity, food spectrum and wide distribution, rats harbor a broad spectrum of GI parasites. The proximity of synanthropic rats to humans and their pets provides ample opportunity for the transmission of parasites (and other diseases) from wild rats to pet rats. However, the range of GI parasites of pet or laboratory rats is quite narrow and includes only species with a direct life cycle that can survive under the simplified conditions of captive rat breeding facilities. Individually housed pet rats usually have an even narrower range of parasites than their counterparts from larger breeding colonies (**Fig. 11**). The identification, diagnosis, and control of rat parasites are well described, mainly due to the frequent use of laboratory rats as experimental models.

Coccidiosis: Eimeria infection
Infection with *Eimeria nieschulzi* is the main cause of rat coccidiosis. The endogenous development of this species takes place in the small intestine, whereas *E separata* parasitizes the large intestine. Unsporulated subspherical oocysts are excreted in the feces, where they can be easily detected by a flotation technique. The infection is usually asymptomatic in adult, immunocompetent rats, but can lead to diarrhea of varying intensity in young and immunocompromised animals. Toltrazuril, diclazuril, or ponazuril (30 mg/kg in 2 treatments 48 hours apart) are effective and safe.[124]

Tritrichomonas muris and other flagellates
The digestive system of rats is frequently colonized by a spectrum of flagellate protists, including *Giardia muris*, *S muris*, *Tritrichomonas muris*, and several others. Infection is asymptomatic in adult, immunocompetent rats and does not require treatment in such cases. Diagnosis is based on the presence of trophozoites in the intestinal contents or the detection of cysts (*Giardia* and *Spironucleus*) in fecal samples by flotation. Treatment is possible with metronidazole (2.5 mg/mL drinking water)[125] as well as with benzimidazoles but is usually not necessary. *G muris* from rats is not zoonotic.

Pinworms
Pinworms are small (2–4 mm) nematodes that inhabit the caudal part of the digestive system. *Aspiculuris tetraptera* has symmetric, ellipsoidal eggs, while the eggs of *Syphacia muris* can be distinguished by their asymmetrical appearance. The latter species differs in that it lays its eggs around the anus, so that they can mainly be detected by perianal swabs using the tape test. In most cases, pinworm infections are asymptomatic and do not require anthelmintic treatment. If control is necessary, benzimidazoles (ie, fenbendazole) are the drugs of choice. As the eggs are resistant to environmental factors, reinfection is very common and long-term administration of fenbendazole-treated feed (150 ppm) is an important approach used in larger rat

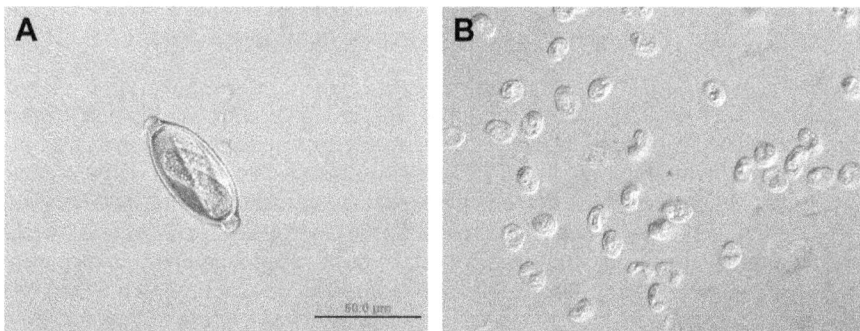

Fig. 11. Endoparasites in rats. *Trichuris muris* (A) and *Cryptosporidium muris* (B) can occasionally be found in young rats with intestinal disease. *C muris* is a sporozoan that attaches to the gastric mucosa. It is only slightly pathogenic. (*Courtesy of* David Modry, DVM.)

colonies.[126] Ivermectin in drinking water (0.007 mg/mL) also cleared the rat colonies of pinworm infection.[127]

Tapeworms

H nana and *H diminuta* are common tapeworms in rodents, including rats. For more information, see "Parasitic Infections" section. Praziquantel (5–15 mg/kg orally, twice 10 days apart) is recommended for treatment. Rats may also serve as intermediate hosts for *Taenia taeniaeformis*.[128] A clinical case was reported of a rat whose abdominal distension was caused by a hepatic sarcoma induced by infection with *T taeniaeformis*.[129] Clinical signs observed in rats infected with hepatic *T taeniaeformis* are nonspecific and may include lethargy, weight loss, anorexia, decrease in reproductive function, and sudden death. The diagnosis of *T taeniaeformis* infection in laboratory rats can be made by ultrasonography and/or radiography.[130] The treatment options for pet rats infected with *T taeniaeformis* are unknown.[3] The safety of praziquantel for the treatment of encysted larvae in rats is not known, and it is possible that killed larvae may elicit a pronounced host immune response that is harmful to the rat. The recommended dose of praziquantel is 30 mg/kg orally every 14 days for 3 treatments.

Neoplasia

Stomach and intestinal neoplasia in pet rats are rare. Gastric fibrosarcoma and carcinoma, intestinal leiomyosarcoma, cecal fibroma, cecal carcinoma, colon adenocarcinoma, and anal leiomyosarcoma have been described.[131–134]

Antibiotic Toxicity

Rats are omnivorous and the potential risk of clostridial enterotoxemia associated with antibiotic ingestion, as in other hindgut fermenter rodents, is low. In a laboratory animal study, antibiotic administration can disrupt the balance of bacteria in the rat intestinal ecosystem, leading to an inflammatory response in their bloodstream and inflammatory changes in the colon.[135] However, the doses of antibiotics were extremely high compared to published doses for pet rats (clindamycin 750 mg/kg, ampicillin 272.1 mg/kg, and streptomycin at a dose of 417.9 mg/kg).

Miscellaneous

Gastric ulceration and erosions

Gastric ulceration and erosions can be identified in the glandular or nonglandular region. There is generally no specific cause, although these conditions are not uncommonly associated with a stress response or trauma from gavage feeding.[63]

Megacolon

Megacolon is a noninfectious inflammatory disease associated with colonic distension, in which neural ganglia and smooth muscle are destroyed while the overlying mucosa remains intact (**Fig. 12**). It is a progressive disease that begins with a marked chronic inflammatory infiltrate in the submucosa and serosa and ends with scarring, degeneration, and loss of smooth muscle with the loss of autonomic ganglia. It can be congenital or acquired. Congenital megacolon is often inherited and occurs in black-eyed whites, huskies, blazed, and some other rat lines, and it has multifactorial inheritance. It can also occur in newborns with anal atresia. Acquired megacolon is usually associated with colonic obstruction/lumen obstruction, spinal damage, and further expansion of the colonic wall. The final stage is associated with malabsorption, enterocolitis, and septicemia.[136,137]

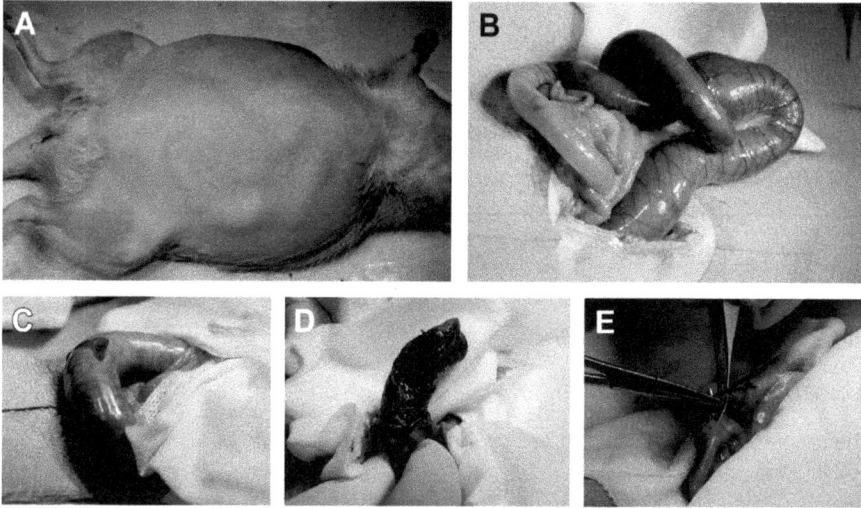

Fig. 12. Rats with megacolon (*A–E*) are commonly presented with abdominal distension (*A*) and constipation. In severe cases, laparotomy may relieve the impaction of the colon (*B–E*). Note the distended colon with fecal material. The incision in the colon was made on the antimesenteric side (*C*), the obstipated material removed (*D*) and the wound sutured with monofilament absorbable material after thorough cleaning (*D*). (*Courtesy of* Vladimir Jekl, DVM.)

Animals present with anorexia, weight loss, abdominal distension, gas accumulation proximal to the obstruction, diarrhea, constipation, and/or failure to thrive. Abdominal palpation, radiography, and ultrasonography reveal a grossly distended colon extending proximally from the recto-sigmoid junction for a variable distance.[137] The lumen of the colon can be up to 8 mm in the transverse section.

Treatment includes an easily digestible diet, fluid therapy, and laxatives/prokinetics. The author (VJ) has had good experience with the use of oral itopride (10 mg/kg q12 h), meloxicam (1–1.5 mg/kg q12 h), and gabapentin (25–50 mg/kg q12 h), but itopride and laxatives are contraindicated in case of colonic impaction. In cases of severe obstruction, surgical intervention to remove impacted material may be considered, but this is only palliative. In the case of congenital megacolon and in more severe cases, euthanasia should be considered. Due to the potential genetical causes, breeding should be discouraged.

SUMMARY

In conclusion, GI tract diseases are one of the most common presentations to veterinarians. As in rabbits, the majority of the patient is seen with GI syndrome secondary to concurrent disease. GI disease diagnosis should follow the same principles as in other animal species.

CLINICS CARE POINTS

- Gastrointestinal syndrome is one of the most commonly seen GI tract disorders in exotic companion rodents due to concurrent illness, stress, or pain.
- GDV in guinea pigs is a life-threatening condition with a poor prognosis and require immediate patient stabilization and, in many cases, also surgery.

- Chinchillas are commonly carriers of the intestinal parasite *G intestinalis*.
- Degus suffer from gas accumulation in the stomach and intestines due to obstructive nasal disease.
- The term "wet-tail" was commonly used in hamsters in the case of infection with *L intracellularis*; however, "wet-tail" (perineal fecal staining) is just a clinical symptom and can be associated with any GI tract disorder resulting in diarrhea.

DISCLOSURE

The authors have nothing to disclose.

FUNDING

The article was partially supported by the grant of VETUNI Brno, Czech Republic (No. 2024ITA15).

REFERENCES

1. Ward ML. Rodents: digestive system disorders. In: Keeble E, Meredith A, editors. BSAVA manual of rodents and ferrets. Gloucester: BSAVA; 2009. p. 123–41.
2. DeCubellis J, Graham J. Gastrointestinal disease in Guinea pigs and rabbits. Vet Clin North Am Exot Anim Pract 2013;16(2):421–35.
3. Huynh M, Pignon C. Gastrointestinal disease in exotic small mammals. J Exot Pet Med 2013;22(2):118–31.
4. Pignon C, Mayer J. Guinea pigs. In: Quesenberry KE, Orcutt CJ, Ch Mans, et al, editors. Ferrets, rabbits, and rodents. Clinical medicine and surgery. St. Luis: Elsevier; 2021. p. 270–97.
5. Parsons JL. Nutritional physiology and feeding of companion rodents. Vet Clin North Am Exotic Anim Pract 2024;27(1):1–12.
6. Oliver VL, Pang DSJ. Pain recognition in rodents. Vet Clin North Am Exot Anim Pract 2023;26(1):121–49.
7. Benedetti F, Pignon C, Muffat-es-Jacques P, et al. Development and validation of a pain scale in Guinea pig (*Cavia porcellus*). J Exot Pet Med 2024;50:36–41.
8. Jekl V. Principles of radiography. In: Harcourt-Brown FM, Chitty J, editors. BSAVA manual of rabbit imaging, surgery and dentistry. Gloucester: BSAVA; 2013. p. 39–58.
9. Gómez MN, Domínguez Miño E, García de Carellán A, et al. Abdominal ultrasound features and reference values in healthy Guinea pigs (Cavia porcellus). Vet Rec 2024;194(2):e3668.
10. Chen JY, Chen HL, Wu SH, et al. Application of high-frequency ultrasound for the detection of surgical anatomy in the rodent abdomen. Vet J 2012;191(2):246–52.
11. Banzato T, Bellini L, Contiero B, et al. Abdominal anatomic features and reference values determined by use of ultrasonography in healthy common rats (Rattus norvegicus). Am J Vet Res 2014;75(1):67–76.
12. Dilek ÖG, Dimitrov R, Stamatova-Yovcheva K, et al. Computed tomography and three dimensional anatomical study of the liver in the chinchilla (Chinchilla lanigera). Anat Histol Embryol 2024;53(2):e13025.
13. Hem A, Smith AJ, Solberg P. Saphenous vein puncture for blood sampling of the mouse, rat, hamster, gerbil, Guinea pig, ferret and mink. Lab Anim 1998;32(4):364–8.

14. Jekl V, Hauptman K, Jeklová E, et al. Blood sampling from the cranial vena cava in the Norway rat (Rattus norvegicus). Lab Anim 2005;39(2):236–9.
15. Heimann M, Käsermann HP, Pfister R, et al. Blood collection from the sublingual vein in mice and hamsters: a suitable alternative to retrobulbar technique that provides large volumes and minimizes tissue damage. Lab Anim 2009;43(3): 255–60.
16. Wesche P. Rodents: clinical pathology. In: Keeble E, Meredith A, editors. BSAVA manual of rodents and ferrets. Gloucester: BSAVA; 2009. p. 42–51.
17. d'Ovidio D, Noviello E, Ianniello D, et al. Survey of endoparasites in pet Guinea pigs in Italy. Parasitol Res 2015;114(3):1213–6.
18. Pellett S, Mancinelli E. Veterinary care of hamsters. Part 2: diagnostics, diseases. Companion Animal 2017;22:743–9.
19. Harrup AJ, Rooney N. Current welfare state of pet Guinea pigs in the UK. Vet Rec 2020;186(9):282.
20. Cameron KE, Holder HE, Connor RL, et al. Cross-sectional survey of husbandry for pet Guinea pigs (*Cavia porcellus*) in New Zealand. N Z Vet J 2023;71(1): 27–32.
21. Holtenius K, Björnhag G. The colonic separation mechanism in the Guinea-pig (Cavia porcellus) and the chinchilla (Chinchilla laniger). Comp Biochem Physiol A Comp Physiol 1985;82(3):537–42.
22. Kohles M. Gastrointestinal anatomy and physiology of selected exotic companion mammals. Vet Clin North Am Exot Anim Pract 2014;17(2):165–78.
23. Spines RL. Anatomy of the Guinea-pig cecum. Anat Embryol 1982;165(1):97–111.
24. Jilge B. The gastrointestinal transit time in the Guinea pig. Z Versuchstierkd 1980;22(4):204–10.
25. Iburg TM, Arnbjerg J, Rueløkke ML. Gender differences in the anatomy of the perineal glands in Guinea pigs and the effect of castration. Anat Histol Embryol 2013;42(1):65–71.
26. Minarikova A, Hauptman K, Jeklova E, et al. Diseases in pet Guinea pigs: a retrospective study in 1000 animals. Vet Rec 2015;177(8):200.
27. Dudley ES, Boivin GP. Gastric volvulus in Guinea pigs: comparison with other species. J Am Assoc Lab Anim Sci 2011;50(4):526–30.
28. Jaax GP, Jaax NK, Petrali JP, et al. Coronavirus-like virions associated with a wasting syndrome in Guinea pigs. Lab Anim Sci 1990;40(4):375–8.
29. Onyekaba CO. Clinical salmonellosis in a Guinea pig colony caused by a new Salmonella serotype, Salmonella ochiogu. Lab Anim 1983;17(3):213–6.
30. Coman S, Băcescu B, Coman T, et al. Aspects of the parasitary infestations of Guinea pigs reared in intensive system. Sc Parasit 2009;10(1–2):97–100.
31. Flausino G, Lopes CW, Teixeira-Fillho WL, et al. Phenotypic and genotypic characterization of *Eimeria caviae* from Guinea pigs (Cavia porcellus). Acta Protozool 2014;53(3):269–76.
32. Hernández-Castro C, Dashti A, Köster PC, et al. First report of rodent-adapted Cryptosporidium wrairi in an immunocompetent child, Spain. Parasitol Res 2022;121(10):3007–11.
33. Rojas-Moncada J, Becerra Terrones M, Torrel Pajares S, et al. First report of antiparasitic resistance to ivermectin in Guinea pigs from Cajamarca, Peru. Rev Investig Vet Perú, Lima 2023;34(2):e23437.
34. Moore RW, Greenlee HH. Enterotoxaemia in chinchillas. Lab Anim 1975;9(2): 153–4.
35. Rothman SW. Presence of Clostridium difficile toxin in Guinea pigs with penicillin-associated colitis. Med Microbiol Immunol 1981;169(3):187–96.

36. Hedley J. Antibiotic usage in rabbits and rodents. Practice 2018;40(6):230–7.
37. Wasson K, Criley JM, Clabaugh MB, et al. Therapeutic efficacy of oral lactoba-cillus preparation for antibiotic-associated enteritis in Guinea pigs. Contemp Top Lab Anim Sci 2000;39(1):32–8.
38. Bennett IV, Yardley JH. Staphylococcal enterocolitis in chinchillas. Bull Johns Hopkins Hosp 1956;98(6):454–63.
39. Lichtenberger M, Lennox A. Updates and advanced therapies for gastrointes-tinal stasis in rabbits. Vet Clin North Am Exot Anim Pract 2010;13(3):525–41.
40. Jekl V, Hauptman K, Knotek Z. Evidence-based advances in rodent medicine. Vet Clin North Am Exot Anim Pract 2017;20(3):805–16.
41. Tsubouchi T, Saito T, Mizutani F, et al. Stimulatory action of itopride hydrochloride on colonic motor activity in vitro and in vivo. J Pharmacol Exp Therapeut 2003; 306(2):787–93.
42. Park SJ, Choi EJ, Yoon YH, et al. The effects of prucalopride on postoperative ileus in Guinea pigs. Yonsei Med J 2013;54(4):845–53.
43. Torres C, Carcelén F, Ara M, et al. Efecto de la suplementación de una cepa pro-biótica sobre los parámetros productivos del cuy (Cavia porcellus). Rev Inv Vet 2013;24:433–40.
44. Bazán V, Bezada S, Carcelén F, et al. Efecto de la infección subclínica de Sal-monella Typhimurium sobre los parámetros productivos en la producción de cuyes de engorde (Cavia porcellus). Rev Investig Vet 2019;30(4):1697–706.
45. Goicochea-Vargas J, Salvatierra-Alor M, Acosta-Pachorro F, et al. Genomic characterization and probiotic potential of lactic acid bacteria isolated from feces of Guinea pig (Cavia porcellus). Open Vet J 2024;14(2):716–29.
46. Lee KJ, Johnson WD, Lang CM. Acute gastric dilatation associated with gastric volvulus in the Guinea pig. Lab Anim Sci 1977;27(5 Pt 1):685–6.
47. Hawkins MG, Graham JE. Emergency and critical care of rodents. Vet Clin North Am Exot Anim Pract 2007;10(2):501–631.
48. Mitchell EB, Hawkins MG, Gaffney PM, et al. Gastric dilatation-volvulus in a Guinea pig (Cavia porcellus). J Am Anim Hosp Assoc 2010;46(3):174–80.
49. Nógrádi AL, Cope I, Balogh M, et al. Review of gastric torsion in eight Guinea pigs (Cavia porcellus). Acta Vet Hung 2017;65(4):487–99.
50. Keith JC, Rowles TK, Warwick KE, et al. Acute gastric distention in Guinea pigs. Lab Anim Sci 1992;42(4):331–2.
51. Abad JL, Lopez-Figueroa C, Martorell J. Acute pancreatic necrosis due to omental torsion in a Guinea pig (Cavia porcellus) with secondary splenic, hepat-ic, and pulmonary necrosis. J Exot Pet Med 2021;36:23–4.
52. Song KK, Goldsmid SE, Lee J, et al. Retrospective analysis of 736 cases of canine gastric dilatation and volvulus. Aust Vet J 2020;98(6):232–8.
53. Theus M, Bitterli F, Foldenauer U. Successful treatment of a gastric trichobezoar in a Peruvian Guinea pig (Cavia aperea porcellus). J Exot Pet Med 2008;17(2): 148–51.
54. Künzel K, Hittmair KM. Ultrasonographic diagnosis of a trichobezoar in a Guinea pig. Wien Tierarztl Monatsschr 2002;89(3):66–9.
55. Deflers H, Gandar F, Etienne A-L, et al. Successful medical management of a bezoar in a Peruvian Guinea pig (Cavia porcellus). J Exot Pet Med 2019;29: 115–8.
56. Gardhouse SM, Sanchez-Migallon Guzman D, Sadar MJ, et al. Partial gastrec-tomy for resection of a gastric leiomyoma in a Guinea pig (Cavia porcellus). J Am Vet Med Assoc 2016;249(12):1415–20.

57. Nespor J, Heczkova K, Skoric M. Incidence of spontaneous tumours in Guinea pigs: a retrospective study of 153 cases. Acta Vet Brno 2023;92(4):375–80.
58. Stan F. Comparative study of the stomach morphology in rabbit and chinchilla. AgroLife Sci J 2013;2(2):73–8.
59. Stan F. Anatomical particularities of the cecum in rabbits and chinchillas. Bulletin UASVM Veterinary Medicine 2014;71(2):406–12.
60. Krishnamurti CR, Kitts WD, Smith DC. The digestion of carbohydrates in the chinchilla (Chinchilla lanigera). Can J Zool 1974;52(10):1227–33.
61. Biiirnhag G, Siiiblom L. Demonstration of coprophagy in some rodents. Swed J Agric Res 1977;7:105–13.
62. Wu Y, Liu B, Ma X, et al. The microbiota architecture of the Chinchilla gastrointestinal tract. Vet Sci 2024;11(2):58.
63. Reavill D. Pathology of the exotic companion mammal gastrointestinal system. Vet Clin North Am Exot Anim Pract 2014;17(2):145–64.
64. Larrivee GP, Elvehjem CA. Disease problems in chinchillas. J Am Vet Med Assoc 1954;124(927):447–55.
65. Martino PE, Bautista EL, Gimeno EJ, et al. Radman, N.E. Fourteen-year status report of fatal illnesses in captive chinchillas (Chinchilla lanigera). J Appl Anim Res 2017;45(1):310–4.
66. Chen J, Wang W, Lin Y, et al. Genetic characterizations of *Cryptosporidium* spp. from pet rodents indicate high zoonotic potential of pathogens from chinchillas. One Health 2021;13:100269.
67. Levecke B, Meulemans L, Dalemans T, et al. Mixed Giardia duodenalis assemblage A, B, C and E infections in pet chinchillas (Chinchilla lanigera) in Flanders (Belgium). Vet Parasitol 2011;177(1–2):166–70.
68. Pantchev N, Broglia A, Paoletti B, et al. Occurrence and molecular typing of Giardia isolates in pet rabbits, chinchillas, Guinea pigs and ferrets collected in Europe during 2006-2012. Vet Rec 2014;175(1):18.
69. Zikmundová V, Horáková V, Tůmová L, et al. Pet chinchillas (Chinchilla lanigera): source of zoonotic Giardia intestinalis, Cryptosporidium ubiquitum and microsporidia of the genera Encephalitozoon and Enterocytozoon. Vet Parasitol 2024; 331:110275.
70. Adam RD. Giardia duodenalis: biology and pathogenesis. Clin Microbiol Rev 2021;34(4):e0002419.
71. Babero BB, Cattan PE, Cabello C. *Trichuris* bradleyi sp. n., a whipworm from Octodon degus in Chile. J Parasitol 1975;1061–3.
72. Mans C, Fink DM, Giammarco HE, et al. 2021. Effects of compounded metronidazole and metronidazole benzoate oral suspensions on food intake in healthy chinchillas (Chinchilla lanigera). J Exot Pet Med 2021;36:75–9.
73. Cardia DFF, Camossi LG, Lux Hoppe EG, et al. An oxyurid nematode identified in a pet Chinchilla (Chinchilla lanigera). J Exot Pet Med 2016;25(4):311–3.
74. Fulk G. Notes on the activity, reproduction, and social behavior of *Octodon degus*. J Mammal 1976;57:495–505.
75. Woods CA, Kilpatrick C. Infraorder hystricognathi. In: Wilson DE, Reeder DM, editors. Mammal species of the world. A taxonomic and geographic reference. 3rd edition. Baltimore: Johns Hopkins University Press; 2005. p. 1538–600.
76. Jekl V, Hauptman K, Knotek Z. 2011 Diseases in pet degus: a retrospective study in 300 animals. J Small Anim Pract 2011;52(2):107–12.
77. González H, Feder F. Variations of position of cecum and colon ascendens of degu (*Octodon degus*, Molina 1782). Anat Histol Embryol 1997;26:305–10 (In German).

78. Langer P. The digestive tract and life history of small mammals. Mammal Rev 2002;32:107–31.
79. Bennet ET. On the genus *Octodon*, and its relation with *Ctenomys*, blainv. And *poephagomys*, F. Cuv: including a description of a new species of *Ctenomys*. Trans Zool Soc Lond 1841;2(1):75–86.
80. Nagy B, Kassai E, Mándoki M, et al. Investigation on the causes leading to death in degu (Octodon degus) between 1998-2009. Magy Allatorvosok Lapja 2012; 134(3):160–5.
81. Digiani MC, Landaeta-Aqueveque C, Serrano PC, et al. Pudicinae (nematoda: heligmonellidae) parasitic in endemic chilean rodents (caviomorpha: Octodontidae and abrocomidae): description of a new species and emended description of pudica degusi (babero and cattan) n. comb. J Parasitol 2017;103(6):736–46.
82. Caccio SM, Beck R, Almeida A, et al. Identification of Giardia species and Giardia duodenalis assemblages by sequence analysis of the 5.8 S rDNA gene and internal transcribed spacers. Parasitology 2010;137(6):919–25.
83. Najecki DL, Tate BA. Husbandry and management of the degu (*Octodon degus*). Lab Anim (NY) 1999;28:54–62.
84. Jekl V. Degus. In: Quesenberry K, Orcutt C, Ch Mans, Carpenter J, editors. Ferrets, Rabbits and rodents. Clinical medicine and surgery. St. Luis: Elsevier; 2021. p. 323–33.
85. Jekl V, Hauptman K, Skoric M, et al. Elodontoma in a degu (Octodon degus). J Exot Pet Med 2008;17:216–20.
86. Jekl V, Zikmund T, Hauptman K. Dyspnea in a degu (*Octodon degu*) associated with maxillary cheek teeth elongation. J Exot Pet Med 2016;25(2):128–32.
87. Nakata M, Wu CC, Chambers JK, Uchida K, Nakayama H. Spontaneous intranasal tumours in degus (Octodon degus): 20 cases (2007-2020). J Small Anim Pract 2022;63(11):829–33.
88. O'Neill DG, Kim K, Brodbelt DC, et al. Demography, disorders and mortality of pet hamsters under primary veterinary care in the United Kingdom in 2016. J Small Anim Pract 2022;63(10):747–55.
89. Bean AD. Hamsters and gerbils. In: Graham JE, Doss GA, Beaufrére H, editors. Exotic animal emergency and critical care. Hoboken, USA: Wiley Blackwell; 2021. p. 349–71.
90. Hoffman RA, Robinson PF, Magalhaes H, editors. The golden hamster – its biology and use in medical research. Ames, IA: Iowa State University Press; 1968. p. 91–109.
91. Fox JG, Dewhirst FE, Fraser GJ, et al. Intracellular Campylobacter-like organism from ferrets and hamsters with proliferative bowel disease is a Desulfovibrio sp. J Clin Microbiol 1994;32(5):1229–37.
92. Gebhart CJ, Guedes RMC. Lawsonia intracellularis. In: Gyles CL, Prescott JF, Songer JG, et al, editors. Pathogenesis of bacterial infections in animals. 4the ed. Oxford, UK: Wiley-Blackwell Publishing; 2010. p. 500–12.
93. Johnson EA, Jacoby RO. Transmissible ileal hyperplasia of hamsters. II: ultrastructure. Am J Pathol 1978;91(3):451–61.
94. Vannucci FA, Borges EL, de Oliveira JS, et al. Intestinal absorption and histomorphometry of Syrian hamsters (Mesocricetus auratus) experimentally infected with Lawsonia intracellularis. Vet Microbiol 2010;145(3–4):286–91.
95. Cooper DM, Gebhart CJ. Comparative aspects of proliferative enteritis. J Am Vet Med Assoc 1998;212(9):1446–51.
96. Fiskett RAM Lawsonia intracellularis infection in hamsters (Mesocricetus auratus). J Exot Pet Med 2011;20(4):277–83.

97. Miwa Y, Mayer J. Hamsters and gerbils. In: Quesenberry KE, Orcutt CJ, Mans C, et al, editors. Ferrets, rabbits and rodents—clinical medicine and surgery. 4th edition. Missouri: Elsevier; 2021. p. 368–84.
98. Sambol SP, Tang JK, Merrigan MM, et al. Infection of hamsters with epidemiologically important strains of Clostridium difficile. J Infect Dis 2001;183(12):1760–6.
99. Keel MK, Songer JG. The comparative pathology of Clostridium difficile-associated disease. Vet Pathol 2006;43(3):225–40.
100. Hart M, O'Connor E, Davis M. Multiple peracute deaths in a colony of Syrian hamsters (Mesocricetus auratus). Lab Anim (NY) 2010;39:99–102.
101. Ryden EB, Lipman NS, Taylor NS, et al. Clostridium difficile typhlitis associated with cecal mucosal hyperplasia in Syrian hamsters. Lab Anim Sci 1991;41(6):553–8.
102. Chang J, Rohwer RG. Clostridium difficile infection in adult hamsters. Lab Anim Sci 1991;41(6):548–52.
103. Delmee M. Laboratory diagnosis of Clostridium difficile disease. Clin Microbiol Infect 2001;7:411–6.
104. Motzel SL, Gibson SV. Tyzzer disease in hamsters and gerbils from a pet store supplier. J Am Vet Med Assoc 1990;197(9):1176–8.
105. Waggie KS, Thornburg LP, Grove KJ, et al. Lesions of experimentally induced Tyzzer's disease in Syrian hamsters, guineapigs, mice and rats. Lab Anim 1987;21(2):155–60.
106. Nagamine CM, Shen Z, Luong RH, et al. Co-infection of the Siberian hamster (Phodopus sungorus) with a novel Helicobacter sp. and Campylobacter sp. J Med Microbiol 2015;64(5):575–81.
107. Burr HN, Paluch L-R, Roble GS, et al. Parasitic diseases. In: The laboratory rabbit, Guinea pig, hamster, and other rodents. Amsterdam; Boston: Elsevier Academic Press; 2012. p. 839–66.
108. Sürsal N, Gökpinar S, Yildiz K. Prevalence of intestinal parasites in hamsters and rabbits in some pet shops of Turkey. Turkiye Parazitol Derg 2014;38(2):102–5.
109. Schagemann G, Bohnet W, Kunstyr I, et al. Host specificity of cloned Spironucleus muris in laboratory rodents. Lab Anim 1990;24:234–9.
110. Pritchett KR, Johnston NA. A review of treatments for the eradication of pinworm infections from laboratory rodent colonies. Contemp Top Lab Anim Sci 2002;41:36–46.
111. Mijatović S, Štajner T, Čalovski IČ, et al. Human infections by Hymenolepis diminuta in Europe: a case report and literature review. Trans R Soc Trop Med Hyg 2024. trae037.
112. Baldrey V. Approaches to common conditions of the gastrointestinal tract in pet hamsters. Comp Animal 2021;26:20–6.
113. Cunnane SC, Bloom SR. Intussusception in the Syrian golden hamster. Br J Nutr 1990;63(02):231–7.
114. Rother N, Bertram CA, Klopfleisch R, et al. Tumours in 177 pet hamsters. Vet Rec 2021;188(6):e14.
115. Greenacre CB. Spontaneous tumors of small mammals. Vet Clin Exot Anim Pract 2004;7:627–51.
116. Bennett RA. Soft tissue surgery. In: Quesenberry KE, Carpenter JW, editors. Ferrets, rabbits, and rodents. 3rd edition. Saint Louis: W.B. Saunders; 2012.
117. Rey F, Bulliot C, Bertin N, et al, REMORA Team. Morbidity and disease management in pet rats: a study of 375 cases. Vet Rec 2015;176(15):385.

118. Vdoviaková K, Petrovová E, Maloveská M, et al. Surgical anatomy of the gastro-intestinal tract and its vasculature in the laboratory rat. Gastroenterol Res Pract 2016;2632368.
119. Otto GM, Franklin C, Clifford CB. Biology and diseases of rats. In: Fox JG, Anderson LC, Loew FM, et al, editors. Laboratory animal medicine. 3rd edition. London, UK: Elsevier, Academic Press; 2015. p. 121–65.
120. Huber AC, Yolken RH, Mader LC, et al. Pathology of infectious diarrhea of infant rats (IDIR) induced by an antigenically distinct rotavirus. Vet Pathol 1989;26(5): 376–85.
121. Barthold SW, Griffey SM, Percy DH. Pathology of laboratory rodents and rabbits. 4th edition. Ames, (USA): Wiley Blackwell; 2016. p. 119–72.
122. Ribas A, Saijuntha W, Agatsuma T, et al. Rodents as a source of Salmonella contam-ination in wet markets in Thailand. Vector Borne Zoonotic Dis 2016;16(8):537–40.
123. Szmolka A, Lancz ZS, Rapcsák F, et al. Emergence and comparative genome analysis of Salmonella Ohio strains from Brown rats, poultry, and swine in Hungary. Int J Mol Sci 2024;25(16):8820.
124. Marroquin SC, Eshar D, Browning GR, et al. (2020). Diagnosis and successful treatment of Eimeria infection in a pair of pet domestic rats (Rattus norvegicus) with ponazuril. J Exot Pet Med 2020;33:31–3.
125. Beyhan YE, Hökelek M. Giardia muris infection in laboratory rats (Rattus norve-gicus) and treatment with metronidazole. Turkiye Parazitol Derg 2014;38(3):181.
126. Huerkamp MJ, Benjamin KA, Webb SK, et al. Long-term results of dietary fen-bendazole to eradicate Syphacia muris from rat colonies. J Am Assoc Lab Anim Sci 2004;43(2):35–6.
127. Zenner L. Effective eradication of pinworms (Syphacia muris, Syphacia obvelata and Aspiculuris tetraptera) from a rodent breeding colony by oral anthelmintic therapy. Lab Anim 1998;32(3):337–42.
128. Lin YC, Rikihisa Y, Kono H, et al. Effects of larval tapeworm (Taenia taeniaefor-mis) infection on reproductive functions in male and female host rats. Exp Para-sitol 1990;70(3):344–52.
129. Irizarry-Rovira A, Wolf A, Bolek M. Taenia taeniaformis induced metastatic he-patic sarcoma in a pet rat (Rattus norvegicus). J Exot Pet Med 2007;16:45–8.
130. Ito A, Sakakibara Y, Ma L, et al. Ultrasonographic and serologic studies of exper-imental cysticercosis in rats infected with Taenia taeniaeformis. Parasite Immunol 1998;20(3):105–10.
131. Grasso P, Creasey M. Carcinoma of the colon in a rat. Eur J Cancer 1969;5(4): 415–9.
132. Burn JI, Sellwood RA, Bishop M. Spontaneous carcinoma of the colon of the rat. J Pathol Bacteriol 1966;91(1):253–4.
133. Majka JA, Sher S. Spontaneous gastric carcinoid tumor in an aged Sprague-Dawley rat. Vet Pathol 1989;26(1):88–90.
134. Bomhard E. Frequency of spontaneous tumors in Wistar rats in 30-months studies. Exp Toxicol Pathol 1992;44(7):381–92.
135. Tong G, Qian H, Li D, et al. Intestinal flora imbalance induced by antibiotic use in rats. J Inflamm Res 2024;17:1789–804.
136. Meehan CJ, Fleming S, Smith W, et al. Idiopathic megacolon in the BB rat. Int J Exp Pathol 1994;75(1):37–42.
137. Nyska A, Waner T, Galiano A, et al. Constipation and megacolon in rats related to treatment with oxodipine, a calcium antagonist. Toxicol Path 1994;22(6):589–94.

Reptile and Amphibian Gastroenterology

Joanna Hedley, BVM&S, DZooMed (Reptilian), DECZM (Herpetology), MRCVS[a],*,
Jessica M. Hornby, BVetMed, PGDip(VCP), MVetMed, MRCVS[b]

KEYWORDS

- Reptile • Amphibian • Gastrointestinal • Digestive

KEY POINTS

- Understanding the normal structure and function of the gastrointestinal (GI) tract will help the reptile clinician recognize and interpret abnormalities.
- A variety of infectious and noninfectious diseases may result in GI signs, so a logical diagnostic approach is vital to identify the initial cause.
- It is important to always fully review husbandry and diet as deficits in captive care can often be important predisposing factors for GI disease.

INTRODUCTION

Reptile and amphibian veterinarians are frequently presented with patients exhibiting clinical signs suggestive of gastrointestinal (GI) disease. Understanding the normal structure and function of the GI tract is essential to aid appropriate diagnosis. This article will focus on the approach to a patient with GI signs and the problems affecting the GI tract from the esophagus to the colon. Alternative texts are available for further information on the oral cavity, liver, gall bladder, pancreas, and cloaca.[1–4]

ANATOMY AND PHYSIOLOGY

The basic structure of the GI tract is similar across reptile species comprising the oral cavity, esophagus, stomach, small intestine, and large intestine (colon) terminating at the cloaca. However, anatomy and physiology can vary significantly among species depending on diet and life stage.

---

[a] Exotic Species and Small Mammal Medicine and Surgery, Beaumont Sainsbury Animal Hospital, Royal Veterinary College, 4 Royal College Street, London, UK; [b] School of Veterinary Medicine and Science, University of Nottingham, Sutton Bonington Campus, Leicestershire, UK
* Corresponding author. RVC Exotics Service, Beaumont Sainsbury Animal Hospital, Royal Veterinary College, 4 Royal College Street, London, UK.
E-mail address: jhedley@rvc.ac.uk

Vet Clin Exot Anim 28 (2025) 295–313
https://doi.org/10.1016/j.cvex.2024.11.003
1094-9194/25/© 2024 Elsevier Inc. All rights reserved, including those for text and data mining, AI training, and similar technologies.
vetexotic.theclinics.com

Abbreviations	
CT	computed tomography
GI	gastrointestinal
PCR	polymerase chain reaction
qPCR	quantitative PCR
UVB	ultraviolet B

Starting at ingestion, food passes from the oral cavity down to the esophagus, which is generally a simple tubular structure. In snakes, the esophagus can have a storage function, as the stomach is often too small to accommodate the entire prey item predigestion, especially in ophiophagic species (eg, king cobra [*Ophiophagus hannah*]). In some species such as egg-eating snakes, the esophagus is an important site of mechanical digestion with eggs being swallowed whole and then forced by axial muscular contractions against modified ventral spinal processes to crush them. The shell fragments are then regurgitated. Sea turtles and some tortoises can also use the esophageal muscles to crush food and in sea turtles, the esophagus is lined by keratinized caudally directed papillae to trap food while seawater is expelled.[5]

From the esophagus, food then passes into the stomach. Digestion usually begins here with secretion of enzymes, hydrochloric acid, and pepsinogen. The low stomach pH is particularly important to kill any live prey and to stop putrefaction while food is held in the stomach, which may be several days. The speed of digestion within the stomach is mainly influenced by temperature with higher temperatures reducing gastric pH and increasing enzyme activity, consequently increasing the rate of digestion. Other factors include the presence of venom, which can also speed digestion, hydration, and health status.[5] In snakes, the stomach can be hard to distinguish from the rest of the GI tract if they have not recently eaten, as there is no defined cardiac sphincter, and some digestion may occur in the distal esophagus. After feeding, however, the stomach and intestines distend and hypertrophy significantly. Gastric pH, which can be high following a period of fasting, reduces rapidly and gastric contractions increase.[6] In crocodilians, gastroliths are a common finding. Their significance is debated; they have been proposed to play a role in mechanical digestion, have a hydrostatic function or just be accidentally swallowed and therefore, an incidental finding.[5]

Following initial digestion in the stomach, food passes into the intestines for further digestion and absorption. As in other species, pancreatic enzymes and bile salts aid the digestive process, including chitinase in insectivores, which is secreted by the stomach and pancreas to break down the hard exoskeleton of invertebrate prey. The small and large intestines can usually be easily distinguished in the herbivorous reptile but are less clearly delineated in the carnivore. In general, herbivores have much longer and more developed intestines than omnivores while carnivores such as snakes have a short simple tubular structure.[7] Some species, however, retain well-developed ceca despite no obvious dietary need. Examples include some boids, the omnivorous black tegu (*Tupinambis teguixin*), and insectivorous maned forest lizard (*Bronchocela jubata*), whereas in herbivorous chelonians, the cecum is not well developed.[5] A well-developed hindgut is a sensible dietary adaptation in those species that eat a high-fiber diet to allow fermentation of food material, particularly given that food is rarely chewed into small parts unlike in mammals. The colon of the green iguana (*Iguana iguana*) is divided into pockets, which allows food to be retained there for up to 3.5 days to ensure adequate time for hindgut fermentation.[5,8] Intestinal motility is influenced by a number of factors including temperature, and it is controlled by the vagal nerve. From the intestine, any indigestible matter passes into the cloaca. Further water reabsorption can occur within the cloaca and urates and feces are often mixed together.

In amphibians, the GI tract has a similar structure but can vary with life stage. For example, juvenile anurans are generally omnivorous and have a poorly developed stomach, which is mainly for food storage with digestion occurring in the intestines. Adults in contrast are generally carnivorous so as juveniles transition into adults, the stomach expands and develops extensive glands for digestion to occur here.[9] As with reptiles, species-specific adaptations may be seen with one of the most striking being that of the now extinct gastric-brooding frogs (*Rheobatrachus* spp). The female ingested her eggs after they had been fertilized and brooded them in her stomach until the young were fully developed. During this time, production of stomach acid was reduced and most digestion occurred in the small intestine. Once young were fully developed, they were regurgitated out and stomach digestion returned to normal.[10]

DIAGNOSTIC APPROACH
History Taking and Physical Examination

Taking a full history and performing a full physical examination are always helpful even for cases where the problem may seem obvious, as so many of the disorders seen in reptiles and amphibians can be multifactorial.

Important points to check on history taking include

- Where the animal was obtained (eg, if wild caught, may suggest an infectious cause).
- Size of enclosure (small enclosures may limit ability to stretch out and exercise predisposing to constipation).
- Substrate (could this be easily ingested and result in impaction?).
- Appropriate temperature range for species (low temperatures can cause reduced GI motility and immunosuppression).
- Appropriate ultraviolet provision for species (insufficient ultraviolet B [UVB] provision may result in hypocalcemia and reduced GI motility).
- Appropriate humidity for species (dehydration may predispose to impaction).
- Any possible toxin exposure.
- Any other animals affected.
- Current and previous diet (what is fed vs what is actually eaten?).
- Any vitamin or mineral supplementation.
- Previous medical history.
- Current medical concerns (there may be specific GI signs—vomiting, diarrhea, constipation, melena, prolapse, or more nonspecific signs such as anorexia, lethargy, and weight loss).

A full physical examination is recommended in every case as GI signs can often be secondary to systemic disease, rather than a primary GI disorder. Assessment of the GI tract may be limited depending on species, but in most snakes and lizards, coelomic palpation can be performed in the conscious animal to help localize the source of the problem.

Diagnostic Imaging

Imaging can be a useful first diagnostic step to rule in or out structural abnormalities. Whole body radiographs are usually easily performed in a conscious patient. Multiple views should be taken, at minimum dorsoventral and lateral views, ideally with a horizontal beam. For amphibians, the use of dental radiography can be considered for finer detail in such small patients. Radiography can help identify organ enlargement, masses, or radiopaque GI foreign bodies in addition to non-GI pathology such as poor bone density, which may be relevant if hypocalcemia is suspected to be a factor. However, to clearly differentiate the GI tract from other structures or identify radiolucent foreign bodies, contrast studies are often required (**Fig. 1**).

For contrast radiographs, barium or an iodine-based contrast media may be administered orally, via a stomach tube or even retrograde per-cloaca. Normal contrast studies are available for comparison in a variety of species, such as green iguana, red-eared slider (*Trachemys scripta elegans*), Greek tortoise (*Testudo hermanni*), and central bearded dragons (*Pogona vitticeps*).[11–14] Radiographs will usually need to be repeated to assess progress of the contrast throughout the GI tract. An extended timeframe is required compared to a mammalian patient as GI transit time can take between 2 days and 5 weeks depending on the species, even at appropriate environmental temperature.

Barium provides better mucosal detail than iodine-based contrast agents but should only be administered if there is no suspicion of GI perforation due to the risk of inflammation and granuloma formation. Barium also takes longer to transit through the GI tract, so there is a risk of solidification and should be avoided if GI surgery is planned. Dose recommendations vary between 5 and 25 mL/kg.[12,13] Iodine-based contrast agents may be preferred for those patients with prolonged GI transit times,

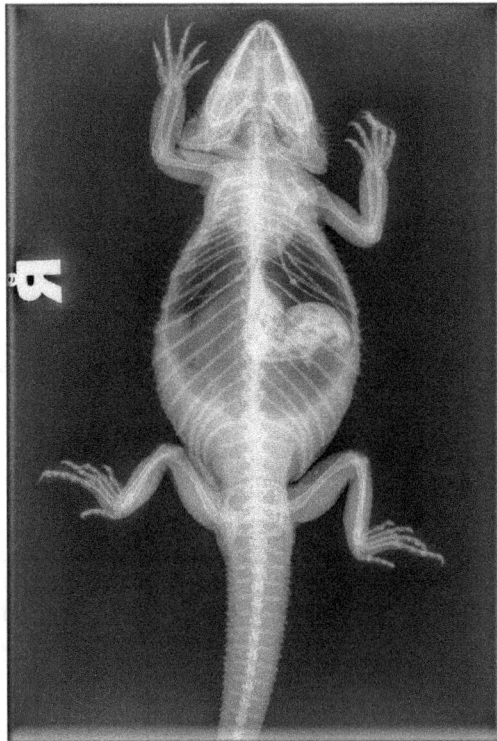

Fig. 1. Dorsoventral radiograph of a central bearded dragon (*P vitticeps*) presented for regurgitation. Contrast was administered via gastric gavage but remained in the stomach indicating an outflow abnormality.

although radiopacity and mucosal detail can be reduced in the distal intestinal tract compared with barium.[13] In dehydrated patients, care should be taken due to their hyperosmolar properties, and they should be either used at lower doses or avoided. Standard dose recommendations vary between 5 and 7.7 mL/kg.[13,14]

Coelomic ultrasound can also be useful to assess the GI tract and identify any thickening or obstruction, in addition to ruling in or out any other cause of clinical signs such as hepatic disease. The normal ultrasonographic appearance and dimensions of the GI tract has been described in multiple species.[15–17] Depending on patient size, a probe size of 7 to 14 MHz can be used. Ultrasound is easiest to perform if the GI tract is either empty or fluid filled. Assessment of the GI tract in an herbivore is often limited due to the presence of gas, and in chelonians, it may be limited by the shell.

Increasingly, advanced imaging techniques such as computed tomography (CT) are being used, especially in patients where radiography and ultrasound are limited as in many chelonian or crocodilian patients. The GI tract can still be difficult to clearly differentiate, but administration of an intravenous contrast agent such as an iodine-based media will help enhance soft tissue structures or contrast agents can be administered directly into the GI tract as previously described. Alternatively, MRI could be considered for select cases, although the logistics of this being performed (price, anesthetic time, and availability) often limits its use in general practice.

Endoscopy is another valuable diagnostic technique, which is increasingly used in both reptile and amphibian patients. Coelioscopy provides a general overview of the coelomic structures and is well described in numerous texts. Alternatively, if the problem has been localized, endoscopy may be performed either via the oral cavity (to access the esophagus or stomach) or via the cloaca (to access the colon) to evaluate the GI tract, collect any diagnostic samples and even for therapeutic purposes such as foreign body removal.[18] A rigid endoscope is usually used with saline infused for insufflation or air if assessing the esophagus in case of aspiration.

Sample Collection

A fecal sample is one of the most useful samples to collect when investigating a suspected GI disease, as long as the animal is still regularly passing feces. Following prolonged anorexia, no fecal material may be available, and in these cases, a cloacal wash can be considered instead although diagnostic value may be limited. Alternatively, the veterinarian may choose to start supportive tube feeding to encourage movement of ingesta and wait for a sample depending on the urgency of diagnosis.

Fecal samples can be examined in-house and, at minimum, a wet preparation and flotation should be performed to check for parasites (**Figs. 2** and **3**). If parasites are present, further analysis (eg, modified McMaster technique) is valuable to provide a quantitative assessment of worm egg count and guide treatment decisions. In certain situations, additional testing such as acid-fast staining may also be indicated (eg, when testing for cryptosporidiosis, although this should always be verified by polymerase chain reaction [PCR] testing) (**Fig. 4**). Fecal culture and sensitivity are rarely indicated as primary bacterial enteritis is uncommon and care should be taken interpreting results as a wide range of commensals may be isolated, including *Salmonella* spp. If specific viruses are suspected, samples should be collected for PCR testing (see "Infectious diseases" section) and veterinarians are encouraged to check submission requirements with their local exotics laboratory to maximize chances of obtaining a positive result. Ultimately, histopathology will provide the most definitive diagnosis in many cases but is usually performed postmortem due to the thin-walled nature of the reptile GI tract and risk of dehiscence.

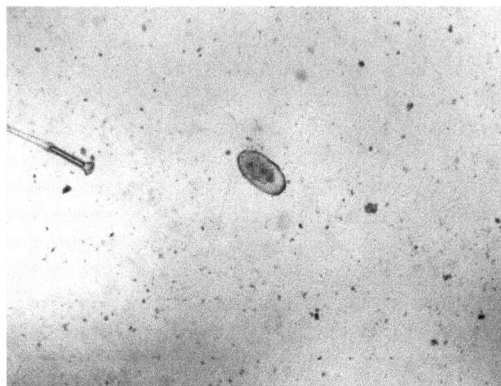

Fig. 2. Oxyurid eggs are a common incidental finding on fecal analysis.

Hematology and Biochemistry

Bloodwork may be performed and can provide information on general health status. For animals acutely vomiting or with profuse diarrhea, electrolyte abnormalities may be seen. Those with inflammatory disease may have an increased white blood cell count with a heterophilia and monocytosis, or anemia in chronic cases. Low albumin levels are suggestive of malabsorption, hepatic disease, or protein-losing enteropathy, although may also just be a consequence of anorexia. However, hematology and biochemistry results are often nonspecific (eg, elevations in aspartate transferase [AST] and creatine kinase [CK]) or even within normal limits in patients with GI disease.

INFECTIOUS DISEASES
Viral

Viral pathogens are increasingly reported as causes of GI disease in reptiles and amphibians. However, the presence of virus does not necessarily confirm that this is the primary etiology and predisposing factors as well as other pathogens should always be considered. Some of the more common viruses that have been implicated in GI disease are summarized in the following sections.

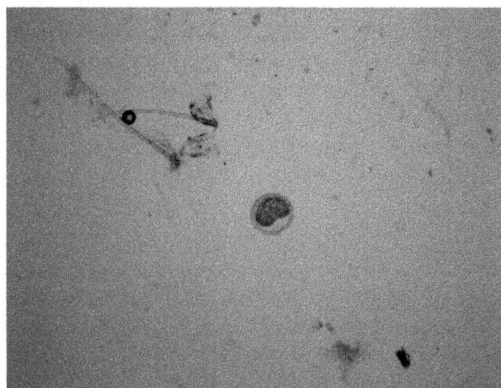

Fig. 3. Ascarid eggs can be identified by their round shape and thick wall.

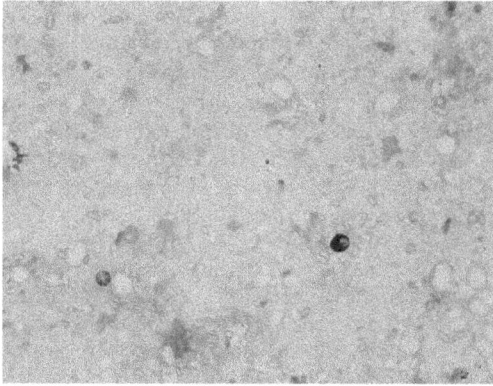

Fig. 4. Cryptosporidia oocysts measure approximately 4 to 8 μm and appear red on a green background with a modified acid-fast stain.

Herpesviridae

Herpesviruses are a significant cause of disease in chelonians affecting a variety of body systems. *Chelonid alphaherpesvirus 5* is associated with fibropapillomatosis of marine turtles, classically associated with dermal masses but internal masses can occur affecting the GI tract, specifically the oral cavity and intestines.[19] It is suspected this virus has been present for millions of years and that the cause of increased clinical disease is likely associated with ecological changes.[20] Diagnosis is often presumed based on clinical signs but can be confirmed by submitting biopsies of the masses for PCR.[21] Treatment is supportive only, and although surgery is often reported to alleviate clinical signs, masses often reoccur.[22] Tortoises and semiaquatic turtles are also affected by herpesviruses that have been specifically associated with stomatitis, glossitis, and esophagitis.[23] In lizards such as varanids, enteritis has been reported associated with a novel herpesvirus (Varanid herpesvirus 3), although within these cases, *Salmonella* spp and trematodes were also present and hence the clinical significance of this was unclear.[24] Currently no curative treatment exists although antivirals and vaccines have been trialed.[25] While herpesviruses have been reported in amphibians, they do not appear to be associated with GI signs.

Adenoviridae

Adenoviruses can also affect multiple body systems in reptiles, often resulting in GI and neurologic signs. Most commonly identified in squamate species, clinical signs include regurgitation, inappetence, and diarrhea.[26–28] In chelonians, adenoviruses have only been detected more recently with anorexia, lethargy, and diarrhea reported in a group of illegally imported Forsten's tortoises (*Indotestudo forstenii*), which tested positive by PCR for a novel *Siadenovirus*. Postmortem findings included oronasal fistula, segmental darkening of the serosa of the intestines and ulceration of the tongue.[29] Severe hyperplastic stomatitis and esophagitis has also been reported in a Mediterranean spur-thighed tortoise (*Testudo graeca*) associated with adenovirus infection.[30] Although adenoviruses are more commonly associated with hepatopathies in crocodilians, necrotizing enteritis has been reported in a young Nile crocodile (*Crocodylus niloticus*).[31] Diagnosis of adenovirus can be confirmed by PCR testing from cloacal swabs and hepatic or intestinal samples. Treatment is supportive only, however, euthanasia often being required.

Ranaviruses

In reptiles, ranaviruses are most often reported in chelonians and result in a range of clinical signs.[32] GI findings include necrotizing stomatitis and esophagitis. Diagnosis is based on PCR of combined oral/cloacal swabs and blood in the live animal or samples of the liver or GI tract postmortem. No curative treatment exists although raising the environmental temperature to above 90°F has been suggested to reduce viral replication. While ranaviruses are frequently reported in amphibians, GI signs are rarely seen with other body systems predominantly affected.

Arenaviridae

Arenaviruses are most commonly associated with inclusion body disease in snakes with species varying in their response to infection. Pythons typically develop neurologic signs and disease develops quickly.[20] In contrast, boas often present with regurgitation and a more chronic course of disease. PCR testing is possible based on samples from blood, esophageal swabs, or liver biopsies in live animals or samples of the brain postmortem. No treatment exists, and if clinical signs are present, then euthanasia is recommended.

Bacterial

As a wide range of bacteria are naturally found as commensals within the GI tract, a positive culture does not necessarily indicate this is the primary cause of disease. A heavy growth of one bacterium may be suggestive but ideally would be combined with additional diagnostics such as histopathology to confirm etiology. However, some of the frequently seen commensals can be opportunistic pathogens such as *Pseudomonas* spp, *Acinetobacter* spp, and *S* spp if primary GI pathology is present. Mycobacterial infections such as *Mycobacterium chelonae*, *Mycobacterium marinum*, and *Mycobacterium fortuitum* should also be considered whenever granulomas are noted especially in cases not responding to appropriate medical management.[33] Atypical bacterial infection has also been reported with *Chlamydia* infection linked with regurgitation in emerald tree boas (*Corallus caninus*). In these snakes, severe changes were observed along the GI tract including included esophagitis, gastritis, gastric atrophy and fibrosis, enteritis, and colitis.[34]

Parasites

A variety of parasites are found in reptiles and amphibians, some which may cause pathology but many being commensals within the GI tract. Knowledge of different groups and how to quantify these is, therefore, important to ascertain if medical intervention is needed.

One of the most common parasite groups identified on fecal analysis is the oxyurids (pinworms). Oxyurids are generally considered commensals of many herbivores and omnivores and rarely associated with clinical disease. Time of day, season, and other factors may influence shedding of eggs, so treatment decisions depend not only on parasite load but also on whether they are associated with clinical signs.[35] If treatment is required, an antiparasitic such as fenbendazole can be used to reduce numbers.

Ascarids (roundworms) are also commonly identified on fecal analysis and can cause more significant pathology because of their ability to migrate through viscera or embed themselves in GI mucosa.[36] Clinical signs can be nonspecific including weight loss, anorexia, and delayed regurgitation (snakes specifically). In Crocodylia, specifically caimans, *Brevimulticaecum* sp has been reported to cause marked focal ulceration to the stomach wall.[37] Despite marked visceral pathology, animals rarely exhibit clinical signs. Alternatively, nematodes can also accumulate to cause GI obstruction. *Kalicephalus* infection has been reported in various colubrids including corn snakes (*Pantherophis guttatus*) and an eastern milk snake (*Lampropeltis triangulum*), associated with anorexia.[38,39] Treatment success with fenbendazole has been variable. Those snakes that did not survive were reported on postmortem examination to have extensive esophageal and gastric pathology (abscessation and ulceration) associated with nematode infection. Both oxyurids and ascarids can usually be easily detected on fecal analysis, and regular screening is advised particularly of any new arrivals, so that parasites can be treated at an early stage.

Cestodes and trematodes are less commonly encountered in captive reptiles and amphibians due to their indirect life cycle but should be considered especially in recently acquired animals or those that might come into contact with an intermediate host.[36] Infections may be subclinical, damage GI mucosa, or result in intestinal obstruction in large numbers. Treatment usually involves praziquantel following diagnosis on fecal assessment.

Protozoa such as ciliates and flagellates are often found on fecal analysis and are rarely associated with pathology, high numbers usually indicating dysbiosis. Coccidia, however, can be associated with significant GI disease, specifically the families Sarcocystidae, Eimeriidae, and Cryptosporidiidae. *Isospora amphiboluri* is of particular concern in juvenile bearded dragons with clinical signs including diarrhea, anorexia, weight loss, or failure to thrive.[40] Oocysts can be identified on fecal analysis by their 2 sporocysts. Treatment options include toltrazuril or trimethoprim/sulphonamides and thorough cleaning of the enclosure is vital to prevent reinfection. *Cryptosporidium* is also of particular concern, specifically *Cryptosporidium serpentis* and *Cryptosporidium testudinis* that are usually found within the intestinal tract and *Cryptosporidium varanii* and *Cryptosporidium ducismarci* found within the stomach.[41] Clinical signs include vomiting, anorexia, and emaciation although some animals may be completely asymptomatic. In snakes, *C serpentis* results in gastric mucosal hypertrophy and a prominent stomach may be palpated on physical examination. Diagnosis is based on either fecal samples or gastric washes or biopsies depending on the site of infection. In Eastern indigo snakes (*Drymarchon couperi*), a recent study revealed that endoscopic biopsy for histology and quantitative PCR (qPCR) analysis were the most reliable diagnostics for disease diagnosis, while gastric lavage and gastric swabs for qPCR are useful for screening for the presence of pathogen.[42] Acid-fast staining can be used as an initial screen but may result in false positives due to the presence of mammalian strains of *Cryptosporidium* from prey animals. PCR testing is, therefore, required to confirm diagnosis. Various treatments have been trialed but no definitive successful treatment has been reported.

NONINFECTIOUS DISEASES
Foreign Bodies

Animals with GI foreign bodies often present with vague clinical signs including anorexia and weight loss before ultimately a reduction or cessation in fecal output. In captivity, common foreign bodies include substrate, especially when animals are fed directly from the enclosure floor. Material often accumulates over time especially if animals are dehydrated or temperatures are suboptimal. For wildlife casualties, foreign bodies may be the reason for presentation or an incidental finding. Specifically, sea turtles are commonly found with a variety of foreign bodies from marine debris such as fishing hooks.[43] Foreign bodies can cause GI irritation, pressure necrosis, obstruction through accumulation, perforation, and even carry the risk of causing volvulus as reported in a hawksbill sea turtle (*Eretmochelys imbricata*).[44] Diagnosis is usually based on imaging or sometimes exploratory surgery is required (**Figs. 5–7**). Treatment may be medical only with oral fluids or laxatives used to encourage the foreign body to pass. Alternatively, in more severe cases, endoscopic or surgical intervention may be required depending on location.

Trauma

Trauma of the GI tract may occur from forces within the lumen such as a perforating foreign body, or from external forces outside the body cavity such as vehicle or machinery strikes. The inciting cause is not always clear, but trauma has been suggested to be associated with some of the volvulus and intussusception cases seen reported in reptiles.[45,46] Diagnosis is based on imaging and treatment is always surgical. The authors have also treated a gastrocutaneous fistula in Horsfield's tortoise (*Testudo horsfieldii*). This patient presented initially with a shell dermatitis. Clinical signs appeared to resolve after medical management but on reexamination 9 months later the problem had returned. Contrast CT revealed a gastrocutaneous fistula, which was surgically corrected (**Fig. 8**). It is hypothesized the infection developed penetrated the shell causing a focal coelomic reaction adjacent to the stomach, which ultimately fused together.

Nutritional Disorders

Dietary deficits are a common cause or contributing factor for GI disease. Inadequate water provision or lack of digestible fiber can result in reduced GI transit times and ultimately constipation, especially if combined with inappropriate environmental temperature and lack of exercise.[47] Unfortunately, problems are often only identified at a late stage when other signs are present such as lethargy, straining, hindlimb weakness, or even cloacal prolapse. Diagnosis is often suspected on coelomic palpation and confirmed on imaging. Endoscopy can also be helpful for visualizing and potentially breaking down impacted fecal material, although this must be carried out carefully to avoid iatrogenic trauma. Medical treatment with fluid therapy may be sufficient to resolve signs as long as husbandry and diet deficits are also corrected. The use of laxatives has been reported as have prokinetics, although evidence of their efficacy is lacking.[48] Should medical management be unsuccessful surgery may be required to remove impacted feces (**Fig. 9**).

Alternatively, more specific dietary deficits such as a lack of appropriate calcium ± vitamin D3 may be seen; often also associated with inadequate UVB provision and environmental temperatures. As calcium is required for GI motility, hypocalcemia can result in ileus. Diagnosis is often based on clinical history and physical examination findings with reduced bone density seen on radiographs. Biochemistry may reveal hypocalcemia in severe cases, but normal calcium levels do not rule out a problem.

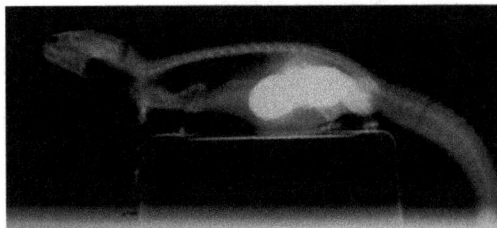

Fig. 5. Horizontal beam lateral radiograph of a leopard gecko (*Eublepharis macularius*) with a sand impaction.

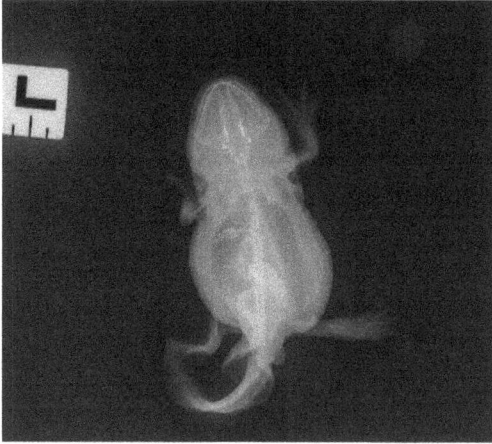

Fig. 6. Dorsoventral radiograph of an axolotl (*Ambystoma mexicanum*), which presented for a spinal deformity and failure to thrive. Foreign material visualized throughout the GI tract was thought to be accumulating secondary to the spinal pathology.

Treatment involves husbandry corrections and providing supplemental calcium, initially parenterally and then orally while husbandry changes take effect. Ongoing parenteral calcium supplementation and vitamin D3 supplementation is not recommended due to the risk of metastatic tissue calcification.

Congenital

Congenital abnormalities of the GI tract have been rarely reported in reptiles although should be considered in juveniles that are failing to thrive or those with external abnormalities. A postmortem of a dicephalic spur-thighed tortoise (*T graeca ibera*) revealed

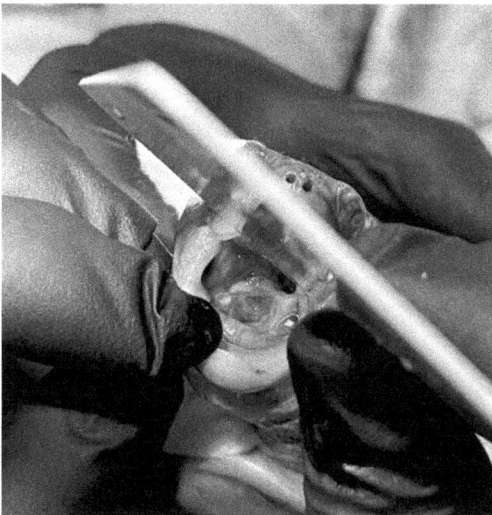

Fig. 7. Red-bellied short-necked turtle (*Emydura subglobosa*) with a fish skull lodged within the cranial esophagus.

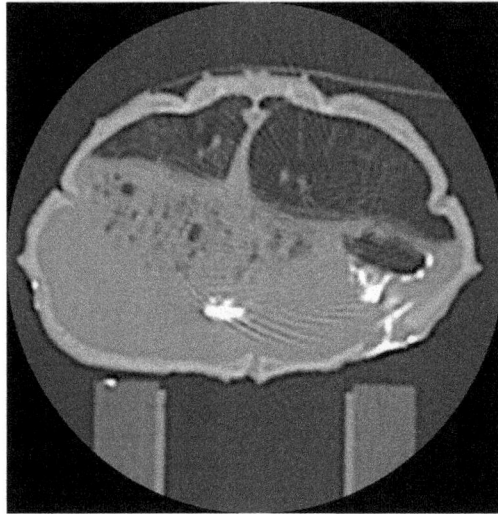

Fig. 8. CT image to show a gastrocutaneous fistula in a Horsfield's tortoise (*T horsfieldii*) highlighted by iodine-based contrast media.

that the entire cranial GI tract from esophagus to stomach was duplicated with food accumulation seen unilaterally prior to a pyloric valve atresia.[49] In addition, focal mild stenosis and segmental dilation of the colon was noted. Genetics and incubation environment are likely causes of congenital disease; therefore, when these occur, the perinatology should be reviewed thoroughly. To the authors' knowledge, no reports exist of congenital malformation of the GI tract that has been successfully treated and no reports exist of congenital GI disease in amphibians.

Toxins

Fenbendazole is a commonly used antiparasitic drug in herpetological medicine with published doses for a variety of species, yet toxicity has been suggested at elevated doses. Postmortem examination of 4 Fea's vipers (*Azemiops feae*) that had deteriorated and died in quarantine after receiving fenbendazole revealed moderate-to-

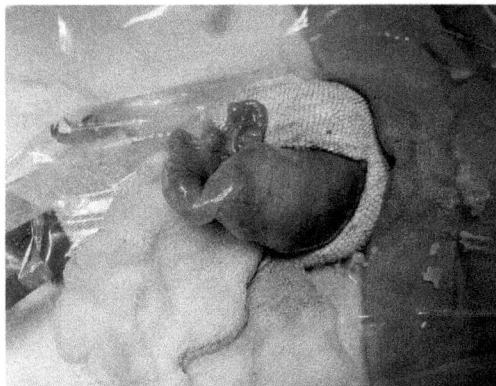

Fig. 9. Surgical treatment of constipation in a central bearded dragon (*P vitticeps*).

severe necrosis along the small intestine epithelium in all snakes.[50] Each animal had received a dose ranging from 428 to 1064 mg/kg far exceeding recommended doses. Hematologic and biochemical changes can occur, however, at lower doses, with extended heteropenia in addition to transient hypoglycemia, hyperphosphatemia, and hyperuricemia being reported in 6 Hermann's tortoises (*T hermanni*) following 2 courses of 50 mg/kg fenbendazole.[51] Although risks are considered low at published doses, care should therefore be taken to dose accurately and monitor for any potential side effects if using repeated treatment courses.

The family of plants Ericaceae (heaths or heather) contains grayanotoxins, which affect membrane-based sodium channels resulting in multisystemic signs including GI dysfunction. Azaela plants (part of the Ericaceae family) have been reported to result in lethargy and bloating as well as ataxia and bradycardia following ingestion in iguanas. Treatment is supportive only with oral fluids resulting in recovery in 1 case.[52]

Oak trees (*Quercus* spp) contain tannic acid, which along with its metabolites gallic acid and pyrogallol cause ulceration of the GI tract and pathology of the liver and kidneys. An African spurred tortoise (*Centrochelys sulcata*) that was kept in an enclosure with oak trees was reported to be found dead after 2 days of polyuria. On postmortem examination, the GI tract was found to contain oak leaves with fibrinonecrotic stomatitis, esophagitis, and thrombi in the stomach with secondary focal ischemic necrosis.[53]

Neoplasia

GI neoplasia has been reported across a variety of species. In reptiles, snakes appear particularly overrepresented and in amphibians, neoplasia appears most common in anurans.[54,55] Neoplasia should be considered as a differential for any coelomic swelling although may also present with more general GI signs (regurgitation, vomiting, diarrhea, melena, and constipation) or even with nonspecific signs such as lethargy, anorexia, or weight loss.

Diagnostic approach usually involves initial imaging, either radiography (±contrast) or ultrasound, to establish the location and extent of the lesion and any metastases. Advanced imaging such as CT can be helpful in providing more detail in these cases. Hematology and biochemistry may be performed to rule out other differentials, but changes in cases of GI neoplasia are usually nonspecific. Histopathology is required for definitive diagnosis with biopsies taken endoscopically, via exploratory celiotomy or postmortem.

Historically cases have often on been diagnosed on post mortem, so reports of successful treatment are limited, but, more recently, complete surgical excision has been reported with a good prognosis in some cases.[56] Early diagnosis is, therefore, vital to identify tumors before spread is too advanced at which point, euthanasia is recommended if quality of life is compromised.

Esophageal Neoplasia

Neoplasia of the esophagus is uncommon, but adenocarcinoma has been reported in a rattlesnake, carpet python (*Morelia spilota*), and mata mata (*Chelus fimbriatus*).[54,57,58] Metastases were not identified in any of these cases but remain a potential risk. Surgical excision was performed in the carpet python, but survival time was only 2.5 months. A hemangioma has also been reported in the esophageal wall of a red-eared slider with the animal presenting for reduced appetite and dysphagia.[59] On clinical examination, a swelling was identified affecting the ventral neck. Imaging and endoscopy identified an esophageal mass and diagnosis was confirmed on post mortem.

Gastric Neoplasia

A variety of gastric tumors have been reported, but recently gastric neuroendocrine carcinomas are increasingly recognized in bearded dragons.[60] These carcinomas are highly malignant and often metastasize to the liver, in addition to the kidneys and other organs. As with other GI neoplasia, clinical signs can be vague or alternatively a mass may be detected on coelomic palpation. Performing bloodwork can actually be useful in these cases as marked hyperglycemia is often present with anemia in some cases. The hyperglycemia is thought to be due to the somatostatin produced by the tumor, which inhibits insulin secretion, resulting in the elevated blood glucose levels. Other differentials for hyperglycemia such as primary pancreatic pathology should be considered but the presence of a gastric mass or thickening is usually suggestive of a neuroendocrine carcinoma. Definitive diagnosis usually requires histopathology, but fine needle aspiration for cytology may provide useful information to rule out other differentials.[61] Successful treatment has not been reported.

In snakes and chelonians, gastric adenocarcinoma appears more commonly reported with a variety of species affected.[62,63] Animals often present with vague signs and a poorly defined thickening of the gastric wall, although interestingly a red-eared slider was reported to have been treated for several days for suspected diabetes mellitus, which suggests that hyperglycemia may have been present. Generally, gastric adenocarcinomas are just locally invasive although metastases have been reported. Even without more extensive spread, they may progress to obstruction of the GI tract or perforation with associated coelomitis, so treatment is recommended. Successful surgical excision has been reported in a diamond python where almost complete subtotal gastric resection was performed and the residual stomach stretched over time to return to function.

Other individual case reports of gastric tumors include a cystic adenoma in a Central African rock python (*Python sebae*) and a gastric sarcoma in a cottonmouth (*Agkistrodon piscivorus*).[64] There are also 2 reports of GI lymphosarcoma in African spurred tortoises and Galapagos tortoises (*Chelonoidis* spp), and in both cases, an infectious agent was speculated to be involved due to the multiple animals involved.[65,66] However, in each case, definitive diagnosis appears to have been post-mortem.

Although less information is available, gastric neoplasia should also be considered as a differential in amphibians, with gastric leiomyomas being reported in the Japanese fire-bellied newt (*Cynops pyrrhogaster*), although clinical significance appears uncertain.[67]

Intestinal Neoplasia

Intestinal neoplasia appears relatively commonly described in snakes especially adenomas and adenocarcinomas in colubrids and crotalids and surgical excision has been attempted although long-term prognosis is unknown (**Fig. 10**).[68] A retroviral etiology has been suggested in boas and pythons.[69] Other intestinal neoplasia reported include leiomyosarcoma or leiomyoma in an indigo snake (*Drymarchon corais couperi*), cornsnake (*P guttatus*), and palm viper (*Bothriechis marchi*) and polyps in a pine snake (*Pituophis melanoleucus*).[63] Lizards can also be affected with reports of colonic adenocarcinoma in a variety of species as well as leiomyomas.[63,70] In chelonians, intestinal leiomyoma has been reported in green sea turtles (*Chelonia mydas*) including one case with associated intestinal volvulus and stricture, which was successfully resolved.[71]

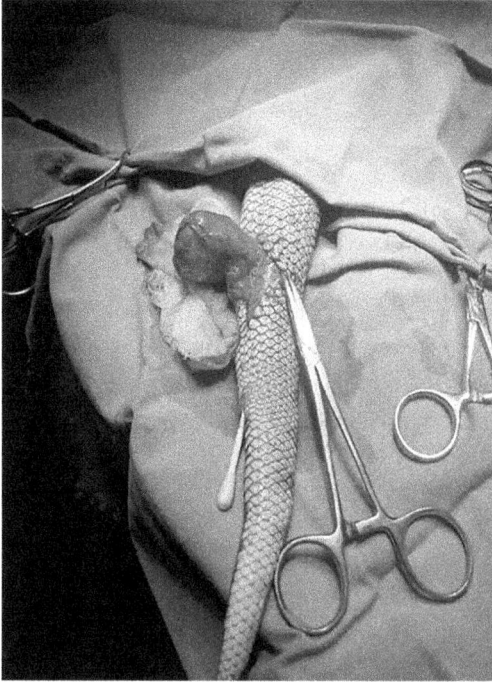

Fig. 10. Intestinal neoplasia in a Western hognose snake (*Heterodon nasicus*).

In amphibians, intestinal adenocarcinoma has been reported in multiple species including Amazon milk frogs (*Trachycephalus resinifictrix*), splendid tree frog (*Pelodryas splendida*), mountain chicken (*Leptodactylus fallax*), and Northern leopard frog (*Lithobates pipiens*).[72–76] It is thought to represent a significant cause of death especially in the captive mountain chicken population with diet or GI irritants resulting in chronic inflammation hypothesized to be predisposing factors.[75]

SUMMARY

GI disorders in reptiles and amphibians are a common presentation to the veterinary clinic. Although new pathogens continue to be identified and more advanced diagnostics are being developed, a thorough history and clinical examination will always provide important information even for cases where the problem may seem obvious, as so many of the disorders seen in reptiles and amphibians can be multifactorial. A logical diagnostic approach is, therefore, vital to identify the underlying cause and guide treatment plan.

CLINICS CARE POINTS

- Many GI disorders can be diagnosed on in-house testing such as faecal analysis, radiography and ultrasound without the need for advanced diagnostics in every case as long as a logical approach is taken.
- Take care to always look for the primary cause(s) of GI signs - many of the bacteria and parasites isolated are commensals so always consider other predisposing factors.

DISCLOSURE

The authors have nothing to disclose.

REFERENCES

1. Hedley J. Anatomy and disorders of the oral cavity of reptiles and amphibians. Vet Clin North Am Exot Anim Pract 2016;19(3):689–706.
2. Divers SJ. Herpatology. In: Divers SJ, Scott SJ, editors. Mader's reptile and Amphibian medicine and surgery. 3rd edition. St Louis, MO: Elsevier Health Sciences; 2019. p. 649–68.
3. Stahl SJ. Diseases of the reptile pancreas. Vet Clin North Am Exot Anim Pract 2003;6(1):191–212.
4. McArthur S, Machin RA. Gastroenterology - cloaca. In: Divers SJ, Scott SJ, editors. Mader's reptile and Amphibian medicine and surgery. 3rd edition. St Louis, MO: Elsevier Health Sciences; 2019. p. 775–85.
5. Skoczylas R. Physiology of the digestive tract. In: Gans C, editor. Biology of the reptilia, 8. London: Academic Press; 1978. p. p589–665. Physiology B.
6. Secor SM. Digestive physiology of the Burmese python: broad regulation of integrated performance. J Exp Biol 2008;211(24):3767–74.
7. Hoppe MI, Meloro C, Edwards MS, et al. Less need for differentiation? Intestinal length of reptiles as compared to mammals. PLoS One 2021;16(7):e0253182.
8. Parsons T, Cameron JE. Internal relief of the digestive tract. In: Gans C, Parsons T, editors. Biology of the reptilia, 8. London: Academic Press; 1977. p. p159–222. Morphology E.
9. Hourdry J, L'Hermite A, Ferrand R. Changes in the digestive tract and feeding behavior of anuran amphibians during metamorphosis. Physiol Zool 1996;69(2):219–51.
10. Tyler MJ, Shearman DJ, Franco R, et al. Inhibition of gastric acid secretion in the gastric brooding frog, Rheobatrachus silus. Science 1983;220(4597):609–10.
11. Taylor SK, Citino SB, Zdziarski JM, et al. Radiographic anatomy and barium sulfate transit time of the gastrointestinal tract of the leopard tortoise (Testudo pardalis). J Zoo Wildl Med 1996;180–6.
12. Smith D, Dobson H, Spence E. Gastrointestinal studies in the green iguana: technique and reference values. Vet Radiol Ultrasound 2001;42(6):515–20.
13. Long CT, Page RB, Howard AM, et al. Comparison of gastrografin to barium sulfate as a gastrointestinal contrast agent in red-eared slider turtles (Trachemys scripta elegans). Vet Radiol Ultrasound 2010;51(1):42–7.
14. Meyer J. Gastrografin® as a gastrointestinal contrast agent in the Greek tortoise (Testudo hermanni). J Zoo Wildl Med 1998;183–9.
15. Bucy DS, Guzman DS, Zwingenberger AL. Ultrasonographic anatomy of bearded dragons (Pogona vitticeps). J Am Vet Med Assoc 2015;246(8):868–76.
16. Holland MF, Hernandez-Divers S, Frank PM. Ultrasonographic appearance of the coelomic cavity in healthy green iguanas. J Am Vet Med Assoc 2008;233(4):590–6.
17. Banzato T, Russo E, Finotti L, et al. Ultrasonographic anatomy of the coelomic organs of boid snakes (Boa constrictor imperator, Python regius, Python molurus molurus, and Python curtus). Am J Vet Res 2012;73(5):634–45.
18. Littman EM, Berg KJ, Goldberg RN, et al. Endoscope-guided marble foreign body removal technique in an inland bearded dragon (Pogona vitticeps). J Herpetol Med Surg 2022;32(4):253–8.

19. Work TM, Balazs GH, Rameyer RA, et al. Retrospective pathology survey of green turtles Chelonia mydas with fibropapillomatosis in the Hawaiian Islands, 1993–2003. Dis Aquat Organ 2004;62(1–2):163–76.
20. Marschang RE, Origgi FC, Stenglein MD, et al. Viruses and viral diseases of reptiles. In: Jacobson ER, editor. Infectious diseases and pathology of reptiles. Boca Raton, FL: CRC Press; 2007. p. 575–704.
21. Lu Y, Wang Y, Yu Q, et al. Detection of herpesviral sequences in tissues of green turtles with fibropapilloma by polymerase chain reaction. Arch Virol 2000;145: 1885–93.
22. Page-Karjian A, Perrault JR, Zirkelbach B, et al. Tumor re-growth, case outcome, and tumor scoring systems in rehabilitated green turtles with fibropapillomatosis. Dis Aquat Organ 2019;137(2):101–8.
23. Sim RR, Norton TM, Bronson E, et al. Identification of a novel herpesvirus in captive Eastern box turtles (Terrapene carolina carolina). Vet Microbiol 2015; 175(2–4):218–23.
24. Hughes-Hanks JM, Schommer SK, Mitchell WJ, et al. Hepatitis and enteritis caused by a novel herpesvirus in two monitor lizards (Varanus spp.). J Vet Diagn Invest 2010;22(2):295–9.
25. Okoh GS, Horwood PF, Whitmore D, et al. Herpesviruses in reptiles. Front Vet Sci 2021;8:642894.
26. Catroxo MH, Pires JR, AMCRPF M, et al. Detection of paramyxovirus, reovirus and adenovirus infection in king snakes (Lampropeltis triangulum spp.) by transmission electron microscopy and histopathology techniques. Int J Environ Agric Res 2018;4:66–75.
27. Garner MM, Wellehan JFX, Pearson M, et al. Pathology and molecular characterization of two novel atadenoviruses in colubrid snakes. J Herpetol Med Surg 2008;18(3):86–94.
28. Raymond JT, Garner MM, Murray S, et al. Oroesophageal adenovirus-like infection in a palm viper, bothriechis marchi, with inclusion body-like disease. J Herpetol Med Surg 2002;12(3):30–2.
29. Rivera S, Wellehan JFX, McManamon R, et al. Systemic adenovirus infection in Sulawesi tortoises (Indotestudo forsteni) caused by a novel siadenovirus. J Vet Diagn Invest 2009;21(4):415–26.
30. Garcia-Morante B, Pénzes JJ, Costa T, et al. Hyperplastic stomatitis and esophagitis in a tortoise (Testudo graeca) associated with an adenovirus infection. J Vet Diagn Invest 2016;28(5):579–83.
31. Jacobson ER, Gardiner CH, Foggin CM. Adenovirus-like infection in two Nile crocodiles. J Am Vet Med Assoc 1984;185(11):1421–2.
32. Johnson AJ, Pessier AP, Wellehan JFX, et al. Ranavirus infection of free-ranging and captive box turtles and tortoises in the United States. J Wildl Dis 2008;44(4): 851–63.
33. Mitchell MA. Mycobacterial infections in reptiles. Vet Clin North Am Exot Anim Pract 2012;15(1):101–11.
34. Lock B, Heard D, Detrisac C, et al. An epizootic of chronic regurgitation associated with chlamydophilosis in recently imported emerald tree boas (Corallus caninus). J Zoo Wildl Med 2003;34(4):385–93.
35. Pike C, Hsieh S, Baling M. Monitoring infection load of oxyurid (nematoda) and Isospora (coccidia) in captive inland bearded dragons (Pogona vitticeps). Perspect. Anim. Health Welf 2023;2:77–90.
36. Walden HDS, Greiner EC, Jacobson ER. Parasites and parasitic diseases of reptiles. Infectious Diseases and Pathology of Reptiles 2020;859–968.

37. Cardoso AMC, de Souza AJS, Menezes RC, et al. Gastric lesions in free-ranging black caimans (Melanosuchus Niger) associated with Brevimulticaecum species. Vet Pathol 2013;50(4):582–4.

38. Klaphake E, Cross C, Patton S, et al. Gastric impaction in a milk snake, lampropeltis triangulum, caused by kalicephalus sp. J Herpetol Med Surg 2005;15(1):21–3.

39. Matt CL, Nagamori Y, Stayton E, et al. Kalicephalus hookworm infection in four corn snakes (Pantherophis guttatus). J Exot Pet Med 2020;34:62–6.

40. Walden M, Mitchell MA. Pathogenesis of isospora amphiboluri in bearded dragons (Pogona vitticeps). Animals (Basel) 2021;11(2):1–14.

41. Bogan Jr JE. Gastric cryptosporidiosis in snakes, a review. J Herpetol Med Surg 2019;29(3–4):71–86.

42. Bogan JE, Mason AK, Mishel K, et al. Comparison of sampling techniques and diagnostic tests for Cryptosporidium serpentis in eastern indigo snakes (Drymarchon couperi). Am J Vet Res 2024;85(10):1–9.

43. Franzen-Klein D, Burkhalter B, Sommer R, et al. Diagnosis and management of marine debris ingestion and entanglement by using advanced imaging and endoscopy in sea turtles. J Herpetol Med Surg 2020;30(2):74–87.

44. Schumacher J, Papendick R, Herbst L, et al. Volvulus of the proximal colon in a hawksbill turtle (Eretmochelys imbricata). J Zoo Wildl Med 1996;27(3):386–91.

45. Applegate JR, Drapp RL, Lewbart GA. Nonfatal traumatic gastric evisceration in two box turtles (Terrapene carolina carolina). J Herpetol Med Surg 2016;26(3–4):80–4.

46. Hornby JM, Hedley J, Spiro S. Intestinal torsion and volvulus through a mesenteric rupture in a bearded dragon (Pogona vitticeps). J Herpetol Med Surg 2023;33(3):139–45.

47. Johnson R, Doneley B. Diseases of the gastrointestinal system. In: Reptile medicine and surgery in clinical practice. 2017. p. 273–85.

48. Tothill A, Johnson J, Branvold H, et al. Effect of cisapride, erythromycin, and metoclopramide on gastrointestinal transit time in the desert tortoise, gopherus agassizii. J Herpetol Med Surg 2000;10(1):16–20.

49. Palmieri C, Selleri P, Di Girolamo N, et al. Multiple congenital malformations in a dicephalic spur-thighed tortoise (testudo graeca ibera). J Comp Pathol 2013;149(2–3):368–71.

50. Alvorado T, Garner MM, Gamble K, et al. Fenbendazole overdose in four fea's vipers (Azemiops feae). Proceedings AAZV 2001;28.

51. Neiffer DL, Lydick D, Burks K, et al. Hematologic and plasma biochemical changes associated with fenbendazole administration in Hermann's tortoises (Testudo hermanni). J Zoo Wildl Med 2005;36(4):661–72.

52. Rossi J Azalea. Rhododendron sp., Toxicity in a Green Iguana, Iguana iguana. Bulletin ARAV 1995;5(2):4–5.

53. Rotstein DS, Lewbart GA, Kristen Hobbie D, et al. Suspected oak, quercus, toxicity in an African Spurred Tortoise, sulcata. J Herpetol Med Surg 2003;13(3):20–1.

54. Garner MM, Hernandez-Divers SM, Raymond JT. Reptile neoplasia: a retrospective study of case submissions to a specialty diagnostic service. Vet Clin North Am Exot Anim Pract 2004;7(3):653–71.

55. Hopewell E, Harrison SH, Posey R, et al. Analysis of published amphibian neoplasia case reports. J Herpetol Med Surg 2020;30(3):148–55.

56. Baron HR, Šlapeta J, Donahoe SL, et al. Compensatory gastric stretching following subtotal gastric resection due to gastric adenocarcinoma in a diamond python (Morelia spilota spilota). Aust Vet J 2018;96(12):481–6.

57. Duke EG, Harrison SH, Moresco A, et al. A multi-institutional collaboration to understand neoplasia, treatment and survival of snakes. Animals 2022;12(3):258.

58. Lombardini ED, Desoutter AV, Montali RJ, et al. Esophageal adenocarcinoma in a 53-year-old mata mata turtle (Chelus fimbriatus). J Zoo Wildl Med 2013;44(3): 773–6.
59. Gál J, Jakab C, Szabó Z, et al. Haemangioma in the oesophagus of a red-eared slider (Trachemys scripta elegans). Acta Vet Hung 2009;57(4):477–84.
60. LaDouceur EE, Argue A, Garner MM. Alimentary tract neoplasia in captive bearded dragons (Pogona spp). J Comp Pathol 2022;194:28–33.
61. Anderson KB, Meinkoth J, Hallman M, et al. Cytological diagnosis of gastric neuroendocrine carcinoma in a pet inland bearded dragon (Pogona vitticeps). J Exot Pet Med 2019;29:188–93.
62. Baron HR, Allavena R, Melville LM, et al. Gastric adenocarcinoma in a diamond python (Morelia spilota spilota). Aust Vet J 2014;92(10):405–9.
63. Frye F. Neoplasia. In: Biomedical and surgical aspects of captive reptile husbandry Volume II. Malabar, Florida: Krieger Publishing Company; 1991. p. p585.
64. Schlumberger HG, Lucke B. Tumors of fishes, amphibians, and reptiles. Cancer Res 1948;8(12):657–753.
65. Duncan M, Dutton CJ, Junge RE. Lymphosarcoma in African spurred tortoise (Geochelone sulcata). Proceedings AAZV 2002;71.
66. Rideout BA, Worley MB, Anderson MP, et al. Alimentary tract lymphomas in Galapagos tortoises. In: Proceedings AAZV. 1993. p. 222–3.
67. Pfeiffer CJ, Asashima M. Gastric leiomyomas in the Japanese newt, Cynops pyrrhogaster; ultrastructural observations. J Comp Pathol 1990;102(1):79–87.
68. Lamglait B, Lemberger K. Colonic adenocarcinomas in a familial group of captive amur rat snakes (Elaphe schrencki). J Zoo Wildl Med 2017;48(2):491–6.
69. Oros J, Lorenzo H, Andrada M, et al. Type A–like retroviral particles in a metastatic intestinal adenocarcinoma in an emerald tree boa (Corallus caninus). Vet Pathol 2004;41(5):515–8.
70. Patterson-Kane JC, Redrobe SP. Colonic adenocarcinoma in a leopard gecko (Eublepharis macularius). Vet Rec 2005;157(10):294.
71. Helmick KE, Bennett RA, Ginn P, et al. Intestinal volvulus and stricture associated with a leiomyoma in a green turtle (Chelonia mydas). J Zoo Wildl Med 2000;31(2): 221–7.
72. Balamayooran G, Snook E, Tocidlowski M, et al. Retrospective survey of amphibian pathology cases at Texas A& University System (2016–2020). J Comp Pathol 2021; 185:87–95.
73. López J, Barbón AR, Smithyman J, et al. High prevalence of intestinal adenocarcinoma in a captive population of Amazon milk frog (Trachycephalus resinifictrix). J Zoo Wildl Med 2016;47(4):1061–8.
74. Vaughan RJ, Vitali SD, Payne KL, et al. A splendid tree frog with edema syndrome and intestinal adenocarcinoma. Vet Clin North Am Exot Anim Pract 2006;9(3): 583–7.
75. Ashpole IP, Steinmetz HW, Cunningham AA, et al. A retrospective review of postmetamorphic mountain chicken frog (Leptodactylus fallax) necropsy findings from European zoological collections, 1998 to 2018. J Zoo Wildl Med 2021;52(1): 133–44.
76. Stilwell JM, Boylan SM, Daniel W, et al. Intestinal adenocarcinoma with cloacal prolapse and reduction in a northern leopard frog (Lithobates pipiens). J Herpetol Med Surg 2021;30(4):237–41.

Fish Gastroenterology

Juliette Raulic, DMV, IPSAV, DES, Dipl ACZM[a],
Karine Béland, DMV, IPSAV, DES, MSc, Dipl ACZM[a],
Claire Vergneau-Grosset, DMV, IPSAV, CES, Dipl ACZM[b],*

KEYWORDS

- Fish • Digestive system • Gastroenterology • Physiology • Anatomy
- Infectious disease • Noninfectious disease

KEY POINTS

- A comprehensive understanding of anatomy, physiology, and nutritional requirements is essential for the effective management of digestive disease. This knowledge facilitates accurate diagnosis and enables the development of tailored therapeutic strategies.
- While gastrointestinal disease of mammals is typically associated with emesis and diarrhea, signs in fish may be nonspecific, such as dysorexia, discoloration, abnormal buoyancy, or presence of fecal casts.
- An increasing number of studies are available regarding imaging of the fish gastrointestinal tract.
- The clinical challenge presented by this system lies in the necessity to consider the potential for systemic disease affecting the digestive tract, and to differentiate among commensal, pathogenic microorganisms, and opportunistic infections from the normal microbiota.

INTRODUCTION

Fish represent the most common companion exotic animal in the United States and Canada in a number of individuals and hold the third place after dogs and cats in terms of the number of households.[1] Beyond companion animals, fish gastrointestinal diseases are particularly relevant for the aquaculture industry as feed represents about 50% to 70% of the costs associated with fish production.[2] Thus, nutrient malabsorption may have dramatic consequences both for the fish health and body condition score, but also for farmers.

In this review, the authors discuss the anatomy, physiology, and pathology of the digestive system of fish. Although the swim bladder is embryologically derived from the digestive tract, it will not be covered here as many excellent reviews are available

[a] Centre Hospitalier Universitaire Vétérinaire, Université de Montréal, St Hyacinthe, Canada;
[b] Zoological Medicine, Department of Clinical Sciences, Faculté de Médecine Vétérinaire, Université de Montréal, St Hyacinthe, Canada
* Corresponding author. 3200 rue Sicotte, Saint-Hyacinthe, QC J2S 2M2, Canada.
E-mail address: claire.grosset@umontreal.ca

Vet Clin Exot Anim 28 (2025) 315–330
https://doi.org/10.1016/j.cvex.2024.11.004
1094-9194/25/© 2024 Elsevier Inc. All rights are reserved, including those for text and data mining, AI training, and similar technologies.

elsewhere.[3,4] Similarly, good reviews are available regarding fish nutrition, which will not be covered here.[5]

ANATOMY AND PHYSIOLOGY OF THE DIGESTIVE TRACT

Among the more than 30,000 species of fish, there is a wide variability in the anatomy of the digestive tract. It is relevant for veterinary practitioner to be familiar with the normal anatomy of the fish they are treating, as this may condition interpretation of imaging techniques, as well as possible treatments. For instance, some fish, such as goldfish (*Carassius auratus*), zebrafish (*Danio rerio*), and koi (*Cyprinus carpio* koi), are agastric, that is, lack a stomach.[4] Certain fish have a pneumostomous swim bladder, displaying a connection, called the pneumatic duct, between their digestive tract and their swim bladder, while pneumoclistous swim bladders lack this connection. In Acipenseridae (sturgeons), gizzard shads (*Dorosoma* spp.), and mullets, the stomach is a grinding organ.[4] In some species, such as Salmonidae, pyloric ceca are present caudally to the fundus of the stomach (**Fig. 1**), while a cecum is not present prior to the colon in fish. The pyloric ceca increase the absorption surface of the stomach and are not fermentative organs. The intestine is usually short and simple in fish. In certain species, such as Acipenseridae, elasmobranchs, lungfishes, and bichir eels (*Polypterus senegalus*), a spiral colon is present, which should not be mistaken for a lesion or a digestive foreign body (**Fig. 2**). Regarding the hepatobiliary system, most fish have a gallbladder, which should not be mistaken for a lesion. Another anatomic difference that may be surprising for small animal veterinarians is that the digestive orifice of fish is located cranially to the urogenital papilla.

Knowing the normal anatomy is also relevant to understand the pathophysiology of some diseases in fish. For instance, the thyroid and heart of fish are located in close vicinity to their esophagus, which explains the occurrence of regurgitation and/or anorexia in case of goiter or cardiomegaly.[6] In particular, in syngnathids, it is not unusual to observe anorexia as the first clinical sign in case of goiter, as their dermal scales present in these species prevents the thyroid mass from being visualized externally.[7] In some shark species, it is physiologic to observe an exteriorization of the stomach through the mouth, as this is a normal process thought to be useful to clean the gastric content. However, exteriorization of the stomach through the gill slits is pathologic.[8] The transit time is highly variable depending on the species and is affected by the temperature of the patient (see "Diagnosing diseases of the digestive tract" section).[4] The gastrointestinal tract of fish is a key component of their immune system. It is involved in the innate immune system via the production of mucus by goblet cells, the quality of the mucosal barrier, and in the adaptative immune system

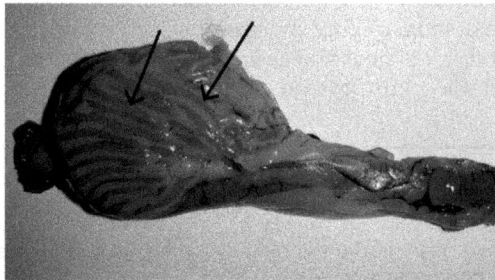

Fig. 1. Normal macroscopic appearance of the pyloric ceca (pointed by the *black arrows*) in a rainbow trout (*Oncorhynchus mykiss*). The oral section is toward the left of the image and the aboral section is toward the right of the image. (*Photo credit* Aquarium du Quebec.)

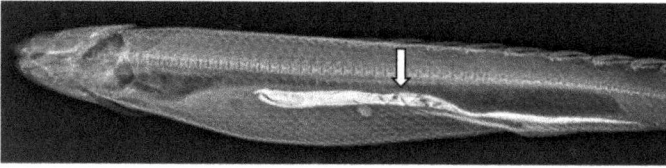

Fig. 2. Normal appearance of the spiral colon (pointed by the *white arrow*) of a bichir eel (*Polyphemus senegalus*) filled with barium: this right lateral radiographs was obtained 4 days after administration or oral barium. (*Source* Aquarium du Québec).

through the gut-associated lymphoid tissues. Thus, any component affecting the intestine, such as heat stress, may affect the systemic health of fish.[9]

Contrary to mammals, clinical signs of gastrointestinal disease may be difficult to detect in fish, due to their aquatic environment. Vomitus or diarrhea are rapidly diluted in a tank and only experienced owners or aquarists may notice abnormalities. On the other end, white fecal casts, which represent the persistence of fecal material at the digestive orifice, may be detectable. These may be due to malabsorption associated with some diseases, such as the infectious pancreatic necrosis virus, or spring viremia of carp, among others.[10] An indirect way to evaluate the gastrointestinal tract is also to evaluate the body condition score of fish and their body weight trend. For some species, body weight scores have been described, like for the spotted eagle ray (*Aetobatus narinari*).[11] More generally, fish body condition score may be evaluated by comparing the width of the head to the width of the body; fish with a proportional larger head being considered thinner.

The brain–gut axis is an emerging topic of research in mammals. The term describes the bidirectional communication between cognitive functions and peripheral intestinal function, which is partly mediated through the microbiota and through cortisol secreted by the hypothalamo-hypophyseal-interrenal axis in fish.[9,12] While the role of the digestive microbiome of fish is still poorly characterized, probiotics and prebiotic supplements are already widely used in the fish aquaculture industry.[13] Using molecular techniques, in particular through the sequencing of the 16S rRNA genes, normal populations of bacteria present in the gastrointestinal tract have been characterized in some teleost fish. Due to the growing need to limit resistance to antibiotics and to the consumer demand, interest has shifted toward the evaluation of prebiotics as a way to improve fish health. Some oral phototherapeutic products, such as oregano oil, have shown promising results to stimulate the immune system of channel catfish (*Ictalurus punctatus*), by increasing antioxidant activity, resulting in increased resistance against *Aeromonas hydrophila* infection.[14] Many oral prebiotics stimulate the production of short-chain fatty acids, which display antioxidant and antimicrobials effects. For instance, oral beta-glucans, nondigestible oligosaccharides, have been shown to enhance the immune system of fish through a prebiotic effect influencing the microbiome composition.[15,16]

DIAGNOSING DISEASES OF THE DIGESTIVE TRACT

Diagnosing diseases of the digestive system in fish is a complex process that requires a combination of clinical examination, laboratory testing, and imaging techniques. These methods are essential for identifying both infectious and noninfectious diseases, which can significantly impact fish health. The initial step in diagnosing digestive diseases in fish involves a thorough clinical examination. This includes observing external signs such as abnormal behavior, increased buoyancy that can indicate a gas-filled gastrointestinal tract, skin discoloration (eg, *Cryptobia* flagellates in discus), emaciation, bloating, and any more specific signs near the oral cavity or the vent. In particular, certain disease of the digestive tract can cause white fecal cast, meaning that fecal material remains attached to the vent of fish. Certain parasites can also cause a red vent (ie, *Anisakis* spp.) and others may be macroscopically detectable exiting the vent (ie, *Camallanus* spp.). A detailed review of the fish's environment, diet, behavior, and recent health changes is also critical in narrowing down potential causes.

Blood tests, including hematology and plasma biochemistry, can provide valuable information about a fish's metabolic state and organ function. Parameters such as liver enzymes (eg, alanine aminotransferase [ALT], aspartate aminotransferase), glucose levels, and electrolytes can indicate digestive disorders, including liver diseases or metabolic imbalances.[17] In terms of biochemistry, the gamma-glutamyl transferase is a specific enzyme of the digestive tract in black sea bass (*Centropristis striata*), while the ALT is the only enzyme specific of the liver tissue.[18]

Imaging techniques, such as radiography, ultrasonography, computed tomography (CT), or MRI, are increasingly used to diagnose digestive diseases in fish.[19,20] Plain radiography can be useful for detecting denser masses, some foreign bodies and visualizing skeletal abnormalities, but less precise for soft tissues. In certain cases, contrast radiography, anterograde or retrograde, can serve as a valuable diagnostic tool.[21] Various studies have evaluated gastric emptying and gastrointestinal transit time in fish using imaging techniques like barium series in spotted wolffish (*Anarhichas minor*)[22] and hybrid tilapia (*Oreochromis niloticus* × *Oreochromis mossambicus*),[23] or simple radiographs in streaked prochilodus (*Prochilodus scrofa*).[24] Digestive barium can also be used in other species, like in this case of colon stenosis (**Fig. 3**). Other methods, such as marker diets in Gulf of Mexico sturgeons (*Acipenser oxyrinchus*) and natural stable isotopes, offer noninvasive, accurate, and practical alternative to traditional approaches for determining gastrointestinal transit time, optimize feeding strategies, and improve fish health.[25,26] Various factors affecting transit time have been highlighted as the frequency and feeding time or water temperature.[27,28] A study assessing the effect of metoclopramide on gastrointestinal motility in cownose rays (*Rhinoptera bonasus*) and whitespotted bamboo sharks (*Chiloscyllium plagiosum*) concluded that it significantly accelerated gastric emptying and reduced gastrointestinal transit time in both species.[29]

Ultrasound provides real-time imaging of soft tissues, allowing for the detection of masses, fluid accumulations, and other abnormalities. Goncin and colleagues showed that contrast-enhanced ultrasound is a promising tool allowing for noninvasive monitoring of organ perfusion in aquatic species.[30] This method is used in patients with atherosclerosis, tumors of the liver, colon, prostate, and gastrointestinal inflammation.[31] Another article highlights the effectiveness of this imaging technique in

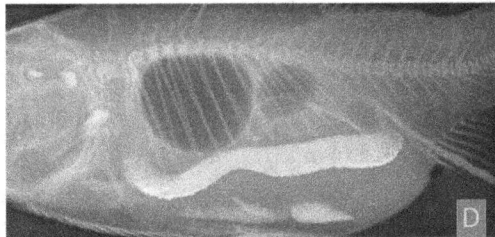

Fig. 3. Contrast radiographs demonstrating a complete colonic stenosis of unknown cause in a goldfish (*Carassius auratus*). This case was confirmed by surgery. (*With permission from* Claire Grosset, DMV, IPSAV, CES, Dipl. ACZM.)

visualizing and quantifying inflammation within the intestinal tissue in rainbow trout (*Oncorhynchus mykiss*), aiding in the early detection and treatment of intestinal disorders in fish.[32] However, ultrasound imaging may have some limitations, especially when imaging very small fish with a low spatial resolution,[33] fish with prominent dermal plates, or when evaluating patients with cutaneous edema, in which repeated application of the ultrasonographic probe can lead to skin ulcerations. In such cases, other imaging modalities should be favored.

Endoscopy is a minimally invasive diagnostic tool that allows for the detection of gastric ulcers, tumors, and other lesions but also facilitates biopsy collection for further analysis. Gastroscopy has been used in the diagnosis and treatment of an electric eel (*Electrophorus electricus*) with a lead wire and in a case of chronic regurgitations with gastric mucus gland hyperplasia in a green moray eel (*Gymnothorax funebris*).[34,35] Coelioscopy has been described as well in some species and is a great tool to evaluate different organs such as gastro-intestinal tract and liver.[36] These publications underscored the importance of endoscopic techniques in aquatic species, facilitating accurate diagnosis and treatment of gastrointestinal disorders.

The use of CT scan for gastrointestinal assessment in fish represents an innovative advancement in aquatic veterinary medicine. Contrast-enhanced CT using intravenous iopamidol provides detailed imaging of the vascular structures and parenchymal organs (liver, etc.).[19] Furthermore, this study showed that fish with hyperattenuating material in their intestines (food particles) aided in distinguishing intestinal segments from liver tissue.[37] The use of CT scan also allows to assess the swim bladder as demonstrated in koi carp.[38] In addition, MRI, although not always accessible and expensive, is known to be superior for early diagnosis of digestive tumors as seen in a case of intestinal adenocarcinoma in a rainbow trout.[39]

Other laboratory test such as smears of digestive content (obtained by enema, gastroscopy, or cloacoscopy), fine needle aspiration of a mass (using acid-fast stains as needed), and fecal sample examination (direct microscopy, flotation), culture, and molecular techniques, such as polymerase chain reaction (PCR), are used to detect and identify specific pathogens, including bacteria, viruses, and parasites. To obtain a stool sample, consider siphoning debris from the bottom of the tank, collecting a sample following fish defecation during anesthesia, gentle pressure on the coelom, or cloacal/rectal washes to collect fecal material.[40] Histopathological examination remains a cornerstone for diagnosing gastrointestinal diseases. Tissue samples from affected areas (eg, stomach, intestines, liver) are collected, fixed, and examined microscopically for cellular changes, such as inflammation, necrosis, tumors, or parasitic infiltration.[41] As described in a case of periventiduct leiomyoma in a koi, immunohistochemistry, which is a crucial tool for qualifying tumor types more precisely, is not always applicable and validated in fish.[42]

INFECTIOUS DISEASES OF THE DIGESTIVE TRACT

Several microorganisms are found in the digestive tract of fish. Determining which microorganisms are commensal and which ones are pathogenic is clinically challenging. Moreover, some commensal microorganisms can cause opportunistic infections that can further complicate our analysis and medical care.

Although we acknowledge that many digestive pathogens are of importance in aquaculture, this section focuses on the most clinically relevant gastrointestinal infectious diseases of pet and aquarium fish. For a more complete review of infectious etiologies in fish, readers are referred to previous numbers of the Veterinary Clinics of North America: Exotic Animal Practice.[43,44]

Risk factors for the development of gastrointestinal infections in fish under human care include malnutrition, suboptimal environmental conditions, social stress, concomitant diseases, poor biosecurity, and suboptimal quarantine protocols. All of those risk factors can render the fish more susceptible to infections and exacerbate clinical signs.

Selected Infectious Disease Affecting the Oral Cavity

Some metazoans like leeches and crustaceans can invade the oral cavity of a wide variety of fishes and can cause lesions ranging from mild to severe. Of those, *Branchellion torpedinis*, a leech species that exclusively infect elasmobranchs, can result in severe oral ulceration and anemia. *B torpedinis* can be especially challenging to control in a large habitat housing numerous demersal elasmobranchs but treatment options and strategies have recently been discussed elsewhere.[45,46] *Lymphocystis disease viruses* are pathogens that infect a large range of freshwater and marine fish including Cichlidae, Poeciliidae, Anabantoidei, spotted scats (*Scatophagous* spp.), and Banggai cardinalfish (*Pterapogon kauderni*). These lymphocystiviruses are usually host-specific and the clinical signs associated with an infection range from asymptomatic to apparition of numerous whitish nodules on various location of the body, including around the oral cavity. The morbidity and mortality rates remain low unless the mass prevents the fish from feeding, and reducing the stressors is the most effective way to control the disease in a population.[10]

Selected Infectious Disease Affecting the Stomach and the Intestines

The *protozoans* covered in this paragraph have a direct life cycle and can spread by direct and indirect contacts. Identification of the protozoans by direct microscopy of a gastric or an intestinal wet mount or by histopathology of the affected gastrointestinal section is the diagnostic tools of choice.[47] *Spironucleus* spp. and *Hexamita* spp. are often found in clinically normal Cichlidae, Cyprinidae, Salmonidae, and Anabantoidei fish and thought to be commensal. However, these diplomonad flagellates appear to be more pathogenic in discus (*Symphysodon* spp.) and angelfish (*Pterophyllum* spp.), in which they can cause inappetence, chronic weight loss, enterocolitis, and coelomic distension, particularly under stressful conditions. Although the mortality rate is usually low, these fish are often referred to as "poor doers."[47] Historically, *Spironucleus vortens* was thought to be associated with lateral line depigmentation but this association, to date, is not confirmed.[48] In fish exhibiting clinical signs associated with a *Spironucleus* spp. or a *Hexamita* spp. infection, oral administration of 50 to 100 mg/kg of metronidazole every 24 hours for 3 to 5 days is a recommended treatment, with concurrent reduction of environmental stressors.[47] Other dosages of metronidazole used in fish are available elsewhere.[16,49] The main differential diagnosis for these flagellates is *Cryptobia* spp. *Cryptobia iubilans* is also a flagellate found in the gastrointestinal tract of healthy Cichlidae including discus and oscars (*Astronotus ocellatus*). However, *C. iubilans* can also cause granulomatous gastritis that can result in lethargy, hyporexia, and weight loss in affected fish, especially under stress. This infection is hard to get rid of and the treatments are rarely effective. The medical management should focus on the improvement of the environmental conditions.[47]

Camallanid nematodes Are Often Referred to as "Red Worms" with *Camallanus cotti* Being Commonly Reported in Several Species of Poeciliidae, Anabantiformes, and Cichlidae.

These nematodes have an indirect life cycle with invertebrates being the intermediate hosts and fish the definitive ones. Fish with intestinal camallanids are usually subclinical but can develop gastrointestinal signs, especially under suboptimal environmental conditions and when the intermediate host can flourish in the habitat. The clinical signs seen in affected fish include hyporexia, coelomic distension, weight loss, and red worms coming out of the cloaca, anus, or body wall. Mortalities associated with camallanid infections are rare. On postmortem examination, hyperemia and ulcerations can be observed in the gastrointestinal tract of affected fish. Subclinical fish with a low parasitic load are usually not treated although reduction of the environmental stressors is always indicated. Fish showing associated clinical signs can be treated with anthelmintics.[50] Clinicians should, however, ensure the safety of these drugs before using them as sensitivity and toxicity have been reported in teleosts and elasmobranchs, especially when using fenbendazole and ivermectin, including at routine dosages.[49,51–53] Ivermectin appears to have a low margin of safety in fish species, presumably due to the reduced blood–brain barrier in fish compared to that of mammals.[4,49] If numerous fish should be treated and little information is available on the safety of a given drug for a given species, it is advisable to treat only a small subset of the population first.

Enteromyxum spp. are coelozoic myxozoans that can infect several species of marine fish in aquarium including tangs, wrasses, blennies, and emperor angelfish (Pomacanthus imperator). Some species of freshwater teleost have also been experimentally infected. Enteromyxum leei is the most common species infecting the intestinal tract, and occasionally the gallbladder, of aquarium-housed marine teleost. The older fish in the group are typically the first to be affected, which is unusual for myxozoan infections, and develop chronic enteritis. The affected fish can be subclinical for months, before experiencing hyporexia, anemia, coelomic distension, cloacal or anal prolapse, and wasting. The mortality rate can reach 100% in stressful environmental conditions although intermittent mortalities are more typical of the disease. The presence of the Enteromyxum spp. characteristic spores on direct microscopy of an intestinal wet mount or on histopathology confirms the diagnosis. An infection by Enteromyxum spp. can also be diagnosed by a PCR or an in-situ hybridization on a rectal swab. On postmortem examination, emaciation and catarrhal enteritis with intralesional spores are classic lesions. Spores are occasionally observed in the esophagus, the stomach, or the gallbladder.[54,55]

Systemic diseases causing gastrointestinal signs in fish are also listed in **Table 1**.

NONINFECTIOUS DISEASES OF THE DIGESTIVE TRACT

Noninfectious diseases of the fish digestive system encompass a range of pathologic conditions resulting from nutritional, environmental, toxic, genetics, or metabolic factors.

Nutritional imbalances are a common cause of digestive diseases in fish. Deficiencies in certain vitamins (eg, vitamins C, E, or B) can lead to gastrointestinal disorders like intestinal atrophy, hemorrhages, and lesions of the intestinal mucosa. For instance, a deficiency in vitamin C can cause connective tissue degeneration, resulting in poor nutrient absorption and intestinal inflammation.[64] Metabolic disorders, such as lipidopathies, typically arise from improper feeding, stress, pathologies, or hormonal imbalances. Excessive lipid accumulation in the liver (hepatic lipidosis) is common in aquaculture fish, leading to liver dysfunction, indirectly affecting the digestive system.[65]

Toxic diseases result from exposure to harmful chemicals, such as pesticides, heavy metals, or certain feed additives. Most toxic substances found in food, or the environment, are absorbed through several entry points, including the digestive system. Often these toxins will have local and/or systemic effects.[66,67] When in contact

Table 1
Selected pathogens that cause systemic diseases with possible concurrent gastrointestinal clinical signs in pet and aquarium fish

Pathogens	Species Affected	Clinical Signs, Lesions
Bacteria		
Yersinia ruckeri[56] (Enteric Redmouth Disease)	Freshwater fish, particularly salmonids	Reddening of the mouth, exophthalmos, enteritis, thick yellow fluid within the intestinal lumen, hemorrhagic septicemia
Edwardsiella spp.[56] (Enteric Septicemia, Edwardsiellosis)	Several species of marine and freshwater fish including catfish, eels, flounders, salmonids	Cutaneous ulcerations, spiral swimming, exophthalmos, gastroenteritis
Erysipelothrix piscisicarius sp. nov.[57,58]	Barbs and tetras Western mosquitofish (*Gambusia affinis*)	Necrotizing facial dermatitis (including around the oral cavity)
Virus[10]		
Infectious pancreatic necrosis virus (IPNV) and IPN-like birnaviruses	Freshwater and marine salmonids (IPNV); other teleosts (IPN like)	White feces, pale yellow fecal pseudocast Acute septicemia
Spring viremia of carp virus[a] Rhabdovirus	Cyprinids	Pale or mucoid fecal cast Cloacal or anal prolapse Hemorrhagic septicemia
Carp edema virus Poxvirus[59]	Common carp, koi	Cutaneous hemorrhagic lesions, especially around the oral cavity Gill necrosis
Parasites		
Scuticociliates[47] Ciliated protozoans	Freshwater and marine teleost Potentially emerging in elasmobranchs and sygnathids[46]	Enteritis ± yellow mucoid feces Various cutaneous and systemic signs including neurologic
Fungus		
Fusasporis stethaprioni[58,60] Microsporidium	Black (*Gymnocorymbus ternetzi*) and cardinal (*Paracheirodon axelrodi*) tetras	Intestine necrosis Necrotizing systemic disease
Exophiala spp.[61]	Sea dragons[62] Lumpfish[63] and other demersal teleost species Salmonids Elasmobranchs	Stomach ± intestine necrosis Necrotizing granulomatous systemic disease

[a] WOAH (World Organization for Animal Health) notifiable disease.

with the digestive mucosa, many toxins cause local damage, including necrosis, as in the case of cadmium, Almix herbicide, or microcystins exposure.[68–70] Compared to mammals, fish may not be as sensitive to the gastrointestinal toxic effects of anti-inflammatory drugs. For instance, a study evaluating the effects of a single intramuscular dose of meloxicam at 5 mg/kg in goldfish did not show any acute digestive adverse effects at necropsy.[71] Similarly, no adverse effects were noted in rainbow trout receiving a single intramuscular dose of 2 mg/kg of robenacoxib.[72] Of note, these studies were performed in clinically normal fish, and caution may be warranted in sick fish affected by intestinal ulcerations, especially with long-term administration. Further studies at different doses, frequencies, in other species, and at different water temperatures are required to rule out full digestive toxicity of non-steroidal anti-inflammatory drugs (NSAIDs) in fishes.

In addition to nutritional or metabolic imbalances and toxic exposure, intraluminal (foreign body, neoplasia, and other mass types, volvulus, intussusception) and extraluminal (coelomic mass, organomegaly, adhesions) mass effects should also be considered potential causes of gastrointestinal disease.

Any foreign body can lead to mucosal lesions (with or without secondary infections), partial or complete digestive obstruction, or even perforation. The release of an ingested toxin can also depend on the composition of a given foreign body. The therapeutic approach differs depending on the type of obstruction and its localization in the digestive tract. Gastric foreign bodies can be removed by gastroscopy, like in a case of a lead wire sub-obstruction with signs of intoxication in an electric eel.[34] Other gastric foreign bodies can be simply removed through the large oral cavity using suitable forceps, like in a case of gastric stones from a red-tailed catfish (*Phractocephalus hemioliopterus*) stomach.[73] In some fish species, such as Salmonidae and sharks, gastric foreign bodies will be naturally regurgitated without veterinary intervention.

Different lesions in the oral cavity can lead to difficulty in prehend food and gastrointestinal signs. First, dental issues in fish, such as malocclusion, periodontal disease, excessive wear, damage, or fracture of teeth can significantly affect fish feeding behavior and result in inadequate nutrition, leading to malnutrition. Second, any jaw fracture, abnormal bone or cartilage development, and oro-pharyngeal mass like goiter can lead to inability to prehend food.[7]

Tumors of the upper digestive tract, including those located in the oral cavity, pharynx, and esophagus, have been reported in various fish species that may present clinical signs such as difficult feeding, visible lesions in the oral cavity, and weight loss. In koi carp, the detection of Cyprinid herpesvirus 1 in oral squamous cell carcinoma warrants further investigation to understand the mechanisms by which the virus may contribute to carcinogenesis.[74] Another tumor that can be found around the oral cavity is a facial myxoma in goldfish. Intralesional bleomycin chemotherapy and then radiation therapy temporarily reduced the tumor size temporary in a case.[75] In cultured angelfish (*Pterophyllum scalare*), odontogenic hamartomas have been described in the frontal region of the mouth (maxilla and mandible) and may be associated with a retrovirus.[76]

Tumors of the lower digestive tract, including the stomach, intestine, and cloaca, have been documented in various fish species. Intestinal adenocarcinomas have been, to date, reported in zebrafish, koi carp, blue gularis (*Fundulopanchax sjostedti*), Atlantic salmon (*Salmo salar*), and rainbow trout.[77–79] In zebrafish, preneoplastic lesions (epithelial hyperplasia or inflammation) are seen in some subpopulations.[80,81] A study suggests an infectious etiology, a *Mycoplasma* species. A previous study ruled out diet, water quality, or genetic background as potential cause.[82] Although no cause was detected in an outbreak of metastatic intestinal adenocarcinoma in rainbow trout from a Slovene hatchery,[79] a study in salmonid fish showed that the inflammation-dysplasia-carcinoma sequence was associated with a certain commercial diet.[83] A study examined the protective effects of tomatine, a glycoalkaloid found in tomatoes, against dibenzo [a,l] pyrene-induced tumors in rainbow trout. Results indicated that tomatine significantly reduced the incidence of liver and stomach tumors in the trouts compared to those that were not given tomatine.[84] Digestive tumors can lead to acutely fatal complications. For instance, intestinal growths have been associated with intestinal intussusception in 40% of affected rainbow trouts.85

Cloacal tumors in fish, although relatively rare, have been reported in various species and can pose significant health risks. These tumors, which may include types such as squamous cell carcinomas and adenocarcinomas, often manifest as growths or lesions near the cloacal region, leading to clinical signs like difficulty in excretion and changes in behavior.[86] Given the critical role of the cloaca in the excretion of waste and reproduction in fish, the presence of tumors can have profound implications for overall health and reproductive success. Early diagnosis and intervention are essential for managing these conditions and improving outcomes for affected fish like in a case of periventiduct leiomyoma (**Fig. 4**) in a koi, where no recurrence was detected 6 months following surgical debulking of the mass (**Fig. 5**) and local administration of bleomycin.[42]

Other common problems include bloating, where trapped gases cause abdominal distension, or swim bladder dysfunction, which affects buoyancy and can interfere with feeding and digestion. Any physostomous species could develop a swim bladder dysfunction secondary to an esophageal disease (neoplasia, foreign body, or inflammation). These mechanical and physical conditions can significantly impact a fish's ability to process food and absorb nutrients, leading to further health complications if not addressed promptly.

Finally, stress from inappropriate environmental conditions (such as poor water quality, temperature fluctuations, or overcrowding) can induce digestive disorders.

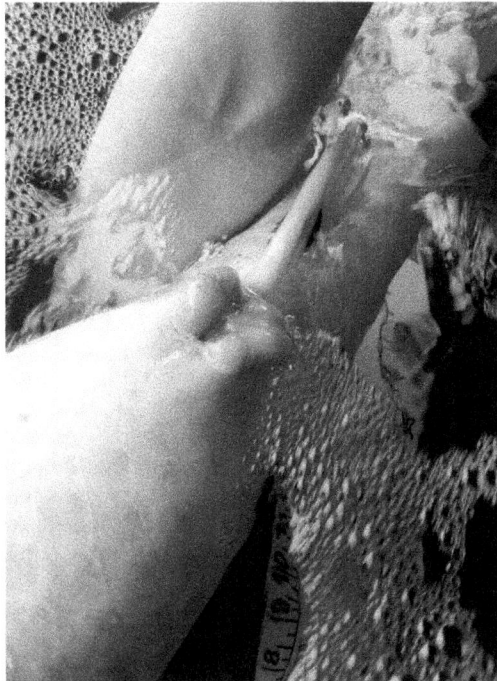

Fig. 4. Periventiductal masses associated with partial prolapse of the genital pore in a 10 year old female koi (*Cyprinus carpio koi*).

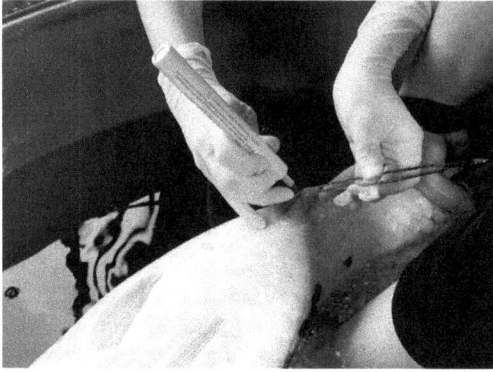

Fig. 5. Peroperative view of the incisional biopsy of the periventiductal mass in a 10 year old female koi (*Cyprinus carpio koi*). Hand-held cautery is used for hemostasis.

These factors can weaken the immune system, promoting the development of noninfectious gastrointestinal lesions like ulcers and hemorrhages.[87] A study explores how inflammation and infection influence the neuroendocrine mechanisms regulating intestinal motility in fish, by altering the secretion of neuropeptides and hormones that are crucial for gut motility. The authors highlight that infections can lead to changes in gut motility, often resulting in gastrointestinal dysfunction, which can further impact nutrient absorption and overall fish health.[88]

SUMMARY

In summary, the digestive system is affected by a range of distinct pathologies, each requiring rigorous diagnostic testing and diverse therapeutic approaches. Consequently, meticulous medical management is paramount. Given the multitude of pathologies that can impact the digestive system, continuous and thorough research is essential to effectively address these conditions. Further investigation is also needed to understand the potential impacts of genetics, diet, environmental factors, microbiota, and how these interactions may influence the development and progression of digestive disorders.

CLINICS CARE POINTS

- Isolation of microorganisms by diagnostic tests should be assess holistically, considering the environmental conditions, the fish species, the fish health status, and its pathogenicity before advancing to the therapeutic stage.

- Advanced medical imaging techniques are essential for accurately diagnosing noninfectious digestive disorders in live fish, providing critical insights that facilitate precise assessment and effective management.

- Histopathology, culture and molecular diagnosis on tissular lesions remains an important tool to diagnose gastrointestinal disease in fish.

DISCLOSURE

The authors have nothing to disclose.

REFERENCES

1. American Veterinary Medical Association. AVMA pet ownership and demographics sourcebook. 2022.
2. Hickey N. Fad medicine. Annual AAFV conference. Springfield (MO), 2023.
3. Strange R. Anatomy and physiology – blood gases and gas bladder function. In: Roberts HE, editor. Fundamentals of ornamental fish health. Ames (IA): Wiley Blackwell; 2010. p. 9–14.
4. Mylniczenko N. Anatomy and taxonomy. In: Hadfield C, Clayton L, editors. Clinical guide to fish medicine. Hoboken (NJ): Wiley Blackwell; 2021. p. 3–34.
5. Corcoran M, Roberts-Sweeney H. Aquatic animal nutrition for the exotic animal practitioner. Vet Clin Exot Anim 2014;17(3):333–46.
6. Vigneault A, Mylniczenko ND, Arnold RD, et al. Management of suspected dilated cardiomyopathy with pimobendan in two leopard sharks (*Triakis semifasciata*). J Zoo Wildl Med 2023;54(2):401–5.
7. Jalenques M, Vergneau-Grosset C, Summa N, et al. A cluster of cases of thyroid hyperplasia in aquarium-housed tropical marine teleosts following a change of salt mix brand. J Zoo Wildl Med 2020;51(3):725–8.
8. Tuttle AD, Burrus O, Burkart MA, et al. Three cases of gastric prolapse through the gill slit in sand tiger sharks, *Carcharhinus taurus* (Rafinesque). J Fish Dis 2008;31(4):311–5.
9. Fox J. Gut Health and Why It Matters. Annual AAFV conference. Springfield (MO), 2023.
10. Hadfield CA. Viral diseases. In: Hadfield C, Clayton L, editors. Clinical guide to fish medicine. Hoboken (NJ): John Willey &Sons Inc; 2021. p. 407–30.
11. Kamerman TY, Davis L, Capobianco J. Development of a body condition scoring tool for the spotted eagle ray, Aetobatus narinari. In: Smith M, Warmolts D, Thoney D, et al, editors. Elasmobranch husbandry manual II. Columbus (OH): Ohio Biological Survey; 2017. p. 147–52.
12. Carabotti M, Scirocco A, Maselli MA, et al. The gut-brain axis: interactions between enteric microbiota, central and enteric nervous systems. Ann Gastroenterol 2015;28(2):203–9.
13. Diwan AD, Harke SN, Gopalkrishna Panche AN. Aquaculture industry prospective from gut microbiome of fish and shellfish: an overview. J Anim Physiol Anim Nutr 2022;106(2):441–69.
14. Zheng ZL, Tan JY, Liu HY, et al. Evaluation of oregano essential oil (*Origanum heracleoticum L.*) on growth, antioxidant effect and resistance against *Aeromonas hydrophila* in channel catfish (*Ictalurus punctatus*). Aquaculture 2009;292(3–4): 214–8.
15. Rodrigues MV, Zanuzzo FS, Koch JFA, et al. Development of fish immunity and the role of beta-glucan in immune responses. Molecules 2020;25(22).
16. Vergneau-Grosset C, Lair S. Medical treatment. In: Hadfield C, Clayton L, editors. Clinical guide to fish medicine. Hoboken (NJ): Wiley and Sons Inc; 2021. p. 233–66.
17. Soto E, Boylan SM, Stevens B, et al. Diagnosis of fish diseases. In: Smith SA, editor. Fish diseases and medicine. Boca Raton (FL): CRC Press; 2019. p. 46–88.
18. Clarke EO III, Christiansen EF, Stoskopf MK, et al. Tissue enzyme activity in black sea bass (*Centropristis striata*) captured off North Carolina, USA. Annual IAAAM conference. Atlanta (GA), 2012.
19. Brust K, Phillips K, Kaufman M, et al. Intravenous contrast-enhanced computed tomography in adult koi (*Cyprinus carpio*). J Zoo Wildl Med 2021;52(2):460–9.

20. Grosset C, Normand-Carmel É, LeNet R, et al. Use of MRI to investigate buoyancy disorders in goldfish: a case series. Annual IAAAM conference. Long Beach (CA), 2018.
21. Huml RA, Khoo LH, Stoskopf MK, et al. Radiographic diagnosis. Vet Radiol Ultrasound 1993;34(3):178–80.
22. Louvard C, Finck C, Lamglait B, et al. Radiographic anatomy and barium sulfate contrast transit time of the gastrointestinal tract in spotted wolffish (*Anarhichas minor*). Annual IAAAM conference. 2021.
23. Heng HG, Ong TW, Hassan MD. Radiographic assessment of gastric emptying and gastrointestinal transit time in hybrid tilapia. Vet Radiol Ultrasound 2007; 48(2):132–4.
24. Barbieri RL, Leite RG, Sterman FDA, et al. Food passage time through the alimentary tract of a brazilian teleost fish, *Prochilodus scrofa* (Steindachner, 1881) using radiography. Braz J Vet Res Anim Sci 1998;35:32–6.
25. Venero JA, Miles RD, Chapman FA. Food transit time and site of absorption of nutrients in Gulf of Mexico sturgeon. N Am J Aquacult 2015;77(3):275–80.
26. De Sandre LCG, Buzollo H, Do Nascimento TMT, et al. Natural stable isotopes for determination of gastrointestinal transit time in fish. J World Aquacult Soc 2016; 47(1):113–22.
27. Gilannejad N, Silva T, Martínez-Rodríguez G, et al. Effect of feeding time and frequency on gut transit and feed digestibility in two fish species with different feeding behaviours, gilthead seabream and Senegalese sole. Aquaculture 2019;513:734438.
28. Mock TS, Alkhabbaz ZH, Rocker MM, et al. Gut transit rate in Atlantic salmon (*Salmo salar*) exposed to optimal and suboptimally high water temperatures. Aquacult Res 2022;53(13):4858–68.
29. Joblon MJ, Flower JE, Thompson LA, et al. Radiographic determination of gastric emptying and gastrointestinal transit time in cownose rays (*Rhinoptera bonasus*) and whitespotted bamboo sharks (*Chiloscyllium plagiosum*) and the effect of metoclopramide on gastrointestinal motility. J Zoo Wildl Med 2020;51(2):326–33.
30. Goncin U, Ton N, Reddy A, et al. Contrast-enhanced ultrasound imaging for assessing organ perfusion in rainbow trout (*Oncorhynchus mykiss*). Sci Total Environ 2021;750:141231.
31. Wilson SR, Burns PN. Microbubble-enhanced US in body imaging: what role? Radiology 2010;257(1):24–39.
32. Horn ME, Brinkmann M, Machtaler S. Contrast-enhanced ultrasound imaging for assessment of intestinal inflammation in rainbow trout. Comp Biochem Physiol C Toxicol Pharmacol 2023;271:109690.
33. Archambault M, Vergneau-Grosset C, Gara-Boivin C, Mélançon V, Binning SA. Testing non-lethal techniques for detecting endoparasites in pumpkinseed sunfish (Lepomis gibbosus), J Fish Dis (in press).
34. Wenger S, Pendl H, Tahas S, et al. Clinical signs, diagnosis, and treatment of lead intoxication in an electric eel (*Electrophorus electricus*). J Zoo Wildl Med 2018; 49(4):1029–31.
35. Meegan J, Sidor IF, Field C, et al. Endoscopic evaluation and biopsy collection of the gastrointestinal tract in the green moray eel (*Gymnothorax funebris*): application in a case of chronic regurgitation with gastric mucus gland hyperplasia. J Zoo Wildl Med 2012;43(3):615–20.
36. Stevens BN, Guzman DS, Phillips KL, et al. Evaluation of diagnostic coelioscopy in koi (*Cyprinus carpio*). Am J Vet Res 2019;80(3):221–9.

37. Kaufman M, Knych H, Brust K, et al. Intravenous iopamidol pharmacokinetics in common carp (*Cyprinus carpio*). J Zoo Wildl Med 2021;51(4):889–95.
38. Pees M, Pees K, Kiefer I. The use of computed tomography for assessment of the swim bladder in koi carp (*Cyprinus carpio*). Vet Radiol Ultrasound 2010;51(3):294–8.
39. Hoitsy M, Hoitsy G, Gal J, et al. Rainbow trout (*Oncorhynchus mykiss*, Walbaum 1792) adenocarcinoma investigation with various diagnostic imaging techniques. J Fish Dis 2024;47(8):e13951.
40. Chapagain P, Arivett B, Cleveland BM, et al. Analysis of the fecal microbiota of fast- and slow-growing rainbow trout (*Oncorhynchus mykiss*). BMC Genom 2019;20(1):788.
41. Roberts RJ. Laboratory methods. In: Roberts RJ, editor. Fish pathology. 4th edition. Chichester: SXW:John Wiley & Sons; 2012. p. 439–81.
42. Vergneau-Grosset C, Summa N, Rodriguez Jr CO, et al. Excision and subsequent treatment of a leiomyoma from the periventiduct of a koi (*Cyprinus carpio koi*). J Exot Pet Med 2016;25(3):194–202.
43. Weber ES 3rd. A veterinary guide to the fish gastrointestinal tract. Vet Clin North Am Exot Anim Pract 2014;17(2):123–43.
44. Weber ES. Gastroenterology for the piscine patient. Vet Clin Exot Anim 2005;8:247–76.
45. Dove ADM, Clauss TM, Marancik DP, et al. Emerging diseases of elasmobranch in aquaria. In: Smith M, Warmolts D, Thoney D, et al, editors. Elasmobranch husbandry manual II. Columbus (OH): Ohio Biological Survey; 2017. p. 263–75.
46. Erlacher-Reid C. Techniques for addressing parasites in saltwater aquariums. In: Miller RE, Lamberski N, Calle P, editors. Fowler's zoo and wild animal medicine, vol. 9. St. Louis, MO: Elsevier; 2019. p. 323–33.
47. Hadfield CA. Protozoal diseases. In: Hadfield C, Clayton L, editors. Clinical guide to fish medicine. Hoboken, NJ: John Willey &Sons Inc; 2021. p. 483–512.
48. Dannemiller NG, O'Connor MR, Van Bonn WG. An integrative review of lateral line depigmentation in marine and freshwater fish. J Am Vet Med Assoc 2021;259(6):617–25.
49. Noga EJ. Pharmacopoeia. In: Noga EJ, editor. Fish disease diagnosis and treatment. 2nd edition. Ames, IA: John Wiley & Sons; 2010. p. 305–31.
50. Hadfield CA. Metazoan diseases. In: Hadfield C, Clayton L, editors. Clinical guide to fish medicine. Hoboken, NJ: John Willey &Sons Inc; 2021. p. 513–68.
51. Reed AN, Clayton LA, Hadfield CA. Morbidity and mortality associated with fenbendazole use in teleost fish at the National Aquarium, Baltimore. Annual IAAAM conference. Altanta (GA), 2012.
52. Myers GE, Garner MM, Barrie MT, et al. Fenbendazole toxicity in sharks. Annual AAZV conference. Dallas (TX), 2007.
53. Mylniczenko ND. Medical management of rays. In: Miller RE, Fowler ME, editors. Fowler's zoo and wild animal medicine. 7th edition. Saint-Louis, MO: Elsevier Saunders; 2011. p. 170–6.
54. Hadfield CA. Myxozoan and coccidial diseases. In: Hadfield C, Clayton L, editors. Clinical guide to fish medicine. Hoboken, NJ: John Willey &Sons Inc; 2021. p. 569–90.
55. Hyatt MW, Waltzek TB, Kieran EA, et al. Diagnosis and treatment of multi-species fish mortality attributed to *Enteromyxum leei* while in quarantine at a US aquarium. Dis Aquat Org 2018;132(1):37–48.
56. Hadfield CA. Bacterial diseases. In: Hadfield C, Clayton L, editors. Clinical guide to fish medicine. Hoboken, NJ: John Willey &Sons Inc; 2021. p. 431–67.

57. Pomaranski EK, Griffin MJ, Camus AC, et al. Description of *Erysipelothrix piscisicarius* sp. nov., an emergent fish pathogen, and assessment of virulence using a tiger barb (*Puntigrus tetrazona*) infection model. Int J Syst Evol Microbiol 2020; 70(2):857–67.

58. Yanong R. Fish medicine updates. In: Miller RE, Calle P, Lamberski N, editors. Fowler's zoo and wild animal medicine, vol. 10. St. Louis, MO: Elsevier; 2023. p. 389–93.

59. Stevens BN, Michel A, Liepnieks ML, et al. Outbreak and treatment of carp edema virus in koi (*Cyprinus carpio*) from Northern California. J Zoo Wildl Med 2018;49(3):755–64.

60. Lovy J, Yanong RPE, Stilwell JM, et al. Tetra disseminated microsporidiosis: a novel disease in ornamental fish caused by *Fusasporis stethaprioni* n. gen. n. sp. Parasitol Res 2021;120(2):497–514.

61. Hadfield CA. Fungal and fungal-like diseases. In: Hadfield C, Clayton L, editors. Clinical guide to fish medicine. Hoboken, NJ: John Willey &Sons Inc; 2021. p. 468–82.

62. Bonar CJ, Garner MM, Weber ES 3rd, et al. Pathologic findings in weedy (*Phyllopteryx taeniolatus*) and leafy (*Phycodurus eques*) seadragons. Vet Pathol 2013;50(3):368–76.

63. McDermott CT, Innis CJ, Nyaoke AC, et al. Phaeohyphomycosis due to *Exophiala* in aquarium-housed lumpfish (*Cyclopterus lumpus*): clinical diagnosis and description. Pathogens 2022;11(12).

64. Mai K, Waagbø R, Zhou XQ, et al. Vitamins. In: Halver JE, Hardy RW, editors. Fish nutrition. 4th edition. San Diego, CA: Academic Press; 2002. p. 57–179.

65. Hadfield CA. Noninfectious diseases (other). In: Hadfield C, Clayton L, editors. Clinical guide to fish medicine. Hoboken, NJ: John Willey &Sons Inc; 2021. p. 378–406.

66. Noga EJ. Problems 89 through 99. In: Noga EJ, editor. Fish disease diagnosis and treatment. 2nd edition. Ames, IA: John Wiley & Sons; 2010. p. 305–31.

67. Hadfield CA. Noninfectious diseases (environmental). In: Hadfield C, Clayton L, editors. Clinical guide to fish medicine. Hoboken, NJ: John Willey &Sons Inc; 2021. p. 357–77.

68. Kruatrachue M, Rangsayatorn N, Pokethitiyook P, et al. Histopathological changes in the gastrointestinal tract of fish, *Puntius gonionotus*, fed on dietary cadmium. Bull Environ Contam Toxicol 2003;71(3).

69. Samanta P, Pal S, Mukherjee AK, et al. Gastrointestinal pathology in freshwater fish, *Oreochromis niloticus* (*Linnaeus*) under almix exposure. J Environ Anal Toxicol 2016;6(1000399). 2161-0525.

70. Ernst B, Hoeger SJ, O'Brien E, et al. Oral toxicity of the microcystin-containing cyanobacterium *Planktothrix rubescens* in European whitefish (*Coregonus lavaretus*). Aquat Toxicol (N Y) 2006;79(1):31–40.

71. Larouche CB, Limoges MJ, Lair S. Absence of acute toxicity of a single intramuscular injection of meloxicam in goldfish (*Carassius auratus auratus*): a randomized controlled trial. J Zoo Wildl Med 2018;49(3):617–22.

72. Raulic J, Beaudry F, Beauchamp G, et al. Pharmacokinetic, Pharmacodynamic, and toxicology study of robenacoxib in rainbow trout (*Oncorhynchus mykiss*). J Zoo Wildl Med 2021;52(2):529–37.

73. Ebrahimzadeh Mosavi HA, Vajihi AR, Hosseini F, et al. Non-surgical removal of some stones from a red tailed catfish (*Phractocephalus hemioliopterus*) stomach as gastric foreign bodies. Iran J Fish Sci 2006;6(1):35–42.

74. Sirri R, Ciulli S, Barbe T, et al. Detection of Cyprinid herpesvirus 1 DNA in cutaneous squamous cell carcinoma of koi carp (*Cyprinus carpio*). Vet Dermatol 2018;29(1):60-e24.
75. Stevens BN, Vergneau-Grosset C, Rodriguez Jr CO, et al. Treatment of a facial myxoma in a goldfish (*Carassius auratus*) with intralesional bleomycin chemotherapy and radiation therapy. J Exot Pet Med 2017;26(4):283–9.
76. Fajardo R, Avendaño-Herrera R, Valladares-Carranza B, et al. Odontogenic hamartomas in cultured angelfish (*Pterophyllum scalare*). J Exot Pet Med 2021; 36:47–51.
77. Magi GE, Di Cicco E, Rossi G. Spontaneous intestinal adenocarcinoma in a blue gularis *Fundulopanchax sjostedti*: an immunohistochemical study. Fish Pathol 2008;43(3):128–31.
78. Bjorgen H, Hellberg H, Loken OM, et al. Tumor microenvironment and stroma in intestinal adenocarcinomas and associated metastases in Atlantic salmon broodfish (*Salmo salar*). Vet Immunol Immunopathol 2019;214:109891.
79. Gombac M, Senicar M, Svara T, et al. Sudden outbreak of metastatic intestinal adenocarcinoma in rainbow trout *Oncorhynchus mykiss*. Dis Aquat Org 2021; 144:237–44.
80. Paquette CE. Intestinal hyperplasia and neoplasms in zebrafish (Danio rerio). [Master of science thesis, Oregon state university]. ScholarsArchive@OSU. 2013. Available at: https://ir.library.oregonstate.edu/concern/graduate_thesis_ or_dissertations/p8418q617.
81. Paquette CE, Kent ML, Buchner C, et al. A retrospective study of the prevalence and classification of intestinal neoplasia in zebrafish (*Danio rerio*). Zebrafish 2013;10(2):228–36.
82. Burns AR, Watral V, Sichel S, et al. Transmission of a common intestinal neoplasm in zebrafish by cohabitation. J Fish Dis 2018;41(4):569–79.
83. Dale OB, Torud B, Kvellestad A, et al. From chronic feed-induced intestinal inflammation to adenocarcinoma with metastases in salmonid fish. Cancer Res 2009;69(10):4355–62.
84. Friedman M, McQuistan T, Hendricks JD, et al. Protective effect of dietary tomatine against dibenzo[a,l]pyrene (DBP)-induced liver and stomach tumors in rainbow trout. Mol Nutr Food Res 2007;51(12):1485–91.
85. Hoitsy M, Hoitsy G, Jakab C, et al. Intussusception caused by intestinal neoplasia in mature rainbow trout (*Oncorhynchus mykiss*, Walbaum 1792). J Fish Dis 2021; 44(7):893–8.
86. Woods LW, Van der Merwe M. Tumors of the cloaca in fish. Vet Clin Exot Anim 2006;9(2):239–56.
87. Anderson DP. Environmental factors in fish health: immunological aspects. In: Iwama G, Hoar WS, Randall DJ, et al, editors. The fish immune system: organism, pathogen, and environment15, 1st edition. Cambridge, MA: Academic Press; 1997. p. 289–310.
88. Serna-Duque JA, Esteban MA. Effects of inflammation and/or infection on the neuroendocrine control of fish intestinal motility: a review. Fish Shellfish Immunol 2020;103:342–56.

Gastrointestinal Endoscopy

Norin Chai, DVM, MSc, PhD, DECZM (Zoo Health Management)*

KEYWORDS

- Endoscopy • Diagnosis • Biopsy • Foreign body

KEY POINTS

- Gastrointestinal endoscopy is a minimally invasive diagnostic and therapeutic tool.
- Indications are diagnostic, such as identifying obstructions, ulcers, neoplasms, infections with biopsy collection, and therapeutic, mainly foreign body removal.
- Challenges and limitations are mainly due to anesthesia risks and technical difficulties due to delicate and often small size of the animals.
- Gastrointestinal endoscopy is a valuable complement to radiography and ultrasonography.

INTRODUCTION

In the field of zoological medicine, the application of diagnostic endoscopy has shown great value in a variety of species. Gastrointestinal (GI) endoscopy is a noninvasive, atraumatic technique that allows visual examination of esophageal, gastric, upper small bowel, and colonic lesions and allows descriptive information of their severity and extent. While its application in small animal medicine is well-documented, the use of gastroscopy in exotic animals seems to be a more specialized field. Endoscopy should be preceded by a careful history and physical examination and by the collection of a laboratory database appropriate to the differentials suggested by the results of the clinical examination. Indications for GI endoscopy in common exotic species are listed in **Table 1**. In the author's experience, GI endoscopy is associated with low morbidity and mortality. However, in unstable patients, GI endoscopy may be contraindicated. Decision between pursuing additional diagnostics, such as GI endoscopy, and stabilizing the patient should be carefully weighed. In this review article, only a handful of select noninvasive procedures will be described for species likely to be encountered in exotic companion animal practice.

EQUIPMENT FOR GASTROINTESTINAL ENDOSCOPY

Depending on the nature of the species and procedures, a variety of instruments may be required. Details are listed in **Table 2**. However, for most procedures, a 2.7 mm, 30° rigid telescope with a 4.8 mm operating sheath offers the greatest versatility and may

Yaboumba, Paris, France
* 10 Boulevard de Picpus, Paris 75012.
E-mail address: norin.chai@yaboumba.org

Vet Clin Exot Anim 28 (2025) 331–345
https://doi.org/10.1016/j.cvex.2024.11.005
vetexotic.theclinics.com
1094-9194/25/© 2024 Elsevier Inc. All rights are reserved, including those for text and data mining, AI training, and similar technologies.

Abbreviations	
FB	foreign body
GI	gastrointestinal

be used in almost all the cases. Reduction in endoscope size may cause a notable decrease in illumination from the same light source and yields a smaller, poorer quality image. The ultimate aim of minimally invasive examination is best accomplished with good visualization. There is no one flexible endoscope that fulfills all the requirements of the upper GI endoscopy in all sizes of veterinary patients. Veterinarians will choose the size according to the indications and the size of the animal treated.

SMALL MAMMALS

The most common endoscopic procedures performed in rabbits and rodents are stomatoscopy (ie, examination of the oral cavity), rhinoscopy, otoscopy, cystoscopy, laparoscopy, and as an aid to endotracheal intubation.[1] Gastroscopy in small herbivores is simply not possible as their stomach is never empty. Rabbit and rodent colonoscopies are mainly performed in laboratory animals for research purposes. Ferrets, a species in which GI diseases are common, are ideal candidates for flexible endoscopy because they have a relatively simple and short GI tract. However, clinicians should remember that ultrasonography is a superior diagnostic imaging method compared with endoscopy for diagnosing and differentiating between submucosal lesions in the GI tract.[2] Thus, gastroscopy should be considered as a complementary examination in addition to the other examinations already performed.

Equipment

Because of the small lumen size of the ferret GI tract, a bronchofiber endoscope of 3 mm in diameter with an operating channel of 1.2 mm and 100 cm long is the most commonly used flexible endoscope in the species. This equipment has only a 2 way tip deflection in a single plane (up and down), but it is typically sufficient for the ferret GI tract.[2] However, for ferrets that are larger than 1 kg body weight, a gastro-

Table 1 Indications for gastrointestinal endoscopy in exotic animals	
Indications for Upper Gastrointestinal Endoscopy (ie, Esophagus, Stomach)	Indications for Proctoscopy, Colonoscopy, and Cloacoscopy
Evaluation of weight loss	Diarrhea
Evaluation of dysorexia and anorexia	Tenesmus (with normal or abnormal fecal consistency)
Evaluation of dysphagia	Hematochezia (with or without normally formed feces)
Evaluation of regurgitation and/or chronic vomiting	Dyschezia
Evaluation of hematemesis	Palpable or visible rectal/cloacal masses and suspected large bowel obstruction
Evaluation of unexplained anemia	Increased fecal mucus
Retrieval of esophageal and gastric foreign bodies	

Table 2
Equipment for gastrointestinal endoscopy in exotics

Equipment	Species/Animals and Remarks
Endovideo camera and monitor Xenon light source and light cable	Most species
1.9 mm integrated telescope	All species <2 kg The vision of the lumen and mucosa may be limited
2.7 mm diameter, 18 cm length, 30° oblique rigid telescope with a 4.8 mm operating sheath	All species between 500 g and 8 kg This equipment offers the greatest versatility
Carbon dioxide (CO_2) insufflator with silicone tubing	All species Care must be taken when using CO_2 insufflation, since it can quickly dry out the organs and the mucosa. In the author experience, the endoscopic procedure should not last more than 10 min. Sometimes, a simple syringe for air or saline infusion is also practical for small animals
1 or 1.7 mm endoscopic biopsy forceps and grasping forceps depending on the size of the telescope	All species
Flexible endoscope with biopsy forceps and grasping forceps	Ferrets, long neck birds, reptiles (aquatic turtles, monitors, and snakes), and amphibians (caudates) Most flexible scopes >2 mm in diameter are equipped with a working channel and a deflectable tip. The diameter and length will be chosen accordingly to the size of the animal

fiberscope with an outside diameter of 8.6 mm, 2.8 mm working channel, 140 cm long may be used. The tip's 2 plane, 4 direction deflection capability (up, down, left, and right) is useful to navigate the GI tract, especially for the more challenging maneuver of advancing through the pylorus into the duodenum.[2] If no pump is available, insufflation in ferrets can be performed with a 60 mL syringe attached to the working channel. Using the latter, the gaseous distension medium is simply room air. If an insufflator is used, care must be taken not to harm the patient or damage the instrument.

Patient Preparation

Before endoscopic evaluation, anti-inflammatory and antibacterial drugs should be stopped for at least 2 weeks to collect proper histologic and microbiologic samples.[2] Removing the food 4 hours before the procedure is enough to perform a gastroscopy in ferrets. Fasting the animal for longer is unnecessary. The endoscopic procedure should not last more than 10 minutes. In the authors' opinion, the best anesthesia for gastroscopy is inhalant anesthesia (isoflurane or sevoflurane), with or without intubation. Ideally, a muscle relaxant should always be administered (eg, midazolam). **Fig. 1**A illustrates a method of securing the endotracheal tube in order to provide anesthesia while performing GI endoscopy. If the clinician expects that the procedure will take longer, intubation should be performed as inflation of the stomach can depress respiratory function by pushing against the diaphragm and limiting the depth of inspiration.[3] Intubation may avoid inadvertent aspiration of fluids during the procedure, but this is rare in ferrets. Premedication with butorphanol (0.03 mg/kg intramuscularly) and midazolam (0.2 mg/kg intramuscularly) will provide analgesia and

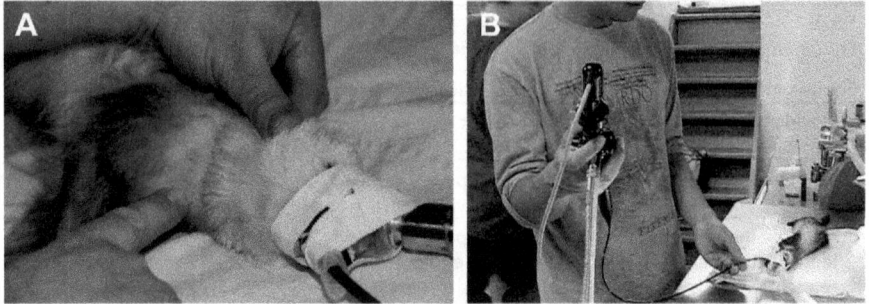

Fig. 1. Gastroscopy in ferrets. (A) Tip to protect the fiberscope. The anesthetic mask is attached to the upper jaw. A fitted syringe body facilitates the introduction of the fiberscope and protects it. (B) For routine upper gastrointestinal endoscopy, the patient is positioned in left lateral recumbency. (*Courtesy of* Norin Chai, France, with permission.)

comfort for the animal. For routine upper GI endoscopy, the patient is positioned in left lateral recumbency (**Fig. 1**B). This position facilitates examination of the pylorus by bringing the pylorus to the top of the abdomen.

Esophagoscopy, Gastroscopy, Duodenoscopy, and Colonoscopy

Generally, the endoscope is advanced to the distal esophagus without any difficulty (**Fig. 2**A, B). **Fig. 2**C illustrates moderate-to-severe inflammation of the esophagus.

To enter the gastroesophageal junction, the tip of the endoscope is deflected approximately 30° to the left of the ferret.[2] After passing the cardia (**Fig. 2**D, E), the gastric mucosa is evaluated (**Fig. 2**F–I). The mucosa should be evaluated for ulcers (see **Fig. 2**I). Biopsies will help to correlate histologic abnormalities with the endoscopic findings. For instance, patients with gastric motility disorders may have mucosal erythema with no histologic abnormalities whereas some will be diagnosed with gastritis and have no gross gastric mucosal lesions.[2] It is essential that the clinician is careful not to perforate the mucosa during the biopsy of an ulcer. Duodenoscopy may be challenging and is not commonly performed. Because the large intestine is anatomically simple, colonoscopy is relatively easy to perform. Interestingly, the visualization is of better quality when the endoscope is slowly withdrawn. Colonoscopy with multiple biopsy specimens was found effective in diagnosing proliferative bowel disease associated with intracellular *Campylobacter* sp in ferrets.[4]

BIRDS

Endoscopy has been used in avian medicine for decades. The air sac system of birds enables the veterinarians to visualize most, if not all, of the major organs of clinical interest.[5] Historically, air sac endoscopy was mainly performed for gender identification; however, in recent years, it has become a popular diagnostic and therapeutic tool. GI conditions are often diagnosed in birds. Common conditions seen include toxicosis, foreign body (FB) ingestion, papillomatosis, neoplasia, and infection due to bacterial, fungal, viral, or parasitic causes.[6] GI endoscopy, in addition to the examination of the buccal cavity, esophagus, crop (if present), proventriculus, and ventriculus, permits application of local therapy and targeted sampling.[7]

Equipment

The esophagus, crop, proventriculus, and ventriculus are anatomically aligned, therefore, for most procedures, a 2.7 mm, 30° rigid telescope offers the greatest versatility.

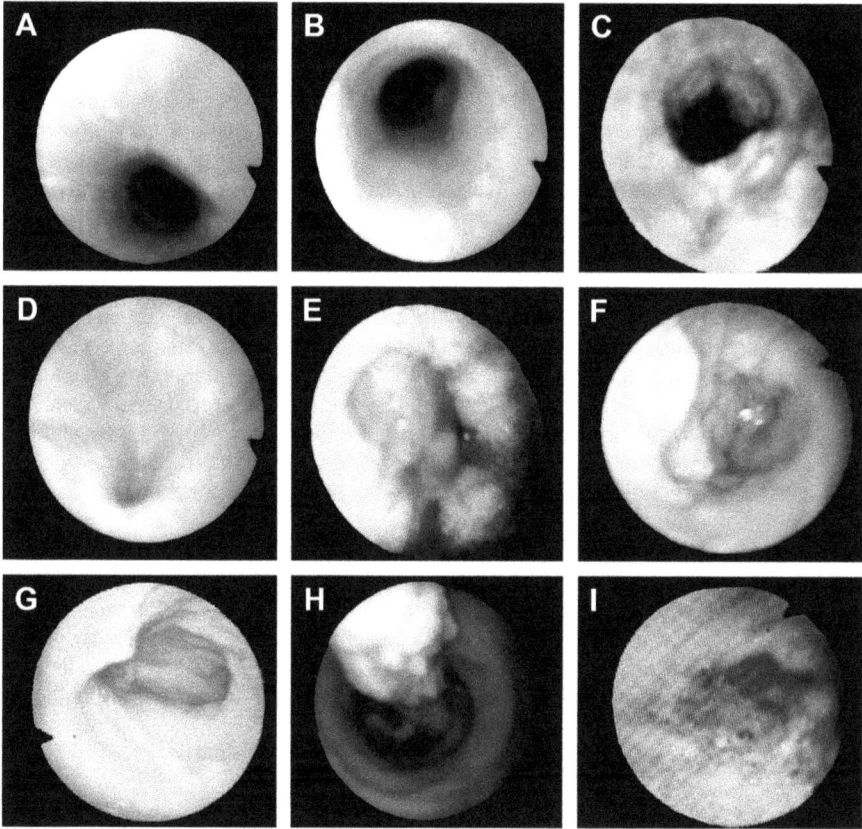

Fig. 2. Upper gastrointestinal endoscopy of a ferret with a 3.7 mm fiberscope. (*A, B*) Appearance of the normal esophagus. Normal mucosa is pale and smooth. (*C*) Esophagitis. (*D*) Visualization of the normal ferret cardia. (*E*) Neoplasia of the cardia (*F*) and (*G*) appearance of the normal stomach (gastric mucosa is usually smooth, bright pink to red) visualized with a smooth insufflation. (*H*) Normal stomach with digestive content. (*I*) Visualization of the gastric ulcers with a raised thickened margin. The accumulated blood gives this usual dark brown color. (*Courtesy of* Christophe Bulliot, France, with permission.)

In birds weighing between 1.5 and 2 kg, the proventriculus can be visualized via the oral cavity using an 18 cm telescope and saline infusion or air insufflation. Flexible endoscope will be used for long neck birds and larger birds (see **Table 2**). FB can be removed using retrieval grasping forceps. Warm fluids offer better visualization of the mucosal surfaces than air insufflation.[5,7]

Patient Preparation

As usual, animals should be stabilized before anesthesia and endoscopy. Exceptions may include emergency procedures like the removal of a life-threatening FB or an urgent debridement of a lesion, mass, or granuloma that obstructs the respiratory tract. Most birds encountered in practice should not be fasted more than 1 hour. Exceptions with raptors that may be fasted for 6 up to 12 hours. General anesthesia is recommended for all endoscopy procedures and all birds should be intubated. The author prefers to place the patient at a 30° to 45° incline (head down) to reduce the risks of aspiration.

Packing the oropharynx with moistened gauze is an additional precaution to prevent aspiration when using large amount of fluids for lavage.[5] In pigeons (*Columba livia*), dorsal recumbency with head at a higher plane was preferred when irrigation with saline solution was performed as this allowed the crop to expand with excess fluid administration.[8] For analgesia, the author uses routinely for psittacines, butorphanol (1 mg/kg), and meloxicam (0.5 mg/kg). The most common contraindication to endoscopic examinations is hemodynamic instability, which would make anesthesia a higher risk procedure.[9]

Esophagus, Crop, and Proventriculus

The esophagus is easily entered by passing the endoscope caudally to the pharynx. The surface of the esophagus is identified by the presented of a series of longitudinal folds (**Fig. 3**A, B). Not all the birds have a crop. Galliformes, Psittaciformes, Columbiformes, and some Passeriformes have a well-developed, true crop. Most diurnal raptors, including scavenging birds, have a crop but owls do not.[7] Endoscopy allows a thorough examination of the crop mucosa (**Fig. 3**C). Lesions can be accurately located (**Fig. 3**D) and foreign objects identified (**Fig. 3**E–H). Endoscopy can also help to refine etiologic hypotheses in the face of certain lesions. **Fig. 4** provides an example of a crop rupture. By examining the mucosa of the crop, a more extensive evaluation of the case can be performed.

In the author's experience, crop or proventricular biopsy is not performed routinely as the risk of perforation is not negligible. However, gastroscopy and biopsy have been evaluated in the pigeon.[8] This study showed that gastroscopy was useful for evaluating the lumen and mucosal surface of the proventriculus and ventriculus in

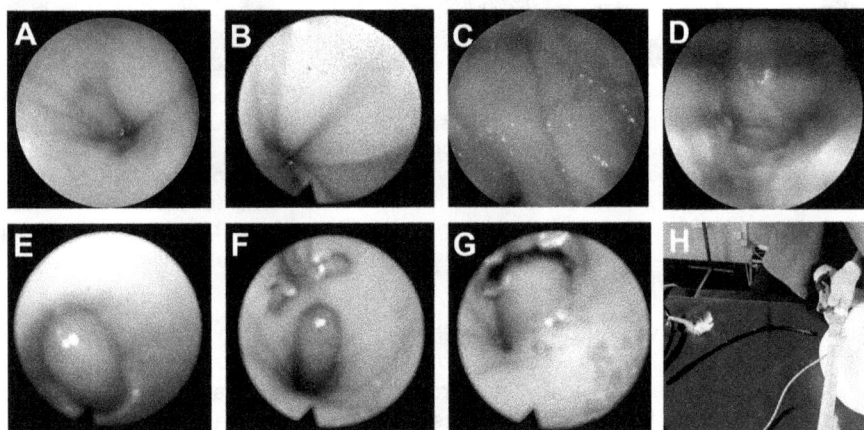

Fig. 3. Upper gastrointestinal endoscopy. (*A*) Appearance of the normal esophagus in a gray parrot (*Psittacus erithacus*; 2.7 mm telescope, air insufflation). Note the size of the folds and the degree of distensibility differ depending on the species. Distension is greater in carnivores (birds of prey) than in granivores such as parrots for example. By examining the surface of the mucosa, any ulceration, inflammation, masses, and so forth will be detected. (*B*) Appearance of the normal esophagus of a mute swan (*Cygnus olor*; 8.6 mm fiberscope, air insufflation). (*C*) Normal crop mucosa of an Alexandrine parakeet (*Palaeornis eupatria*; 2.7 mm telescope, saline infusion). (*D*) Mild crop mycosis, in an Alexandrine parakeet (2.7 mm telescope, air insufflation). (*E–G*) Feeding tube foreign body in the distal esophagus in a mute swan removed with a flexible grasping forceps (8.6 mm fiberscope, air insufflation). (*H*) Size of the removed tube. (*Courtesy of* Norin Chai, France, with permission.)

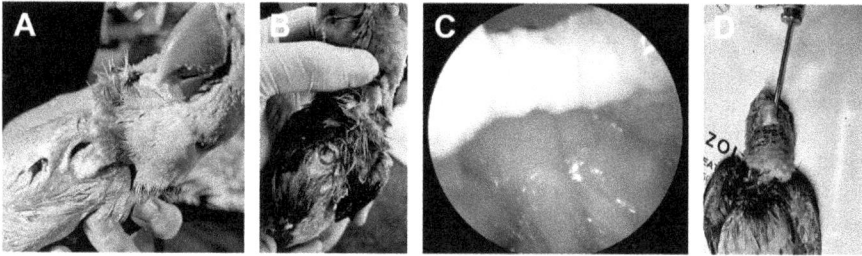

Fig. 4. Crop trauma in an Alexandrine parakeet. (*A*) This Alexandrine parakeet is presented for the presence of food coming out of its throat during force-feeding. (*B*) After cleaning and disinfection, a rupture of the crop is clearly visible. (*C*) Endoscopy confirms the absence of any lesion on the crop and, therefore, concludes that there was an iatrogenic trauma. We can notice the thickening of the edges of the mucosa, which suggests that the trauma does not date from the day of the examination but may be several days before. (*D*) After surgery, a quick endoscopy can help evaluate the seal. (*Courtesy of* Norin Chai, France, with permission.)

pigeons. Biopsy of those organs was safely performed with the appropriate technique (oral infusion of saline solution to achieve lumen dilation and visibility before proventriculus and ventriculus mucosal biopsy with a 1.7 mm endoscopic biopsy forceps), but further evaluation of this technique is needed in birds with clinical disease and birds of other species.

Although the scope of this review is gastroscopy, it is important to remember that in birds, exploration of the digestive tract can and must be complemented with coelioscopy. The digestive tract can be visualized using a standard left caudal thoracic air sac approach (**Fig. 5**A). The approach can detect lesions that are either not visible or impossible to detect by gastroscopy, such as abscesses (**Fig. 5**B) or granulomas (**Fig. 5**C) of the digestive serous membranes. Information on coelioscopy can be found elsewhere.[5]

Cloaca

Indications for cloacoscopy include diarrhea, tenesmus (with normal or abnormal fecal consistency), hematochezia (with or without normal-formed feces), tenesmus (diarrhea or constipation), and palpable or visible rectal/cloacal masses.[5] Chronic prolapse may also be an indication. Using a saline infusion to dilate the cloaca enables highly

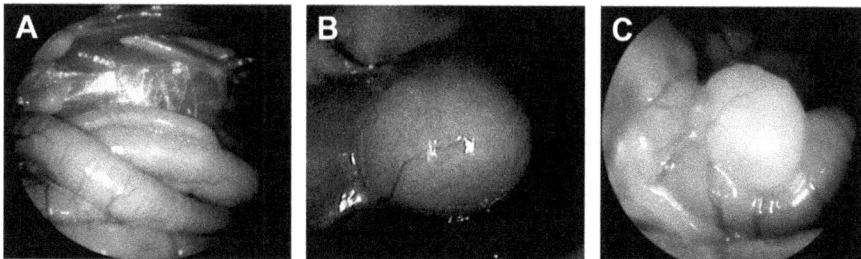

Fig. 5. Exploration of the digestive tract by coelioscopy. The left side is the regular approach. (*A*) Digestive tract of an *Anser* sp. (*B*) Digestive abscess in a Bonelli's eagle (*Aquila fasciata*). (*C*) Digestive mycobacterial granuloma in an Edwards's pheasant (*Lophura edwardsi*). (*Courtesy of* Norin Chai, France, with permission.)

detailed examination of its 3 chambers, the coprodeum (which receives feces from the rectum), urodeum, and proctodeum. Care must be taken to prevent excessive fluid pressure that may lead to retrograde filling of the GI tract and even oral regurgitation. Due to this risk, intubation should be performed in all cases. Cloacal neoplasias can be ablated using radiosurgical or diode laser probes introduced via the sheaths' working canal.[5] The coprodeum is often dilated in idiopathic cloacal prolapse of cockatoos.[7] Note that the serosal surface of the cloaca can be viewed from the left or right abdominal air sacs. The cloaca is typically best viewed from the left side.[5]

Foreign Body Removal

FBs, generally, are encountered in ratites, gallinaceous birds, waterfowl, and psittacine birds. However, any species can present with FB regardless of sex or age. Items ingested can include hair, cloth fibers, parts of toys, plastic tube, feeding tube, and heavy metals. Although most foreign objects are found frequently in the proventriculus and ventriculus, they can be found anywhere along the length of the GI tract. Clinical signs of FB ingestion may be nonspecific such as lethargy, anorexia or hyporexia, dehydration, weight loss, polyuria, dyspnea, ataxia, and paresis (may be caused by the pressure of the FB on the kidney and/or ischiatic nerve roots).[10–12] Physical examination findings are variable as well and can include a low body condition score or a distended coelom (mostly caused by functional ileus and gaseous dilatation proximal to the obstruction). GI signs suggestive of a FB include regurgitation, vomiting, diarrhea, hematochezia, changes in fecal appearance and consistency, and passing undigested food. In cases of perforation, affected birds may exhibit signs of shock or severe depression, or death.[13,14] GI FB may pose a challenge to practitioners, as the clinical signs are vague and not specific for FB. In previous reports of birds with GI FB, hematology and biochemical changes are nonspecific.[10] Diagnosis is based on history, clinical examination, imaging such as radiographs (useful for visualizing foreign material, particularly radiopaque objects, such as metal), and, of course, endoscopy. Endoscopy, in addition to aiding on the diagnosis of FB, may also allow the removal of the FB. The advantage of endoscopic removal is that no incisions to the body wall, air sacs, or GI system are required (see **Fig. 3E–G**).

Retrieval of FB from the ventriculus via the oral cavity is challenging and often not possible. Ingluviotomy is then needed to help the endoscopic removal. The technique has been described for several species.[10,12] The ingluviotomy incision is generally small (1.5 cm). After the procedure, the crop and skin are closed in separate layers in a simple continuous pattern. The approach to ventricular FB in birds is also affected by the type of FB. Sometimes, the density and size of the FB prevents its removal in a single surgery. Staged endoscopic removal may be a viable option, as described by Lloyd and colleagues.[12] Periods of up to 3 weeks were left between procedures to allow time for surgical wounds to heal. This option resulted in a favorable outcome for the bird. Repeated ingluviotomies appeared to cause no significant problems. Lastly, certain small-size FB, potentially admixed with the stomach contents, may be difficult to locate via endoscopy and/or due to the lack of suitable size instrument for retrieval. In these cases, ventriculotomy is indicated.

REPTILES

There are a number of articles that describe endoscopic equipment, approaches, and techniques used for reptile patients.[15] Gastroscopy, in addition to the examination of the esophagus and stomach, allows the application of local therapy, removal of FB from the upper GI, and collection of diagnostic samples for histopathology, bacterial and fungal cultures, and molecular testing. Additionally, surgery like enterotomy may be assisted by endoscopy. For instance, a case of removal of an FB located in the ileum by endoscopy-assisted enterotomy has been described in a leopard tortoise (*Stigmochelys pardalis*).[16] Note that coelioscopy allows visualization of the serosal surfaces or the GI tract and has been described largely elsewhere.[15]

Equipment

As with birds, the 2.7 mm, 30° rigid telescope offers the greatest versatility for the evaluation of the upper GI tract, coelom, cloaca, and rectum. For snakes (**Fig. 6**A), monitors (**Fig. 6**B), and larger reptiles (**Fig. 6**C), flexible endoscopy should be used for GI endoscopic examinations. Air insufflation or saline infusion may be used for better visualization.[15]

Patient Preparation

General anesthesia is recommended for all GI endoscopy procedures and analgesia must be provided. In the author's experience, regional spinal anesthesia (lidocaine, 2 mg/kg, intrathecal) without general anesthesia may be adequate for cloacal examinations in chelonians. As previously mentioned, patients must be stabilized before anesthesia. Since most of the time, the animals are presented sick and, therefore, often anorexic for several days, weeks, or even months, fasting is not typically necessary. However, on an animal that is still eating or when in doubt, the general rule of withholding food for a single feeding cycle is recommended.[15] For short procedures, the author typically induces anesthesia with alfaxalone (12 mg/kg, intramuscular (IM) or 8 mg/kg, intravenous), intubates, and maintains on isoflurane or sevoflurane. The author also routinely uses the combination of ketamine (10 mg/kg) and medetomidine (0.1 mg/kg) given as a single intramuscular injection. Meloxicam (0.4 mg/kg, subcutaneous) and tramadol (10 mg/kg, IM) is used for all species. The animal should be intubated. To minimize the risk of aspiration due to saline infusion, the head is typically placed at a lower position than the body.

Esophagus and Stomach

The esophagus and stomach are easily explored in snakes with a flexible endoscope and insufflation. While exploring the esophagus (**Fig. 7**A), special attention should be given to the esophageal tonsils (**Fig. 7**B, C). Esophageal tonsils are the most common sites, along with the liver, for antemortem histopathological diagnosis of inclusion body disease.[17] After passing the cardia (**Fig. 7**D), the gastric mucosa is evaluated (**Fig. 7**E). Common abnormal findings include mucosal lesions (**Fig. 7**F) and FB (**Fig. 7**G–I). Biopsy of the stomach is the most sensitive technique for detecting *Cryptosporidium serpentis* in snakes. Endoscopic biopsies from 3 gastric sites collected

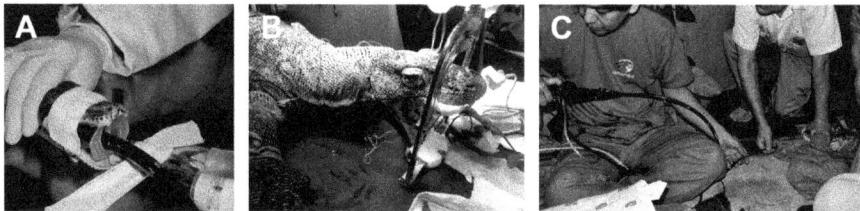

Fig. 6. Flexible gastroscopy in a *Boa constrictor* (*A*), a Komodo dragon (*Varanus komodoensis*; *B*) and in black caiman (*Melanosuchus niger*; *C*). (*Courtesy of* Lionel Schilliger, France, with permission for [*A*], Norin Chai, France, with permission for [*B*, *C*].)

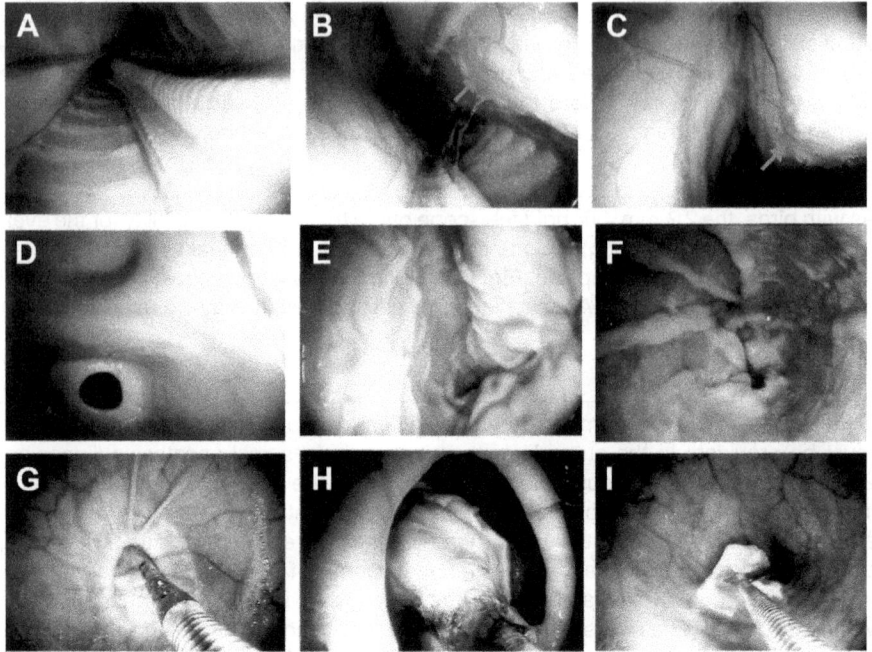

Fig. 7. Esophagoscopy and gastroscopy in snakes. (*A*) Air-distended esophagus of an Indian rock python (*Python molurus*; 9 mm fiberscope, air insufflation). (*B, C*) Visualization of esophageal tonsils (*red arrow*) in an Indian rock python (9 mm fiberscope, air insufflation). (*D*) Cardia of an Indian rock python (9 mm fiberscope, air insufflation). (*E*) Stomach of an Indian rock python with normal folds (9 mm fiberscope, air insufflation). (*F*) Gastric hypertrophy in a carpet python (*Morelia spilota*; 9 mm fiberscope, air insufflation). (*G–I*) Retrieval of a gastric foreign body in a Burmese python (*Python bivittatus*) with a flexible grasping forceps (9 mm fiberscope, air insufflation). (*Courtesy of* Lionel Schilliger, France, with permission.)

3 days after feeding yielded a sensitivity and a specificity of 71.4% and 100%, respectively.[18] Moreover, gastroscopy can help distinguish true infections (ie, gross changes to the gastric mucosa) from nonpathological, non–snake-related cryptosporidia (ie, from the prey) present in fecal samples.[18] When evaluating snakes for gastric cryptosporidiosis, some authors collect 15 to 20 biopsies from the stomach.[19]

With the head and neck extended, the esophagus and stomach of small lizards (**Fig. 8**A, B) and chelonians (**Fig. 8**E) can easily be explored with a rigid telescope. For monitors (**Fig. 8**C, D) and larger reptiles (**Fig. 8**H), flexible endoscopy is needed. Common abnormal findings during endoscopy include parasites (**Fig. 8**F) and mucosal lesions (**Fig. 8**G, H).

Cloaca

In chelonians, the procedure is easier with the animal on dorsal recumbency (**Fig. 9**A). When indicated, the animal can also be placed on ventral recumbency (**Fig. 9**B). A 2.7 mm, 30° rigid endoscope is routinely used, even in larger species (see **Fig. 9**B). However, in some situations, using a flexible endoscope may be easier and more convenient (**Fig. 9**C). Saline-infusion cloacoscopy has been used for a variety of procedures in reptiles, and benefits include excellent visualization of the cloacal mucosa, cloacal compartments, and the detailed examination of the distal colon (**Fig. 9**D).

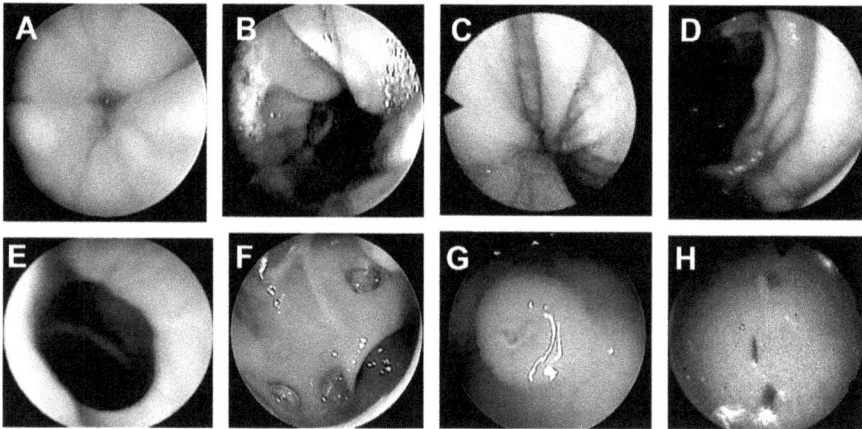

Fig. 8. Esophagoscopy and gastroscopy. (A) Esophagus of a green iguana (*Iguana iguana*; 2.7 mm telescope, air insufflation). (B) Cardia of a green iguana (2.7 mm telescope, air insufflation). (C) Esophagus of a Komodo dragon (*Varanus komodoensis*) using a 9 mm fiberscope and air insufflation. (D) Stomach of a Komodo dragon with normal folds (9 mm fiberscope, air insufflation). (E) Cardia of a South African helmeted terrapin (*Pelomedusa subrufa*; 2.7 mm telescope, air insufflation). (F) Gastric parasitic cyst in a South African helmeted terrapin (2.7 mm telescope, air insufflation). (G) Asymptomatic gastric leiomyoma in a South African helmeted terrapin (2.7 mm telescope, air insufflation). (H) Gastric ulcers in a black caiman (9 mm fiberscope, air insufflation). (*Courtesy of* Norin Chai, France, with permission.)

Cloacoscopy followed by colonoscopy, in addition to other imaging techniques, may also be a useful tool to explore and treat GI obstructions (**Fig. 9**E). A noninvasive, transcloacal technique has been described to assist on breaking down an enterolith located in the distal colon of an Argentine black and white tegu (*Salvator merianae*) under sedation and spinal anesthesia. Saline-infusion cloacoscopy using a 2.7 mm, 30° rigid endoscope confirmed the presence of an enterolith within the distal colon. Then, portions of the enterolith were removed using a dental diamond burr with a soft-tissue shield attached to a low-speed dental handpiece, under endoscopic guidance. Long, atraumatic grasping forceps were also used to grasp, crush, and extract portions of the calculus.[20] Cloacoscopy also allowed the removal of eggshell and egg material from the distal oviducts, and as a guide for the exteriorization of partially prolapsed tissue and resection, or cloacal calculi removal.[21] **Fig. 9**C–F highlight the value of cloacoscopy in a case of hematochezia.

Foreign Bodies

Reptiles are reported to accidentally or intentionally ingest environmental foreign material. Clinical signs associated are often nonspecific and include decreased fecal output, anorexia, dehydration, and lethargy. Regurgitation or vomiting is an uncommon clinical sign. The foreign material may pass through the GI tract without causing proximal obstruction but may lead to constipation or obstipation. Diagnosis is based on anamnesis, physical examination with palpation, and diagnostic imaging such as radiography, computed tomography, and/or ultrasonography.[22] Biopsy and endoscopic grasping forceps may be used for the FB removal (see **Fig. 7**G–I). However, the procedure may be limited by the foreign object's size, shape, and texture. Additionally, if the object has been present for a long time, the wall of the digestive tract may be weakened to the point that adding gas or saline to facilitate endoscopic visualization may lead to perforation or rupture. Therefore, endoscopy should be

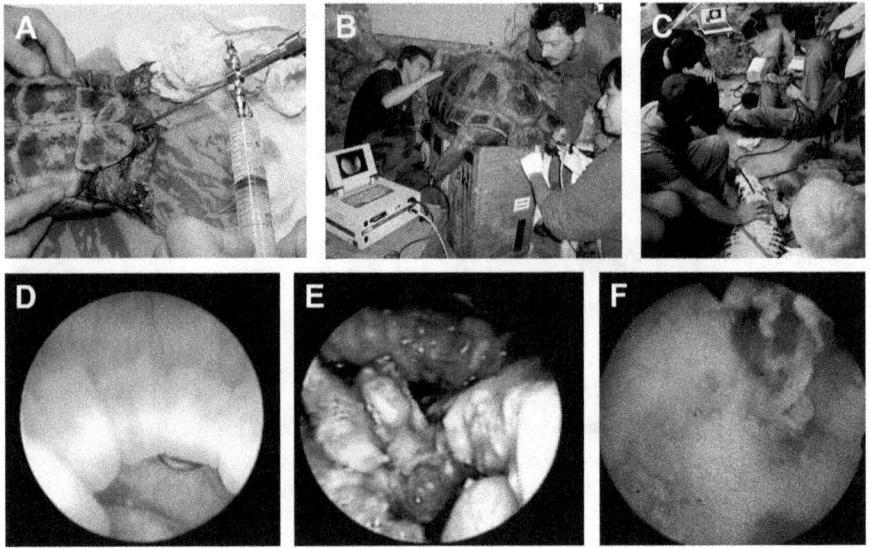

Fig. 9. Cloacoscopy. (*A*) Cloacoscopy of a Greek tortoise (*Testudo graeca*) in dorsal recumbency using saline infusion. (*B*) Cloacoscopy of an Aldabra giant tortoise (*Aldabrachelys gigantea*) in ventral recumbency using saline infusion. (*C*) Cloacoscopy and cloacal mucosa biopsy on a black caiman using air insufflation. (*D*) Saline-infusion view of distal colon of a Greek tortoise showing normal spiral folds and normal feces matter. (*E*) Saline-infusion view in the colon with a notable amount of fecal matter on this Greek tortoise presented with constipation. (*F*) Bleeding ulcer on the cloacal mucosa of this black caiman presented with hematochezia. The colon was not involved. Several biopsies had been done for histopathology and cultures. (*Courtesy of* Norin Chai, France, with permission.)

considered on a case-by-case basis.[23] The clinician must also consider which additional material to use: Magill forceps, Foley catheters, and retrieval basket. Littman and colleagues[23] have proposed a novel suction-creating technique using a red rubber catheter and a syringe to remove spherical gastric FB. The wide end of the catheter was applied directly to the surface of the FB via endoscopic guidance.[23] Negative pressure was applied to the FB using suction created by the attached 20 mL syringe, producing an airtight seal between the catheter and the item.[23]

AMPHIBIANS

The greatest limiting factor of endoscopy in amphibians is probably equipment compatibility owing to the small size of most commonly encountered species. In addition, anesthesia can also be challenging. Nevertheless, valuable information may be gained by passing a small, rigid endoscope through the oropharynx into the stomach. The main indications of gastroscopy in amphibians are the same as in other taxons. A review on endoscopy in amphibians has been published.[24]

Equipment

A 2.7 or 1.9 mm, 30° rigid telescope offers the greatest versatility for gastroscopy in amphibians. Air insufflation or saline infusion may be used for better visualization.

Patient Preparation

In all cases, the amphibian patient should always be handled with care (**Fig. 10**A). For a better visualization, it is better not to feed large frogs and toads for 24 to 48 hours

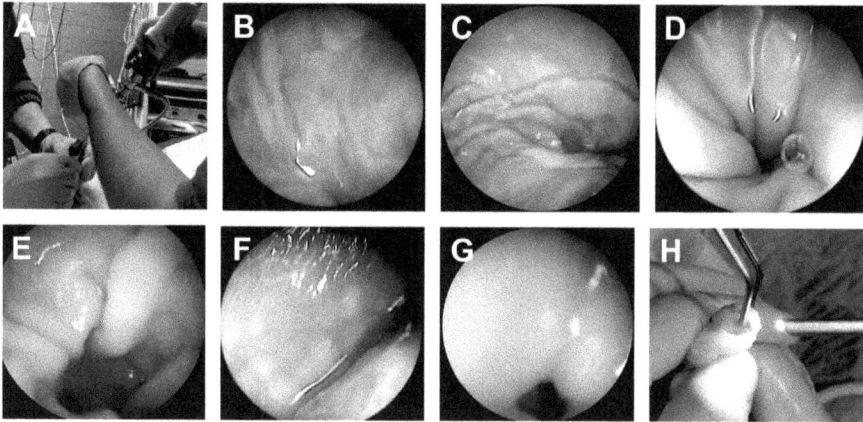

Fig. 10. Esophagoscopy and gastroscopy in amphibians. (*A*) Animal may be handled carefully by an assistant during all the procedure. (*B*) Visualization of the esophagus of an African clawed frog (*Xenopus laevis*). (*C*) Visualization of the esophagus of a blue-and-yellow frog (*Phyllomedusa bicolor*). (*D*) Visualization of the cardia of an African clawed frog. (*E*) Normal stomach of a blue-and-yellow frog. (*F*) Transmural visualization of the follicles in an African clawed frog. (*G*) Visualization of the pylorus of a blue-and-yellow frog. (*H*) Removal of a gastric foreign body in an axolotl (*Ambystoma mexicanum*) after endoscopic assessment of any adhesions of the object to the gastric mucosa and any lesions to it. (*Courtesy of* Norin Chai, France, with permission.)

before endoscopic procedures. Fasting is not required for esophageal endoscopy. Anesthesia is essential for upper GI endoscopy. Analgesia potentiates the effects of anesthetic drugs and reduces recovery time. The drug of choice for sedation or anesthesia is tricaine methanesulfonate (MS-222), which has also been demonstrated to have analgesic potential. Additional anesthetic protocols can be found elsewhere.[24,25]

Esophagus and Stomach

The oral cavity should be gently opened using atraumatic material such as a radiograph film or a rubber spatula.[24] A rigid telescope-sheath system can be used to examine the buccal cavity, esophagus, and stomach. Slight air insufflation is often needed. The oral cavity is separated from the esophagus by a strong sphincter that may be difficult to identify. Once the upper esophageal sphincter is passed, the esophageal mucosa (**Fig. 10**B, C) can be evaluated. The short, wide esophagus makes gastric endoscopy easy to accomplish. The lower esophageal sphincter (**Fig. 10**D) is less resistant than the upper one and can be easily passed. The stomach (**Fig. 10**E–G) can be evaluated for ulcers and FB, and the latter can often be removed with endoscopic assistance (**Fig. 10**H). For Caudates, an endotracheal tube may be used as a mouth-gag to facilitate the insertion of a flexible ureteroscope.

COMPLICATIONS AND POTENTIAL ADVERSE OUTCOMES FOR EXOTICS GASTROINTESTINAL ENDOSCOPY

If endoscopy is performed appropriately, complications are rare but may occur; most common complications are listed under **Box 1**. Of these complications, gastric overdistention due to excessive insufflation is the most common. The abdomen during endoscopic examination should feel distended but should not be tympanic. In the absence of a suction pump, gentle manual compression of the abdomen may help

Box 1
Most common complications of gastrointestinal endoscopy

Gastrointestinal perforation

Laceration of major blood vessels

Laceration of organs adjacent to the gastrointestinal tract

Decreased venous return due to gastric overdistention

Acute bradycardia

Gastric-dilation volvulus

Mucosal hemorrhage

to relieve gastric dilation. It is also essential to remember that the endoscope itself may cause trauma to the mucosa of the organs, potentially resulting in misdiagnosis. Unexperienced clinicians may perforate the esophagus, especially if the lumen is not visualized and excessive pressure is applied. Most commonly, duodenal or gastric perforation results from aggressive biopsy or retrieval technique.

SUMMARY

GI endoscopy in exotic animals, like in cats and dogs, is minimally invasive. However, it is largely underused in exotics. This article may help practitioners consider the benefits and the application of endoscopy for the diagnosis of GI diseases and for the retrieval of gastric FB.

ACKNOWLEDGMENTS

The authors specially thank Christophe Bulliot DVM, DECZM (Small Mammal) and Lionel Schilliger DVM, DECZM (Herpetology), ABVP, for their kind authorization to use their pictures.

DISCLOSURE

The author has nothing to disclose.

REFERENCES

1. Divers SJ. Exotic mammal diagnostic endoscopy and endosurgery. Vet Clin North Am Exot Anim Pract 2010;13(2):255–72.
2. Pignon C, Huynh M, Husnik R, et al. Flexible gastrointestinal endoscopy in ferrets (*Mustela putorius furo*). Vet Clin Exot Anim 2015;18(3):369–400.
3. Weil AB. Anesthesia for endoscopy in small animals. Vet Clin North Am Small Anim Pract 2009;39(5):839–48.
4. Krueger KL, Murphy JC, Fox JG. Treatment of proliferative colitis in ferrets. J Am Vet Med Assoc 1989;194(10):1435–6.
5. Divers SJ. Avian diagnostic endoscopy. Vet Clin North Am Exot Anim Pract 2010;13(2):187–202.
6. Morrisey JK. Gastrointestinal diseases of psittacine birds. J Exot Pet Med 1999;8(2):66–74.
7. Taylor M, Murray MJ. Endoscopic examination and therapy of the avian gastrointestinal tract. Seminars Avian Exot Pet Med 1999;8(3):110–4.

8. Sladakovic I, Ellis AE, Divers SJ. Evaluation of gastroscopy and biopsy of the proventriculus and ventriculus in pigeons (*Columba livia*). Am J Vet Res 2017; 78(1):42–9.
9. Desmarchelier MR, Ferrell ST. The value of endoscopy in a wildlife raptor service. Vet Clin Exot Anim 2015;18(3):463–77.
10. Cotton RJ, Divers SJ. Endoscopic removal of gastrointestinal foreign bodies in two African grey parrots (*Psittacus erithacus*) and a hyacinth macaw (*Anodorhynchus hyacinthinus*). J Avian Med Surg 2017;31(4):335–43.
11. Perpinan D, Curro TG. Gastrointestinal obstruction in penguin chicks. J Avian Med Surg 2009;23(4):290–3.
12. Lloyd C. Staged endoscopic ventricular foreign body removal in a Gyr falcon (*Falco rusticolus*). J Avian Med Surg 2009;23(4):314–9.
13. Hoppes S. Foreign body perforation of the proventriculus of an umbrella cockatoo (*Cacatua alba*). In: Proceedings of the annual conference of the association of avian veterinarians 2017. 29 July - 2 August 2017, Washington DC, USA, p. 137–138.
14. Hoefer H, Levitan D. Perforating foreign body in the ventriculus of an umbrella cockatoo (*Cacatua alba*). J Avian Med Surg 2013;27(2):128–35.
15. Divers SJ. Reptile diagnostic endoscopy and endosurgery. Vet Clin North Am Exot Anim Pract 2010;13(2):217–42.
16. Kik MJL, Nickel RF. Removal of a foreign body from the intestine of a leopard tortoise (*Geochelone pardalis*) via laparoscopy. Der Prakt Tierarzt 2001;82(3):174.
17. Schilliger L, Rossfelder A, Bonwitt J, et al. Antemortem diagnosis of multicentric lymphoblastic lymphoma, lymphoid leukemia, and inclusion body disease in a boa constrictor (Boa constrictor imperator). J Herpetol Med Surg 2014;24(1):11–9.
18. Cerveny SN, Garner MM, D'Agostino JJ, et al. Evaluation of gastroscopic biopsy for diagnosis of Cryptosporidium sp. infection in snakes. J Zoo Wildl Med 2012; 43(4):864–71.
19. Bogan JE Jr. Gastric cryptosporidiosis in snakes, a review. J Herpetol Med Surg 2019;29(3–4):71–86.
20. Epstein JJ, Doss G, Yaw T, et al. Diagnosis and successful medical management of a colonic, urate enterolith in an argentine black and white tegu (*Salvator merianae*). J Herpetol Med Surg 2020;30(1):21–7.
21. Mans C, Sladky K. Endoscopically guided removal of cloacal calculi in three African spurred tortoises (*Geochelone sulcata*). J Am Vet Med Assoc 2012;240(7): 869–75.
22. Eatwell K, Richardson J. Gastroenterology - small intestine, exocrine pancreas, and large intestine. In: Divers SJ, Stahl SJ, editors. Mader's reptile and Amphibian medicine and surgery. St Louis (MO): Elsevier; 2019. p. 761–74.
23. Littman EM, Berg KJ, Goldberg RN, et al. Endoscope-guided marble foreign body removal technique in an inland bearded dragon (*Pogona vitticeps*). J Herpetol Med Surg 2022;32(4):253–8.
24. Chai N. Endoscopy in amphibians. Vet Clin Exot Anim 2015;18(3):479–91.
25. Carpenter JW, Harms CA. Exotic animal formulary. 6th edition. St Louis (MO): Elsevier; 2023.

Pain Management for Gastrointestinal Conditions in Exotic Animals

Dario d'Ovidio, DVM, MS, SpecPACS, PhD, DECZM (Small Mammal)[a],*, Chiara Adami, DMV, FRCVS, FHAE, PhD, Dip ACVAA, Dip ECVAA[b]

KEYWORDS

- Exotic animals • Gastroenterology • Pain recognition • Pain management
- Analgesia • Therapies

KEY POINTS

- Gastrointestinal (GI) disorders are very common in exotic animals and can be extremely painful.
- Major differences in pain mechanisms and manifestations occur across different taxonomic groups.
- The veterinary clinicians should consult up-to-date formularies and recent published studies for specific analgesic dosage recommendations for each species.
- Pain management and patient's response monitoring is crucial in animals experiencing GI pain.

INTRODUCTION

Gastrointestinal (GI) disorders occur very commonly in exotic animal patients. Primary or secondary (eg, toxic, traumatic) GI diseases frequently affect amphibians, reptiles, birds, and small mammals, causing painful conditions associated with inflammation, cramping, gut distention from obstruction, and tympanic abdomen.[1–3]

Pain recognition in exotic species can be challenging as major differences in pain mechanisms and manifestations occur across different taxonomic groups making clinical signs of visceral pain subtle and easily neglected. With regard to treatment, it should be taken into account that GI disorders can affect the absorption of drugs that are to be administered orally, an inconvenience that poses further challenges to pain management. Furthermore, some medications typically used for the treatment of GI diseases, namely opioids and nonsteroidal anti-inflammatory drugs (NSAIDs), can further affect GI function by causing vomiting, anorexia, diarrhea, GI ulcerations,

[a] European College of Zoological Medicine (Small Mammals); Private practitioner, Via C. Colombo 118, 80022 Arzano, Naples, Italy; [b] Department of Veterinary Medicine, University of Cambridge, CB3 0ES, Cambridge, UK
* Corresponding author.
E-mail address: dariodovidio@yahoo.it

Vet Clin Exot Anim 28 (2025) 347–363
https://doi.org/10.1016/j.cvex.2024.11.006
1094-9194/25/© 2024 Elsevier Inc. All rights reserved, including those for text and data mining, AI training, and similar technologies.
vetexotic.theclinics.com

Abbreviations	
COX	cyclooxygenase
CRI	continuous rate infusion
ECM	exotic companion mammal
GDV	gastric dilatation volvulus
GI	gastrointestinal
IBD	inflammatory bowel disease
IM	intramuscular
IV	intravenous
NK1	neurokinin 1
NSAID	nonsteroidal anti-inflammatory drug
SC	subcutaneous

and reduction in daily fecal output.[1,4–7] In addition, due to the lack of information on the pharmacodynamics and pharmacokinetics of the main analgesic drugs in exotic animals, extrapolation of analgesic efficacy across orders and species remains a major limitation.[8] Therefore, although analgesia represents a crucial part of GI disorder management, yet more investigation is needed in order to improve pain management in exotic animal species.

VISCERAL PAIN

Visceral innervation is sparse compared with the sensory innervation of skin, muscles, bones, and associated tissues. As a result, in human patients', visceral sensations tend to be diffuse in character, and because they are generally referred to nonvisceral somatic anatomic structures, verbal patients find them difficult to localize, with visceral differentiation often relying on diagnosis and detection of changes in organ function.[9,10]

With respect to hollow organs, various animal models showed that the peripheral projections of spinal afferents not only innervate distinctly their wall layers, with mucosal, submucosal, intraganglionic, and intramuscular (IM) endings, but also wrap around blood vessels, including those located in the mesentery. All these nociceptors respond to noxious levels of distension, as well as to variety of inflammatory and immune mediators, and there is evidence that they can be inhibited by both gamma-aminobutyric acid (GABA) type B and μ-opioid receptor agonists.[11,12]

Various clinical conditions such as ischemia, thrombosis, acute enlargement of solid viscera associated with stretching of the capsule (organomegaly), and/or organ inflammation, all have the potential to cause visceral pain.[3,13] In human patients, GI dysfunctions and inflammatory bowel diseases (IBDs) are the most prevalent disorders associated with visceral pain.[14–16]

Signals emanating from visceral organs project to the dorsal horn of the spinal cord, where postsynaptic signaling activates spinal and supraspinal autonomic reflexes. For this reason, human patients affected with true visceral pain, besides perceiving a diffuse and poorly defined sensation that is usually subjectively localized in the midline of their body, also reportedly show signs associated with a marked autonomic response such as pallor, profuse sweating, nausea, acute vomiting/diarrhea, and changes in body temperature, blood pressure, and heart rate.[14,17]

Overall, recognition of visceral pain is more challenging than that of somatic pain because of the lack of overt clinical signs. With respect to animal patients, while in mammals some postural/behavioral changes have been associated with visceral pain (eg, hunched posture and reluctance to move in rabbits with GI stasis, back arch in rodents following laparotomy), in birds and herptiles such changes are often nonspecific and occur as generalized lethargy, decreased interaction with their environments, hyporexia/anorexia, change in feeding behavior, and weight loss.[18–20] Death may occur as a consequence of untreated acute pain in all species, and as a result of enterotoxemia/intestinal dysbiosis caused by decreased GI motility in rabbits and herbivore rodents.[21–23]

A multimodal analgesic approach is generally recommended to reduce inflammation and discomfort, as well as to reduce morbidity and mortality in exotic animal patients, with opioids, NSAIDs, and gabapentinoids being the most commonly used classes of drugs for the treatment of both acute and chronic visceral pain.[3,6,24–27]

AMPHIBIAN AND REPTILES

The main GI disorders in amphibians and reptiles include oral cavity, esophageal and gastric infectious or noninfectious diseases, prolapse, gastric ulceration and neoplasia, GI foreign bodies, constipation, tympany and GI stasis, food impaction and maldigestion due to improper management and cloacal dysfunction (see article on Amphibian and Reptile GI disease in this issue).[2,28,29] Several abdominal nondigestive conditions causing secondary compression/alteration of the GI function (follicular stasis) may contribute to cause visceral pain.

Pain Assessment

There are no validated methods to quantify pain in herptile patients, therefore, pain assessment is done mainly through observation of deviations from physiologic species-specific behaviors.[18,30] Evaluation of physiologic parameters (eg, heart and respiratory rate, blood pressure, temperature) should be used in association to behavioral assessment to evaluate pain in amphibians and reptiles.[24,30] Nevertheless, the species-specific anatomic peculiarities (eg, the presence of shell in chelonians), the stress associated to handling and manipulation, as well as the difficulties to gain objective and reliable measurements (eg, indirect blood pressure) across different orders, suborders, and species, make pain assessment extraordinarily challenging in amphibians and reptiles.[8,30]

Despite the paucity of literature regarding pain recognition in reptiles, the available data on the subject identify the following as main indicators of pain: (1) changes in physiologic parameters, (2) demonstration of nocifensive behaviors, (3) decreased interaction within their environments, (4) changes in mentation and/or feeding behavior, and (5) return to normal behaviors once the pain is alleviated.[18,31] However, it should be emphasized that these signs are rather generic and none of them is specific for visceral pain.

Treatment

Opioids

There is evidence suggesting that the opioidergic system plays a role in the control of nociception in many reptile species, and therefore, indicating opioids as the most effective analgesics in reptiles, particularly the μ-opioid agonists compounds. Nevertheless, it is worth considering that most of the published work focused on nociceptive models reproducing somatic, rather than visceral pain, and that compounds proven to be effective for a specific type of pain may not necessarily be as useful for the treatment of other pain syndromes.[25,32]

Many opioid compounds have been investigated in different herptile species, following various routes of administration and in diverse nociceptive models.

The application of transdermal fentanyl patches releasing 12.5 μg/h was investigated in healthy corn snakes (*Pantherophis guttatus*) with respect to behavioral effects and serum fentanyl concentrations.[33] The authors concluded that fentanyl patches may be a suitable and safe analgesic option for this species; however, the gap in knowledge with respect to effective analgesic fentanyl serum concentrations in snakes makes it difficult to translate these findings into useful clinical recommendation.[33] Still regarding pure μ-agonists, in a model of thermal nociception, intraperitoneal administration of both morphine and pethidine seemed to provide a certain degree of pain relief to Nile crocodiles (*Crocodylus niloticus*).[34]

In oriental fire-bellied toads (*Bombina orientalis*), morphine was found to provide better mechanical antinociception than butorphanol, while the addition of dexmedetomidine to an alfaxalone-based solution for immersion anesthesia provided some analgesia, although it appeared to lighten the anesthetic depth.[35,36] Other studies also suggested that the analgesic efficacy of both mixed-opioid, k-agonist/mu-receptor antagonists (ie, butorphanol or nalbuphine), and partial μ-opioid agonists (ie, buprenorphine) is questionable in green iguanas (*Iguana iguana*), central bearded dragons (*Pogona vitticeps*), corn snakes, and red-eared slider turtles (*Trachemys scripta elegans*) exposed to either electrical or thermal noxious stimulation.[25,37,38]

Tramadol is considered a valid alternative to μ-opioid agonists, with proven analgesic properties and reduced adverse respiratory and cardiovascular effects, particularly in aquatic chelonian species such as red-eared slider turtles and sea turtles.[25,39,40]

Nonsteroidal anti-inflammatory drugs

Very few reports evaluated the pharmacokinetics and pharmacodynamics of NSAIDs in reptiles and, to the authors' knowledge, no study investigated any NSAID compound with respect to their effects on visceral nociception in reptile species.[25,41] Doses and routes recommended for mammals may not necessarily be safe and effective when used in reptiles and, therefore, should not be extrapolated and applied to them.

A study evaluating cyclooxygenase (COX) protein expression in traumatized versus normal tissues from eastern box turtles (*Terrapene carolina carolina*) found that traumatized muscles had significantly greater COX-1, but not COX-2 protein concentrations, than normal muscles, suggesting that traditional NSAIDs that block both COX isoforms might be more effective than COX-2-selective drugs.[41] Another study evaluating the role of the COX signaling pathway during inflammation in skin and muscle tissues of ball pythons (*Python regius*) found that the production of COX-1, but not COX-2, was significantly greater in inflamed versus noninflamed skin specimens.[42] The pharmacokinetic behavior of meloxicam has been investigated in various species of sea turtles as well as in red-eared slider turtles. However, pharmacodynamic data are lacking or inconclusive. One report evaluating autonomic responses and catecholamines plasma concentrations failed to demonstrate the analgesic efficacy of meloxicam in ball pythons undergoing surgical cannulation of the vertebral artery, suggesting that therapeutic doses for this species have not been identified yet.[43] In conclusion, and despite NSAIDs are widely used in reptile patients to treat a variety of painful syndromes, there is very little evidence supporting their actual effectiveness and usefulness to treat visceral pain in these species.[25]

BIRDS

The main GI disorders in birds are infectious and noninfectious conditions affecting the oral cavity, crop, esophagus, stomachs (proventriculus and ventriculus), gut and cloaca causing inflammation, erosion/ulceration, perforation (eg, GI foreign bodies), and constipation. Furthermore, both intestinal neoplasms and nondigestive disorders causing secondary compression/alteration of the GI function (eg, reproductive disorders) are supposedly associated with visceral pain in birds (see article on Avian GI disease in this issue).[44,45]

Pain Assessment

Differences between species and their species-specific physiologic behaviors should be considered when assessing pain in birds. Although numeric rating scales have been used in some species (eg, pigeons), there is a lack of validated methods to measure pain and nociception in birds. As a result, pain recognition relies mainly on evaluation of both behavioral changes and alterations in physiologic parameters, such as heart rate, respiratory rate, blood pressure, plasma corticosterone, fecal corticosterone, leukograms, and electroencephalogram readings (**Fig. 1**).[19,46,47]

Treatment

Opioids

Owing to variable distribution of opioid subtypes receptors within the nervous system, the effects of specific opioid agents vary considerably between avian species.[7]

According to the most recent studies on the distribution, quantity, structure, and function of opioid receptors in birds, parenteral κ-agonist/μ-receptor antagonists (eg, butorphanol tartrate at 1–5 mg/kg) may be considered a suitable analgesic option for psittacines, but not for raptors such as American kestrel (*Falco sparverius*) and other birds of the *Falco* genus.[7] However, owing to its short half-life, the administration of either frequent boluses or continuous rate infusions (CRIs) of butorphanol would be necessary to achieve adequate clinical analgesia in psittacines.[48–51] In red-tailed hawks (*Buteo jamaicensis*) undergoing supramaximal electrical stimulation, fentanyl infusion produced a dose-related decrease in isoflurane minimum anesthetic concentration with minimal effects on measured cardiovascular parameters, suggesting that pure μ-agonists may be preferable for raptor avian species.[52] Conversely, hydromorphone is known to produce dose-dependent analgesia in American kestrels even at low doses (0.1–0.6 mg/kg), whereas in cockatiels (*Nymphicus hollandicus*) and orange-winged Amazon parrots (*Amazona amazonica*) higher doses (1–2 mg/kg) are

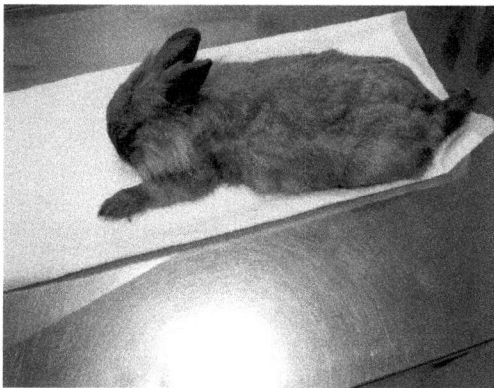

Fig. 1. Pet rabbit (*Oryctolagus cuniculus*) affected with acute complete obstruction of the duodenum caused by a hairball. The rabbit is showing abnormal mentation and appears severely depressed, reluctant to move, minimally responsive and listless.

required to produce antinociception and associated to adverse effects namely agitation, nausea, ataxia, and pupillary constriction.[53,54]

Nonsteroidal anti-inflammatory drugs

NSAIDs are widely used in avian species to treat visceral as well as somatic, acute, or chronic pain being meloxicam the most common NSAID used in avian medicine.[7] Although meloxicam is generally regarded as safe and has a large therapeutic range, a high variability in dosages, elimination half-life, clearance and bioavailability exists across different avian species and must be taken into account when extrapolating doses from one species to another.[7] Carprofen, celecoxib, robenacoxib, mavacoxib, and piroxicam have also been anecdotally evaluated in different species for the treatment of several conditions.[7,55–58] In particular, celecoxib (at 10 mg/kg orally once daily for 6–12 weeks) has been anecdotally associated to a marked clinical improvement in the treatment of inflammation associated with proventricular dilation disease in both pet psittacine and non-psittacine birds.[59–62] To date, the administration of oral coxibs relies on feeding, as in most cases the presence of food in the GI tract increases the bioavailability of these drugs.[63]

EXOTIC COMPANION MAMMALS

Exotic companion mammals (ECMs) are frequently diagnosed with several noninfectious and infectious GI diseases. Common conditions include *Helicobacter mustelae* gastritis, IBD, pancreatic disorders, GI lymphoma, systemic coronavirus, coccidiosis, and liver disease in ferrets; GI motility disorders (ileus/hypomotility), obstructive GI disease/trichobezoars, liver lobe torsion, bacterial and parasitic enteritis (coccidiosis), and GI neoplasia in rabbits; gastric dilatation volvulus (GDV), ileus, gas distention of stomach or intestinal system (tympany), intussusception and obstructive GI disease and trichobezoars in guinea pigs and chinchillas, and parasitic (*Taenia taeniaeformis*) and bacterial (*Clostridium difficile*) enteritis in rats and hamsters, respectively (see articles on Ferret, Rabbit and Rodent GI diseases in this issue).[1,64]

Pain Assessment

Although assessing pain is considered challenging in any ECM species, and particularly in prey species, recent studies have tremendously advanced our understanding of pain recognition in ferrets, rabbits, and rodents.[20,22,26,65–70] Behavioral changes, alterations in physiologic variables, and species-specific pain scales (Grimace scales, composite pain scales) have been reported as useful indicators/tools to recognize pain in several ECM species (**Figs. 2** and **3**).[20,22,70]

Treatment

Opioids

Similarly to reptiles and birds, also in ECM there are species and individual differences with respect to both the distribution of opioid receptors and the response to opioids. As a result, it is crucial that clinicians select the opioid agents carefully and adapt their dose to the target species.[22,70]

Buprenorphine, a partial μ-agonist, is considered the most appropriate option for moderate pain in several ECM species (**Table 1**). In rabbits, its effectiveness for visceral analgesia has been demonstrated when administered either solely or in combination with other drugs.[77,89] However, although the recommended dose for buprenorphine (0.01–0.05 mg/kg) is the same regardless of the route of administration, the latter would significantly affect its duration of the effects, plasma concentrations and bioavailability, suggesting that parenteral administration, and particularly the

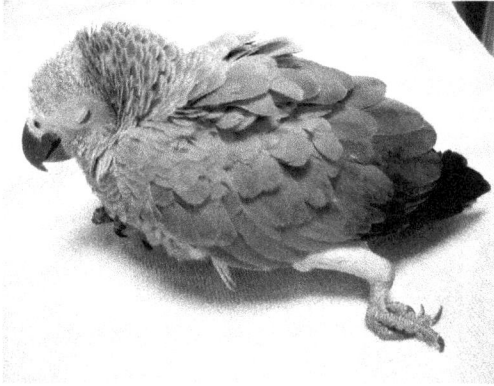

Fig. 2. Gray parrot (*Psittacus erithacus*) with GI (foreign body) obstruction after ingestion of a rubber feeding tube. The bird is lethargic, anorectic, and is showing changes in eye expression (palpebral fissure size).

intravenous (IV) and IM routes, are the most appropriate for immediate pain relief.[71,74] Also in rodents, both the duration of the effects and analgesic efficacy of buprenorphine depend on dose, route of administration, and species, with a considerable variability in dosages and dosing intervals across species.[75] In ferrets, pharmacokinetic data showed that frequent administrations of buprenorphine (ie, every 4–6 hours) are needed to produce plasma levels comparable to those that were found to be analgesic in other species, although no evidence of thermal antinociception was found following subcutaneous (SC) administration of doses ranging from 0.02 to 0.04 mg/kg.[90,91] On the contrary, SC administration of hydromorphone (at 0.2 mg/kg) provided antinociception from 1 to 4 hours postinjection, along with behavioral alterations, mostly characterized by increased and uncoordinated locomotor activity, lip licking, or digging, in ferrets.[90–92]

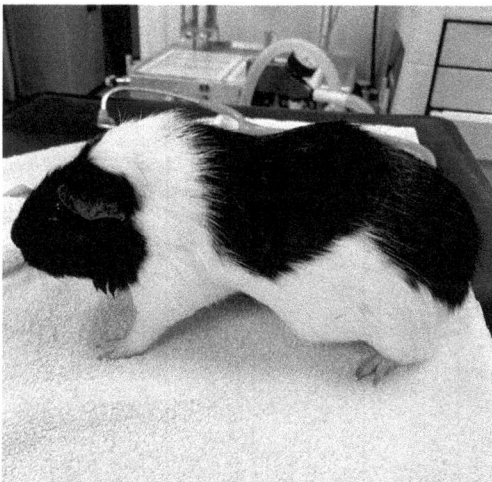

Fig. 3. Guinea pig (*Cavia porcellus*) with GDV. The rodent is showing a rigid posture with the abdomen raised from the table. (*Courtesy of* Imal Khelik.)

Table 1
Analgesic drugs for visceral pain in exotic companion mammal

	Buprenorphine	Hydromorphone	Meloxicam	Lidocaine	Maropitant	Metamizole	Paracetamol
Ferrets	0.01–0.05 q6–12h SC, IV, IM[6,71-73]	0.2 q1-4h IV, SC[74,75]	0.1–0.3 q24 h SC, PO, IM[76]				
Rabbits	0.03–0.1 q4–6h IV, IM, SC[4,70,77]		0.1–1 q12–24 PO[72,78,79]	100 µg/kg/h for 2 d IV (CRI)[80,81]	4 SC once[82]	65 once IV[83]	
Rodents	0.01–0.05 q6–12h SC, IM[a] 0.01–0.05 q8–12h SC[b] 0.05–0.1 q12 h SC[c,72,84]		0.1–0.5 q24 SC, PO[a] 1–2 q12–24 SC, PO[b] 5 q24 SC, PO[c,72,85]		20 mg/kg IV[b,86]	60 mg/kg/day PO[b,87]	200 PO[c,88]

Abbreviations: CRI, constant rate infusion; IM, intramuscular; IV, intravenous; PO, per os (oral administration); q/h, every hour; SC, subcutaneous.
Dose expressed as mg/kg.
[a] Rodents = Guinea pig, Chinchilla, Gerbil, Hamster.
[b] Rodents = Rat.
[c] Rodents = Mouse.

A large number of experimental studies focusing on human GI conditions used rodents as animal model.[72,84,88,93,94] Although visceral pain was experimentally induced and not the result of a naturally occurring disease, the knowledge gathered from these studies is species-specific and pain model-specific, and may potentially be applied to companion rodents suffering from GI disease.

Single-housed rodents and rabbits may be administered analgesics in drinking water, especially after discharge from the hospital. Both tramadol and buprenorphine have been administered by this route to mice with experimentally induced pancreatitis and colitis for 4 to 7 days, targeting oral effective doses of 1 mg/kg and 25 mg/kg, respectively.[84,94] Based on both these analgesic doses and a daily expected water intake of at least 3 mL per mouse, concentrations of buprenorphine and tramadol equal to 0.01 mg/mL and 1 mg/mL, respectively, are usually recommended. However, it should be considered that not only the sickness itself, but also the opioid analgesics, may considerably reduce the mice's water intake, making this route of administration less reliable than the parenteral ones. In contrast to buprenorphine and tramadol, parenteral morphine worsened the outcome of both pancreatitis and colitis in mice, by negatively affecting morbidity and mortality.[88,93]

An experimental study aimed at evaluating the usefulness of fentanyl during cholangiopancreatography in humans, found that fentanyl at 1 μg/kg effectively relaxed the rabbits' sphincter of Oddi, suggesting potential therapeutic applications of this drug for treating pain associated to biliary tract and pancreatic diseases in rabbits.[85]

Nonsteroidal anti-inflammatory drugs

NSAIDs are widely used in ECM to treat a variety of GI conditions.[76,78,79] Meloxicam is the most common anti-inflammatory drug used in ECM.[1] Clinicians should pay attention to the huge differences in meloxicam dosing across different ECM species (see **Table 1**). Pharmacokinetic studies suggest that, in ferrets, meloxicam useful doses (0.2 mg/kg SC) are closer to those of cats and dogs than that of rabbits and rodents, and that sex differences are significant in this species, with females showing higher volume of distribution, faster drug elimination, and lower plasma concentrations than males.[87,95,96]

Metamizole, also known as dipyrone, is a nonselective NSAID with both analgesic and spasmolytic properties and has been used to treat pain associated to experimentally induced colitis in mice as well as to intestinal anastomosis in Wistar rats.[94,97] Its mechanism of action is not yet fully understood; however, the inhibition of prostaglandin synthesis via iso-enzyme cyclooxygenase-3 and activation of both the opioidergic and cannabinoid systems have been theorized.[83] Parenteral doses ranging from 65 mg/kg (IV, in rabbits) to 300 mg/kg (SC, in rats) have been reported to produce some pain relief with minimal cardiovascular effect, although hyperalgesia occurred in rats.[98–100] However, in mice with colitis, metamizole administered in the drinking water with a strength of 1.25 mg/mL significantly reduced water intake.[84]

Paracetamol, also known as acetaminophen, is generally considered an atypical NSAID because it has only minor anti-inflammatory activity and acts almost exclusively within the brain, mainly by blocking COX-2 and inhibiting endocannabinoid reuptake.[101] In mice with colitis, oral paracetamol at the dose of 200 mg/kg helped relieving visceral pain while promoting the overall wellbeing of the animals.[84] Of note, similarly to cats, the hepatic metabolism of acetaminophen via glucuronidation in ferrets is relatively slow; as a result, any dose of acetaminophen in ferrets should be considered potentially toxic.[102,103]

OTHER DRUGS
Maropitant

Maropitant is a neurokinin 1 (NK1) receptor antagonist approved for the use in the treatment and prevention of vomiting and motion sickness in dogs and cats.[104,105] The NK1 receptor antagonists have been shown to increase colonic peristalsis and decrease the number of abdominal contractions in response to colorectal stimulation in rabbits.[80,82,86] In New Zealand White rabbits, administration of maropitant at a dose of 1 mg/kg (SC and IV) resulted in plasma concentrations, detected for up to 24 hours, that were similar to those measured in dogs following administration of comparable doses.[80] Although rabbits cannot vomit and whether they can experience nausea it is currently unknown, it has been postulated that maropitant may play a role in the alleviation of visceral pain in this species.[80] Although doses up to 10 mg/kg of SC maropitant failed to reduce pain in rabbits undergoing surgical neutering, another recent study showed that 4 mg/kg of SC maropitant was effective in decreasing pain-related behaviors (5–8 hours) and behavioral pain scores (12–24 hours) in rabbits after ovariohysterectomy or orchiectomy (see **Table 1**).[81,106] More research is needed to evaluate the effectiveness of maropitant to reduce visceral pain in rabbits and other ECM.[107]

Lidocaine

Lidocaine is a sodium channel blocker whose visceral analgesic properties have been demonstrated in rabbits.[73] Recommended CRI dosages in rabbits range from 75 to 100 μg/kg/min for 1 to 3 days, usually following a loading dose of 2 mg/kg, IV (see **Table 1**).[73,108] In this species, lidocaine CRI represents a valid alternative to opioids for alleviating postoperative pain as it seems to promote GI motility, food intake, and fecal output, while reducing blood glucose concentrations in rabbits undergoing abdominal surgery, when compared with buprenorphine.[73] In addition, a recent study demonstrated that in rabbits with GI obstruction lidocaine CRI decreased morbidity and mortality.[108]

Although data on analgesic effects are still pending in birds, lidocaine CRIs (up to 6 mg/kg/h) have been used in Galliformes, Anseriformes, Psittaciformes, Strigiformes, and Accipitriformes without obvious complications (J. Brandão, personal communication). However, administration of lidocaine at either 3 or 6 mg/kg/h (after loading dose) did not significantly change isoflurane MAC in chickens.[109] Nevertheless, no adverse reactions have been reported in chickens when administered lidocaine IV up to 6 mg/kg, and the total toxic IV dose required to produce systemic toxicity was reported to be 28.96 ± 6.21 mg/kg.[110–113]

Corticosteroids

Corticosteroids (dexamethasone, prednisone, and prednisolone) are commonly used as anti-inflammatories and/or analgesics in canine and feline patients. Similarly, they can be used to treat some inflammatory conditions in exotic animals.[79,114–116] However, corticosteroids should be used cautiously in the vast majority of exotic animal species (reptiles, birds, and steroid-sensitive ECM) because of the potential side effects, associated with the immunosuppressive function. Avian patients as well as rabbits and rodents may develop systemic fungal (eg, aspergillosis) and bacterial disease (eg, *Pasteurella* infection), following the prolonged use of corticosteroids.[1]

SUMMARY

Several exotic animal species (eg, reptiles, birds, ECMs, etc.) are affected by a variety of GI disorders. Similar to dogs and cats, these conditions may cause pain and pain-associated potentially life-threatening adverse effects. Pain recognition in exotic species can be challenging as major differences in pain mechanisms and manifestations occur across different taxonomic groups making clinical signs of visceral pain subtle and easily neglected. In most cases, the information about the pharmacokinetics and pharmacodynamics of several drugs is lacking and extrapolation is commonly performed.

CLINICS CARE POINTS

- Gastrointestinal (GI) diseases cause visceral pain associated with inflammation, cramping, gut distention from obstruction, and tympanic abdomen.
- Recognition of visceral pain is more challenging than that of somatic pain because of the lack of overt clinical signs.
- Opioids, nonsteroidal anti-inflammatory drugs and gabapentinoids are the most commonly used drugs to treat both acute and chronic visceral pain.
- Analgesia represents a crucial part of GI disorder management, although more investigation is needed in order to improve pain management in exotic animals.

DISCLOSURE

The authors have nothing to disclose.

REFERENCES

1. Ritzman TK. Diagnosis and clinical management of gastrointestinal conditions in exotic companion mammals (rabbits, Guinea pigs, and chinchillas). Vet Clin North Am Exot Anim Pract 2014;17(2):179–94.
2. Eatwell K, Richardson J. Gastroenterology—small intestine, exocrine pancreas, and large intestine. In: Divers SJ, Stahl SJ, editors. Mader's reptile and Amphibian medicine and surgery. 3rd edition. St Louis (MO): Elsevier; 2019. p. 761–74.e3.
3. Hawkins MG, Paul-Murphy J, Sanchez-Migallon Guzman D. Recognition, assessment, and management of pain in birds. In: Current therapy in avian medicine and surgery. St Louis, MO: Elsevier; 2016. p. 616–30.
4. Andrews DD, Fajt VR, Baker KC, et al. A comparison of buprenorphine, sustained release buprenorphine, and high concentration buprenorphine in male New Zealand white rabbits. J Am Assoc Lab Anim Sci 2020;59:546–56.
5. Deflers H, Gandar F, Bolen G, et al. Effects of a single opioid dose on gastrointestinal motility in rabbits (Oryctolagus cuniculus): comparisons among morphine, butorphanol, and tramadol. Vet Sci 2022;9:28.
6. Petritz OA, de Matos R. Treatment of pain in ferrets. Vet Clin North Am Exot Anim Pract 2023;26(1):245–55.
7. Sanchez-Migallon Guzman D, Hawkins MG. Treatment of pain in birds. Vet Clin North Am Exot Anim Pract 2023;26(1):83–120.
8. Sladky KK, Mans C. Analgesia. In: Divers SJ, Stahl HL, editors. Mader's and amphibian reptile medicine and surgery. 3rd edition. St Louis (MO): Elsevier-Saunders; 2019. p. 465–74.e3.
9. Cervero F. Visceral versus somatic pain: similarities and differences. Dig Dis 2009;27(Suppl 1):3–10.
10. Gebhart GF, Bielefeldt K. Physiology of visceral pain. Compr Physiol 2016;6(4):1609–33.

11. Sadeghi M, Erickson A, Castro J, et al. Contribution of membrane receptor signalling to chronic visceral pain. Int J Biochem Cell Biol 2018;98:10–23.

12. Grundy L, Erickson A, Brierley SM. Visceral pain. Annu Rev Physiol 2019;81: 261–84.

13. Johnson AC, Greenwood-Van Meerveld B. The pharmacology of visceral pain. In: Barrett JE, editor. Advances in pharmacology. 1st edition. St Louis (MO: Academic Press, Elsevier; 2016. p. 273–301.

14. Sikander S, Dickenson AH. Visceral pain: the ins and outs, the ups and downs. Curr Opin Support Palliat Care 2012;6:17–26.

15. Zeitz J, Ak M, Muller-Mottet S, et al. Pain in IBD patients: very frequent and frequently insufficiently taken into account. PLoS One 2016;11(6):e0156666.

16. Drewes AM, Olesen AE, Farmer AD, et al. Gastrointestinal pain. Nat Rev Dis Primers 2020;6:1.

17. Procacci P, Zoppi M, Maresca M. Visceral sensation. In: Cervero F, Morrison JFB, editors. Progress in pain research. Amsterdam: Elsevier; 1986. p. 21–8.

18. La'Toya VL. Pain recognition in reptiles. Vet Clin North Am Exot Anim Pract 2023; 26(1):27–41.

19. Mikoni NA, Guzman DS, Paul-Murphy J. Pain recognition and assessment in birds. Vet Clin North Am Exot Anim Pract 2023;26(1):65–81.

20. Oliver VL, Pang DSJ. Pain recognition in rodents. Vet Clin North Am Exot Anim Pract 2023;26(1):121–49.

21. Moeremans I, Devreese M, De Baere S, et al. Pharmacokinetics and absolute oral bioavailability of meloxicam in Guinea pigs (*Cavia porcellus*). Vet Anal Anesth 2019;46:548–55.

22. Miller AL, Leach MC. Pain recognition in rabbits. Vet Clin North Am Exot Anim Pract 2023;26(1):187–99.

23. Sadar MJ, Mans C. Hystricomorph rodent analgesia. Vet Clin North Am Exot Anim Pract 2023;26(1):175–86.

24. Sladky KK, Mans C. Clinical analgesia in reptiles. J Exot Pet Med 2012;21(2): 158–67.

25. Sladky KK. Pain recognition in reptiles. Vet Clin North Am Exot Anim Pract 2023; 26(1):43–64.

26. Benato L, Murrell JC, Blackwell EJ, et al. Analgesia in pet rabbits: a survey study on how pain is assessed and ameliorated by veterinary surgeons. Vet Rec 2020; 186(18):603.

27. Ozawa S, Cenani A, Sanchez-Migallon Guzman Lv D. Treatment of pain in rabbits. Vet Clin North Am Exot Anim Pract 2023;26(1):201–27.

28. Clayton LA. Amphibian gastroenterology. Vet Clin Exot Anim 2005;8:227–45.

29. Mans C. Clinical update on diagnosis and management of disorders of the digestive system of reptiles. J Exot Pet Med 2013;22(2):141–62.

30. Stevens CW. Analgesia in amphibians: preclinical studies and clinical applications. Vet Clin North Am Exot Anim Pract 2011;14(1):33–44.

31. Williams CJA, James LE, Bertelsen MF, et al. Tachycardia in response to remote capsaicin injection as a model for nociception in the ball python (*Python regius*). Vet Anaesth Analg 2015;43:429–34.

32. Wambugu SN, Towett PK, Kiama SG, et al. Effects of opioids in the formalin test in the Speke's hinged tortoise (*Kinixy's spekii*). J Vet Pharmacol Ther 2010;33(4): 347–51.

33. Walter B, Johnson S, Sladky K, et al. Serum fentanyl concentrations and behavior associated with transdermal fentanyl application on healthy corn snakes (*Pantherophis guttatus*). J Zoo Wildl Med 2024;54(4):738–45.

34. Kanui TI, Hole K. Morphine and pethidine antinociception in the crocodile. J Vet Pharmacol Ther 1992;15(1):101–3.

35. Adami C, d'Ovidio D, Casoni D. Alfaxalone-butorphanol versus alfaxalone-morphine combination for immersion anaesthesia in oriental fire-bellied toads (*Bombina orientalis*). Lab Anim 2016;50(3):204–11.

36. Adami C, d'Ovidio D, Casoni D. Alfaxalone versus alfaxalone-dexmedetomidine anaesthesia by immersion in oriental fire-bellied toads (*Bombina orientalis*). Vet Anaesth Analg 2016;43(3):326–32.

37. Greenacre CB, Schumacher JP, Tacke G, et al. Comparative antinociception of morphine, butorphanol, and buprenorphine versus saline in the green iguana, Iguana iguana, using electrostimulation. J Herpetol Med Surg 2006;16:88–92.

38. Mans C, Lahner LL, Baker BB, et al. Antinociceptive efficacy of buprenorphine and hydromorphone in red-eared slider turtles (*Trachemys scripta elegans*). J Zoo Wildl Med 2012;43:662–5.

39. Baker BB, Sladky KK, Johnson SM. Evaluation of the analgesic effects of oral and subcutaneous tramadol administration in red-eared slider turtles. J Am Vet Med Assoc 2011;238:220–7.

40. Norton TM, Cox S, Nelson SE Jr, et al. Pharmacokinetics of tramadol and o-des-methyltramadol in loggerhead sea turtles (*Caretta caretta*). J Zoo Wildl Med 2015;46(2):262–5.

41. Royal LW, Lascelles BD, Lewbart GA, et al. Evaluation of cyclooxygenase protein expression in traumatized versus normal tissues from eastern box turtles (*Terrapene carolina carolina*). J Zoo Wildl Med 2012;43:289–95.

42. Sadler RA, Schumacher JP, Rathore K, et al. Evaluation of the role of the cyclooxygenase signaling pathway during inflammation in skin and muscle tissues of ball pythons (*Python regius*). Am J Vet Res 2016;77(5):487–94.

43. Ting AKY, Tay VSY, Chng HT, et al. A critical review on the pharmacodynamics and pharmacokinetics of non-steroidal anti-inflammatory drugs and opioid drugs used in reptiles. Vet Anim Sci 2022;17:100267.

44. Olesen MG, Bertelsen MF, Perry SF, et al. Effects of preoperative administration of butorphanol or meloxicam on physiologic responses to surgery in ball pythons. J Am Vet Med Assoc 2008;233(12):1883–8.

45. Brandao J, Beaufrere H. Clinical update and treatment of selected infectious gastrointestinal diseases in avian species. J Exot Pet Med 2013;2(22):101–17.

46. Desmarchelier M, Troncy E, Beauchamp G, et al. Evaluation of a fracture pain model in domestic pigeons (*Columba livia*). Am J Vet Res 2012;73:353–60.

47. Mikoni NA, Guzman DS, Fausak E, et al. Recognition and assessment of pain-related behaviors in avian species: an integrative review. J Avian Med Surg 2022;36(2):153–72.

48. Riggs SM, Hawkins MG, Craigmill AL, et al. Pharmacokinetics of butorphanol tartrate in red-tailed hawks (*Buteo jamaicensis*) and great horned owls (*Bubo virginianus*). Am J Vet Res 2008;69:596–603.

49. Sanchez-Migallon Guzman D, Flammer K, Paul-Murphy JR, et al. Pharmacokinetics of butorphanol after intravenous, intramuscular, and oral administration in Hispaniolan Amazon parrots (*Amazona ventralis*). J Avian Med Surg 2011;25:185–91.

50. Singh PM, Johnson C, Gartrell B, et al. Pharmacokinetics of butorphanol in broiler chickens. Vet Rec 2011;168(22):588.

51. Guzman DS, Drazenovich TL, KuKanich B, et al. Evaluation of thermal antinociceptive effects and pharmacokinetics after intramuscular administration of butorphanol tartrate to American kestrels (*Falco sparverius*). Am J Vet Res 2014; 75:11–8.

52. Pavez JC, Hawkins MG, Pascoe PJ, et al. Effect of fentanyl target-controlled infusions on isoflurane minimum anaesthetic concentration and cardiovascular function in red-tailed hawks (*Buteo jamaicensis*). Vet Anaesth Analg 2011; 38(4):344–51.

53. Guzman DS, Drazenovich TL, Olsen GH, et al. Evaluation of thermal antinociceptive effects after intramuscular administration of hydromorphone hydrochloride to American kestrels (*Falco sparverius*). Am J Vet Res 2013;74:817–22.

54. Sanchez-Migallon Guzman D, Douglas JM, Beaufrere H, et al. Evaluation of the thermal antinociceptive effects of hydromorphone hydrochloride after intramuscular administration to orange-winged Amazon parrots (*Amazona amazonica*). Am J Vet Res 2020;81:775–82.

55. McGeowen D, Danbury TC, Waterman-Pearson AE, et al. Effect of carprofen on lameness in broiler chickens. Vet Rec 1999;144:668–71.

56. Danbury TC, Weeks CA, Chambers JP, et al. Self-selection of the analgesic drug carprofen by lame broiler chickens. Vet Rec 2000;146:307–11.

57. Keiper NL, Cox SK, Doss GA, et al. Pharmacokinetics of piroxicam in cranes (family *gruidae*). J Zoo Wildl Med 2017;48:886–90.

58. Dhondt L, Devreese M, Croubels S, et al. Comparative population pharmacokinetics and absolute oral bioavailability of COX-2 selective inhibitors celecoxib, mavacoxib and meloxicam in cockatiels (*Nymphicus hollandicus*). Sci Rep 2017;7(1):12043.

59. Dahlhausen B. Resolution of clinical proventricular dilatation disease by cyclogenase inhibition. J American Fed Aviculture 2001;28(4):49.

60. Dahlhausen R, Aldred S, Colaizzi E. Resolution of clinical proventricular dilatation disease by cyclooxygenase 2 inhibition. Proc Annu Conf Assoc Avian Vet 2002;9–12.

61. Perpinan D, Fernandez-Bellon H, Lopez C, et al. Lymphocytic myenteric, subepi- cardial and pulmonary ganglioneuritis in four nonpsittacine birds. J Avian Med Surg 2007;21:210–4.

62. Hoppes SM, Tizard I, Shivaprasad HL. Avian bornavirus and proventricular dilatation disease. Vet Clin North Am Exot Anim Pract 2013;13:339–55.

63. Cox SR, Lesman SP, Boucher JF, et al. The pharmacokinetics of mavacoxib, a long-acting COX-2 inhibitor, in young adult laboratory dogs. J Vet Pharmacol Ther 2010;33:461–70.

64. Huynh M, Pignon C. Gastrointestinal disease in exotic small mammals. J Exot Pet Med 2013;2(22):118–31.

65. Hampshire V, Robertson S. Using the facial grimace scale to evaluate rabbit wellness in post-procedural monitoring. Lab Anim (NY) 2015;44(7):259–60.

66. Reijgwart ML, Schoemaker NJ, Pascuzzo R, et al. The composition and initial evaluation of a grimace scale in ferrets after surgical implantation of a telemetry probe. PLoS One 2017;12(11):e0187986.

67. Banchi P, Quaranta G, Ricci A, et al. Reliability and construct validity of a composite pain scale for rabbit (CANCRS) in a clinical environment. PLoS One 2020; 15(4):e0221377.

68. Haddad Pinho R, Luna SPL, Esteves Trindade PH, et al. Validation of the rabbit pain behaviour scale (RPBS) to assess acute postoperative pain in rabbits (*Oryctolagus cuniculus*). PLoS One 2022;17(5):e0268973.

69. Cohen S, Ho C. Review of rat (Rattus norvegicus), mouse (Mus musculus), Guinea pig (Cavia porcellus), and rabbit (Oryctolagus cuniculus) indicators for welfare. Assessment Animals (Basel) 2023;13(13):2167.

70. van Zeeland Y, Schoemaker N. Pain recognition in ferrets. Vet Clin North Am Exot Anim Pract 2023;26(1):229–43.

71. Deflers H, Gandar F, Bolen G, et al. Influence of a single dose of buprenorphine on rabbit (Oryctolagus cuniculus) gastrointestinal motility. Vet Anaesth analgesia 2018;45:510–9.

72. Michalski CW, Laukert T, Sauliunaite D, et al. Cannabinoids ameliorate pain and reduce disease pathology in cerulein-induced acute pancreatitis. Gastroenterology 2007;132:1968–78.

73. Schnellbacher RW, Divers SJ, Comolli JR, et al. Effects of intravenous administration of lidocaine and buprenorphine on gastrointestinal tract motility and signs of pain in New Zealand White rabbits after ovariohysterectomy. Am J Vet Res 2017;78(12):1359–71.

74. Askar R, Fredriksson E, Manell E, et al. Bioavailability of subcutaneous and intramuscular administrated buprenorphine in New Zealand White rabbits. BMC Vet Res 2020;16:1–10.

75. Myers PH, Goulding DR, Wiltshire RA, et al. Serum buprenorphine concentrations and behavioral activity in mice after a single subcutaneous injection of simbadol, buprenorphine SR-LAB, or standard buprenorphine. J Am Assoc Lab Anim Sci 2021;60(6):661–6.

76. Mayer J, Pignon C. Rodents. In: Carpenter JW, Harms CA, editors. Carpenter's exotic animal formulary. 6th edition. St Louis (MO): Elsevier; 2023. p. 767–837.

77. Shafford HL, Schadt JC. Effect of buprenorphine on the cardiovascular and respiratory response to visceral pain in conscious rabbits. Vet Anaesth Analg 2008; 35(4):333–40.

78. Allweiler SI. How to improve anesthesia and analgesia in small mammals. Vet Clin North Am Exot Anim Pract 2016;19(2):361–77.

79. Applegate JR, Harms CA. Ferrets. In: Carpenter JW, Harms CA, editors. Carpenter's exotic animal formulary. 6th edition. St Louis (MO): Elsevier; 2023. p. 930–85.

80. Ozawa SM, Hawkins MG, Drazenovich TL, et al. Pharmacokinetics of maropitant citrate in New Zealand White rabbits (*Oryctolagus cuniculus*). Am J Vet Res 2019;80(10):963–8.

81. Roeder M, Boscan P, Rao S, et al. Use of maropitant for pain management in domestic rabbits (*Oryctolagus cuniculus*) undergoing elective orchiectomy or ovariohysterectomy. J Exot Pet Med 2023;47:14–20.

82. Okano S, Ikeura Y, Inatomi N. Effects of tachykinin NK1 receptor antagonists on the viscerosensory response caused by colorectal distention in rabbits. J Pharmacol Exp Ther 2002;300:925–31.

83. Lebkowska-Wieruszewska B, Kim TW, Chea B, et al. Pharmacokinetic profiles of the two major active metabolites of metamizole (dipyrone) in cats following three different routes of administration. J Vet Pharmacol Therapeut 2017;41:334–9.

84. Spalinger M, Schwarzfischer M, Niechcial A, et al. Evaluation of the effect of tramadol, paracetamol and metamizole on the severity of experimental colitis. Lab Anim 2023;57(5):529–40.

85. Güitrón-Cantú A, Segura-López FK, Limones-Ortiz G, et al. Efecto del fentanilo a diferentes dosis y de la butilhioscina en el esfínter de Oddi del conejo [Effect of different doses of fentanyl and butylhyoscine on the rabbit's sphincter of Oddi]. Rev Gastroenterol Mex 2011;76(2):89–96.

86. Onori L, Agio A, Taddei G, et al. Peristalsis regulation by tachykin NK1 receptors in the rabbit isolated distal colon. Am J Physiol Gastrointest Liver Physiol 2003; 285:G325–31.

87. Fredholm DV, Carpenter JW, KuKanich B, et al. Pharmacokinetics of meloxicam in rabbits after oral administration of single and multiple doses. Am J Vet Res 2013;74:636–41.

88. Cheatham SM, Muchhala KH, Koseli E, et al. Morphine exacerbates experimental colitis-induced depression of nesting in mice. Front Pain Res (Lausanne) 2021;2:738499.

89. Murphy KL, Roughan JV, Baxter MG, et al. Anaesthesia with a combination of ketamine and medetomidine in the rabbit: effect of premedication with buprenorphine. Vet Anaesth Analg 2010;37(3):222–9.

90. Katzenbach JE, Wittenburg LA, Allweiler SI, et al. Pharmacokinetics of single-dose buprenorphine, butorphanol, and hydromorphone in the domestic ferret (*Mustela putorius furo*). J Exot Pet Med 2018;27:95–102.

91. Desprez I, Crookes A, Di Girolamo N, et al. Subcutaneous administration of hydromorphone (0.2 mg/kg) provides antinociception in ferrets (*Mustela putorius furo*). Am J Vet Res 2023;84(10):1–7.

92. Hech B, Knych H, Desprez I, et al. Pharmacokinetics of hydrorphone hydrochloride after intravenous and subcutaneous administration in ferrets (*Mustela putorius furo*). Vet Anaesth Analg 2024;51(2):152–9.

93. Barlass U, Dutta R, Cheema H, et al. Morphine worsens the severity and prevents pancreatic regeneration in mouse models of acute pancreatitis. Gut 2018;67(4):600–2.

94. Durst M, Graf TR, Graf R, et al. Analysis of pain and analgesia protocols in acute cerulein-induced pancreatitis in male C57BL/6 mice. Front Physiol 2021;12:744638.

95. Chinnadurai S, Messenger K, Papich M, et al. Meloxicam pharmacokinetics using nonlinear mixed-effects modeling in ferrets after single subcutaneous administration. J Vet Pharmacol Ther 2014;37:382–7.

96. Delk KW, Carpenter JW, KuKanich B, et al. Pharmacokinetics of meloxicam administered orally to rabbits (*Oryctolagus cuniculus*) for 29 days. Am J Vet Res 2014;75:195–9.

97. Purnomo E, Nugrahaningsih DAA, Agustriani N, et al. Comparison of metamizole and paracetamol effects on colonic anastomosis and fibroblast activities in Wistar rats. BMC Pharmacol Toxicol 2020;21(1):6.

98. Ruiz-Pérez D, Benito J, Largo C, et al. Metamizole (dipyrone) effects on sevoflurane requirements and postoperative hyperalgesia in rats. Lab Anim 2017;51(4):365–75.

99. Baumgartner CM, Koenighau H, Ebner JK, et al. Cardiovascular effects of dipyrone and propofol on hemodynamic function in rabbits. Am J Vet Res 2009;70:1407–15.

100. Baumgartner C, Koenighaus H, Ebner J, et al. Comparison of dipyrone/propofol versus fentanyl/propofol anaesthesia during surgery in rabbits. Lab Anim 2011;45(1):38–44.

101. Freo U, Ruocco C, Valerio A, et al. Paracetamol: a review of guideline recommendations. J Clin Med 2021;10(15):3420.

102. Court MH. Acetaminophen UDP-glucuronosyltransferase in ferrets: species and gender differences, and sequence analysis of ferret UGT1A6. J Vet Pharmacol Ther 2001;24(6):415–22.

103. Overman MC. A review of ferret toxicoses. J Exot Pet Med 2015;24:398–422.

104. Benchaoui HA, Cox SR, Schneider RP, et al. The pharmacokinetics of maropitant, a novel neurokinin type-1 receptor antagonist, in dogs. J Vet Pharmacol Ther 2007;30:336–44.

105. Hickman MA, Cox SR, Mahabir S, et al. Safety, pharmacokinetics and use of the novel NK-1 receptor antagonist maropitant (Cerenia) for the prevention of emesis and motion sickness in cats. J Vet Pharmacol Ther 2008;31:220–9.

106. Grayck M, Sullivan MN, Boscan P, et al. Use of subcutaneous maropitant at two dosages for pain management in domestic rabbits (Oryctolagus cuniculus) undergoing elective ovariohysterectomy or orchiectomy. Top Companion Anim Med 2024;61:100888.

107. Karna SR, Kongara K, Singh PM, et al. Evaluation of analgesic interaction between morphine, dexmedetomidine and maropitant using hot-plate and tail-flick tests in rats. Vet Anaesth Analg 2019;46(4):476–82.

108. Huckins GL, Tournade C, Patson C, et al. Lidocaine constant rate infusion improves the probability of survival in rabbits with gastrointestinal obstructions: 64 cases (2012-2021). J Am Vet Med Assoc 2023;262(1):61–7.

109. Escobar A, Dzikiti BT, Thorogood JC, et al. Effects of two continuous infusion doses of lidocaine on isoflurane minimum anesthetic concentration in chickens. Vet Anaesth Analg 2023;50(1):91–7.

110. Da Cunha AF, Messenger KM, Stout RW, et al. Pharmacokinetics of lidocaine after a single intravenous administration in chickens (*Gallus domesticus*) anesthetized with isoflurane. Vet Pharmacol Ther 2012;35:604–7.

111. Brandao J, da Cunha AF, Pypendop B, et al. Cardiovascular tolerance of intravenous lidocaine in broiler chickens (*Gallus gallus domesticus*) anesthetized with isoflurane. Vet Anaesth Analg 2015;42:442–8.

112. Schnellbacher R, Comolli J. Constant rate infusions in exotic animals J Exot Pet. Med 2020;35:50–7.

113. Imani H, Vesal N, Mohammadi-Samani S. Evaluation of intravenous lidocaine overdose in chickens (*Gallus domesticus*). Iran J Vet Surg 2013;8(1):9–15.

114. Fisher P, Graham J. Rabbits. In: Carpenter JW, Harms CA, editors. Carpenter's exotic animal formulary. 6th edition. St Louis (MO): Elsevier; 2023. p. 838–928.

115. Frohlich J, Mayer J. Rodents. In: Carpenter JW, Harms CA, editors. Carpenter's exotic animal formulary. 6th edition. St Louis (MO): Elsevier; 2023. p. 379–415.

116. van Zeeland YR, Schoemaker NJ. Analgesia, anesthesia, and monitoring. In: Graham JE, Doss GA, Beaufrere H, editors. Exotic animal emergency and critical care medicine. Hoboken (NJ): Wiley Blackwell; 2021. p. 234–56.

Zoonotic Gastroenteric Diseases of Exotic Animals

Caitlin M. Hepps Keeney, DVM, DACZM[a],
Olivia A. Petritz, DVM, DACZM[b],*

KEYWORDS

- Zoonoses • Gastroenteric • Salmonella • Campylobacter • Giardia

KEY POINTS

- Yearly outbreaks of reptile-associated salmonellosis (RAS) have been reported in the United States since 2019. Factors such as antimicrobial resistance, diet, husbandry, and the growing popularity of reptiles as household pets are all possible contributing factors in the ongoing spread of RAS infections.
- Contact with backyard poultry has been associated with more salmonellosis outbreaks in the United States than any other species of animal, and children aged less than 5 years have been disproportionately affected.
- *Giardia* sp. is a parasite commonly found in the gastrointestinal tract of various mammalian species. However, many Giardia assemblages are host specific, with the majority of human-related cases coming from species that frequently shed Giardia assemblages that have broader pathogenicity. Chinchillas are the exotic pet most frequently reported to cause Giardiasis in humans.
- People at higher risk of illness from all zoonotic diseases, gastrointestinal or other, include children younger than 5 years, adults aged 65 years or older, pregnant women, and people with weakened immune systems due to disease and/or immunosuppressive drugs.

INTRODUCTION

As exotic pet ownership increases in the United States and abroad, so have the reports of zoonoses from those nontraditional pets. There are several routes of transmission for gastrointestinal zoonotic diseases, with fecal-oral being one of the most prevalent. This is also a significant human health concern, as direct contact with the animal is not required for infection if the pathogen can be spread via feces and thus contaminated environments. Of the gastrointestinal zoonoses, *Salmonella* spp. is the most concerning and infected animals are often asymptomatic carriers that intermittently shed the bacteria. It has a wide host range, and among exotic pets, the most

[a] Columbus Zoo and Aquarium, Powell, OH, USA; [b] Department of Clinical Sciences, North Carolina State University, College of Veterinary Medicine, Raleigh, NC, USA
* Corresponding author.
E-mail address: oapetrit@ncsu.edu

Vet Clin Exot Anim 28 (2025) 365–379
https://doi.org/10.1016/j.cvex.2024.11.007   vetexotic.theclinics.com

Abbreviations	
CDC	Centers for Disease Control
FDA	Food and Drug Administration
RAS	reptile-associated salmonellosis

commonly infected species are reptiles, backyard poultry, and hedgehogs. However, both live pet and deceased feeder rodents have also been associated with Salmonella outbreaks in the United States. Campylobacter and Giardia are also important zoonotic agents of exotic pets that often do not cause clinical signs in infected animals. This article reviews the current literature on these and other gastrointestinal zoonoses originating from nontraditional pets, including summaries of recent outbreaks and mitigation strategies to prevent infection in owners and veterinary personnel.

BACTERIAL ZOONOSES
Salmonellosis

Salmonella is a genus of Gram-negative, rod-shaped bacteria belonging to the family *Enterobacteriaceae*.[1] The genus is divided into 2 species, *Salmonella enterica* and *Salmonella bongori*, with *S enterica* being divided into 6 subspecies.[1] Salmonella is also classified based on its propensity to produce clinical disease in humans, with more pathogenic serovars being classified as typhoidal, and less pathogenic as non-typhoidal.[1] Most cases of zoonotic Salmonella are caused by non-typhoidal serovars and result in gastrointestinal signs in people, though more severe disease can occur particularly in immunocompromised individuals.[2] Globally, Salmonella causes up to 1.3 billion cases of clinical disease and 3 million deaths annually, with 1.2 million infections and 450 deaths occurring in the United States alone.[1] Although the majority of these cases are linked to contaminated food, the role of pets is not insignificant and is expanded upon by taxa below.

Reptiles and amphibians
Salmonellosis is the most commonly contracted zoonosis from pet reptiles.[3] The first case of reptile-associated salmonellosis (RAS) in a human was reported in 1943, originating from a turtle.[2] Case frequency has increased over the intervening decades as the ownership of reptiles has increased, with a 2019 to 2020 survey finding approximately 4.5 million reptile owners in the United States.[1,4] In the 1970s, the Food and Drug Administration (FDA) implemented several programs with the intention of eliminating Salmonella in pet reptiles.[2] These programs included verification of Salmonella-free status in order to travel across state lines, prophylactic treatment of turtles with antimicrobials, and dipping eggs in antimicrobial solutions.[2] All of these methods ultimately proved ineffective, with patterns of antimicrobial resistance developing in direct response to these practices.[2] In 1975, the FDA placed a ban on the sale of turtles with a carapace length of less than 4 inches in order to mitigate Salmonella transmission from young turtles, a ban that remains in place to this day.[3]

Salmonella spp. are considered to be a normal part of the gut flora in reptiles, though they are also capable of causing disease in the host.[5] Reptiles can be infected with Salmonella via multiple routes, including transovarial, direct contact with other infected reptiles, and/or consumption of contaminated food.[3] Infected reptiles can shed the bacteria intermittently, with or without associated clinical signs, and some species of snakes have been documented to carry more than one serotype of Salmonella at a time.[3] RAS is caused by non-typhoidal Salmonella serovars and typically results in self-limiting gastrointestinal signs in people, though more serious infections leading to meningitis, sepsis, and death have been reported.[1] These potentially life-threatening infections are commonly seen in children, the elderly, or people with compromised immune function.[1] Despite the overall low prevalence of severe infections, patients with RAS have a higher rate of hospitalization compared to patients without RAS, indicating that reptile-associated infections are more likely to result in severe clinical presentation.[1]

The most commonly reported RAS isolate in human infections is *S enterica* subsp *enterica* (I), accounting for approximately 90% of human cases.[5] Other subspecies that have been reported to cause RAS include *S enterica* subsp. *salamae* (II), *S enterica* subsp. *arizonae* (IIIb), *S enterica* subsp. *diarizonae* (IIIb), *S enterica* subsp. *houtenae* (IV), and *S enterica* subsp. *indica* (VI).[1] The most significant outbreaks of RAS in the United States occurred in 2015 and 2016 and were linked to pet turtles.[3] The majority of patients were children, with 40% of affected individuals requiring hospitalization, but no mortalities were recorded.[1] RAS-linked outbreaks in the United States have occurred at least once yearly since 2019, with 2 outbreaks being reported in 2024.[6] One outbreak was linked to pet central bearded dragons (*Pogona vitticeps*) and the other to small turtles. Both outbreaks and associated investigations are considered ongoing at the time of writing.[6] Overall, the majority of RAS infections are considered sporadic, with few outbreaks of epidemiologic significance.

Reports of Salmonella prevalence in reptiles are mixed, with ranges from 2.1% to 87.5% depending on region and species sampled.[1] Overall trends indicate that Salmonella is most commonly detected in snakes, followed by lizards, chelonians, and crocodilians.[5] These findings are in contrast with reported sources of RAS infections, with chelonians being the most common, followed by lizards and snakes.[5] This discrepancy is likely due to multiple factors, one of which is that Salmonella shedding is often intermittent, and a negative result at any given time point is not necessarily truly representative of the presence or lack of Salmonella in that individual.[5] Additional factors, such as husbandry and stress, can also influence shedding, both of which may vary widely between studies done underlying differing conditions.[5] Temperature in particular may influence both the replication and shedding of Salmonella, with higher temperatures promoting bacterial growth, favoring virulence factors of specific Salmonella serovars, as well as potentially influencing the immune response of the host.[5] An additional factor that should be considered when evaluating the sources of RAS infections is the popularity of different reptile taxa as pets, as this may be a stronger influencing factor than simple prevalence of Salmonella.[5] Similarly, the amount of direct contact that owners have with different species may vary, as well as contact with their environment. For example, aquatic turtles may be more likely to spread Salmonella due to its persistence in water and the increased contact of humans with the environment during cleaning and handling.[5] Therefore, although studies regarding prevalence and shedding of Salmonella in various species are helpful for monitoring trends, they should also be evaluated within the context of a multitude of factors that can lead to zoonotic transmission.

One important factor impacting the likelihood and severity of RAS infections is the changing and growing patterns of antimicrobial resistance in Salmonella species. Early attempts at control strategies are thought to have catalyzed initial patterns of resistance, but antibiotic overuse in pet reptiles, as well as in the food chain, has continued to influence and generate the development of resistant serovars.[2] A 2016 study evaluating antimicrobial resistance in non-typhoidal Salmonella found resistant and multidrug-resistant isolates comprising less than 20% and less than 10% of human cases, respectively.[7] However, the authors emphasize that patterns of resistance demonstrate serovar-specific differences, as well as location-specific differences, making it difficult to assess overall patterns.[7]

A 2022 study looking specifically at Salmonella prevalence and antimicrobial resistance in reptiles species found that 68% of isolated Salmonella species were resistant to at least one antimicrobial.[8] Multidrug-resistant strains were isolated multiple times from clinically normal individuals, regardless of their origin (ie, wild or domesticated).[8] Of note, a higher prevalence of Salmonella was found in domesticated individuals when compared with wild ones.[8] Clinicians should be aware of the potential for augmenting resistance when making any decisions regarding the treatment of Salmonella in a reptile. Reducing zoonotic transmission of Salmonella requires a One Health approach including maintaining animal health, biosecurity, food decontamination, and hygienic practices to reduce human infection.[4] Antibiotics should be used judiciously and may be inappropriate even in certain symptomatic cases of reptilian Salmonella. Probiotics have been suggested as a means of combating Salmonella overgrowth in reptile gastrointestinal tracts without increasing the risk of antibiotic resistance.[5] Positive health outcomes have been reported in reptiles treated with probiotics, but none linked specifically to salmonellosis at this time.[5] It is worth noting that, although probiotics may play a role in reducing the growth and shedding of Salmonella in asymptomatic reptiles, it is unlikely to be a successful sole therapeutic for an animal exhibiting clinical signs of salmonellosis. The uses of prebiotics and bacteriophages are also potential avenues for reduction of Salmonella replication and shedding from the gastrointestinal tract, though few studies have been done in reptile species at this time.[5]

The role that diet may play in Salmonella infections is an emerging area of study. Some have postulated that there may be a higher prevalence of Salmonella based on the feeding strategy of the reptiles, whether they be herbivorous, omnivorous, or carnivorous.[1] A 2016 study looking at zoo-housed reptiles found that although prevalence was not necessarily impacted by diet, the likelihood of developing Salmonella-related illness was significantly associated with a carnivorous diet, as well as a history of prior confiscation.[9] Another study found that changing diet items within the same individuals of the same species can significantly alter the gut microbiota that is present, including the likelihood of detecting Salmonella and other opportunistically pathogenic bacteria.[10] Further research is warranted to determine what recommendations can be made regarding the influence of diet in preventing the growth and shedding of Salmonella in reptiles.

Although amphibians are a less common source of salmonellosis, comprising less than 1% of human cases, their potential for disease transmission should not be overlooked.[1] A 2015 study linked 3 cases of salmonellosis to amphibian ownership in children.[11] Additionally, prevalence of Salmonella spp. in farmed amphibians has been reported to be as high as 90%, indicating the possibility for increases in Amphibian-associated salmonellosis depending on the source of the pet amphibians.[1] The importance of the international wildlife trade should also be considered a cause of increasing cases of Salmonella in both amphibian and reptile species. Illegal trading of wildlife is the world's fourth largest illegal business, and the majority of illegally traded reptiles and amphibians being imported into the United States are sold as pets.[1] These animals are typically transported, held, and managed in suboptimal conditions, creating a higher likelihood of stress-induced shedding of Salmonella.[1] International regulations and management of illegal pet trade will continue to be a necessity for prevention and management of reptile and amphibian-associated cases of salmonellosis.

Backyard poultry

Chickens can be infected with several serotypes of *Salmonella* spp., and these are typically categorized as host-adapted and non-host-adapted, the latter of which are also termed paratyphoid infections. Host-adapted Salmonella are nationally reportable diseases in the United States and include *S enterica* Gallinarum biovars Gallinarium and Pullorum that cause Fowl typhoid and Pullorum disease, respectively.[12] Both Fowl typhoid and Pullorum disease cause systemic disease mainly in young birds, characterized by anorexia, dehydration, weight loss, and diarrhea. Both diseases can cause acute high mortality rates in young birds and they have largely been eradicated from commercial poultry flocks in the United States and abroad. However, these diseases persist in commercial flocks from certain countries as well as in-game bird and backyard flocks in the United States.[12] The National Poultry Improvement Plan was established in the United States in the 1930s to help reduce the incidence of Pullorum Disease (*S enterica* Gallinarum biovar Pullorum), and this has expanded to include Fowl typhoid as well as several other poultry diseases including mycoplasmosis and avian influenza—additional information on this national organization can be found on their Web site (https://www.poultryimprovement.org/). This is a great resource for prevention strategies, not just for commercial poultry operations, but also for owners of smaller backyard poultry farms. Even though all these diseases, host-adapted and non-host-adapted, are part of the *S enterica* complex, the host-adapted species pose minimal zoonotic risk; therefore, the remainder of this section will focus on non-host-adapted Salmonella.[12]

Paratyphoid or non-host-adapted Salmonella can infect many different species across taxa, including humans. Asymptomatic infections in chickens are common, with colonization of the intestinal tract and subsequent shedding within the feces.[12] The bacteria can subsequently invade the intestinal epithelium and disseminate to other internal organs. While national data for backyard poultry are lacking, in commercial broiler flocks, 35% of sampled spleens, livers, and gall bladders were positive for *Salmonella* at the age of 6 to 8 weeks.[13] The reported worldwide prevalence of Salmonella in commercial poultry flocks worldwide is quite variable depending on the flock, purpose (ie, broilers vs egg-layers) and year sampled; ranging from 9% to 57%.[12,14–16] Significant variability has also been reported with backyard flocks, which likely reflects sampling bias and potentially intermittent shedding of the bacteria.[17] Similar to pet reptiles, all backyard poultry should be treated as if they may be positive for Salmonella and proper biosecurity measures followed.[3]

Fecal contamination of the eggshell is the main form of transmission to juvenile birds; however, some serovars can also be transmitted transovarially.[12] Young birds can uncommonly develop clinical signs of disease, including lethargy, reduced weight gain, diarrhea, and dehydration; morbidity and mortality are highest in chicks at the age of 2 to 3 weeks.[12] There are numerous commercially available diagnostic tests for Salmonella in poultry including conventional cultures and more rapid tests such as enzyme immunoassay and polymerase chain reaction (PCR).[12,18] Killed and live Salmonella vaccines have been shown to reduce infection of commercial chickens and subsequent contamination of their eggs; however, the efficacy of these vaccines is not well studied in backyard flocks.[19,20]

Systemic antibiotics, including fluoroquino, were once routinely used for treatment and prevention of Salmonella in commercial poultry worldwide.[21,22] However, this and other indiscriminate use of antibiotics have led to increasing incidences of antibiotic resistance in commercial poultry and poultry products, in addition to reduced antibiotic efficacy.[23–25] In the United States and in many other countries, fluroquinolones are illegal to use in major food-producing species, including chickens and turkeys, regardless of their intended use (egg-laying, broilers, pets, etc.). In some cases, antibiotic therapy increased the susceptibility of chickens to Salmonella infections, suspected to be secondary to derangements of their normal gastrointestinal flora.[26] Therefore, treatment of salmonellosis in commercial poultry is no longer recommended.[12] Biosecurity and sanitation are key preventative measures for reduction of Salmonella infection in both commercial and backyard poultry flocks. If not already infected at the time of purchase, Salmonella can be introduced into a flock via contaminated feed, exposure to wild animals, and/or peridomestic rodents (see Rodent section). Salmonella is also incredibly resistant to the environment, and it has been isolated from an empty poultry house for upward of 1 year in dust despite disinfection.[27]

Humans can acquire Salmonella from exposure to live poultry and poultry products, such as chicken meat and/or eggs. Greater than 70% of all human Salmonella infections in the United States are connected to ingestion of contaminated chicken, turkey, or eggs, and an estimated 11% are due to exposure to live poultry.[28,29] In fact, contact with backyard poultry has been associated with more Salmonella outbreaks in the United States than any other species of animal.[29,30] From 2015 to 2022, there have been 88 multistate outbreaks of Salmonella associated with backyard poultry within the United States, with 7866 reported human illnesses; children aged less than 5 years were disproportionately impacted with these outbreaks compared with other age classes.[29] This represents a nearly 3 times increase in outbreak-associated illnesses compared with data from 1990 to 2014, which could in part reflect the growing population of backyard poultry within the United States.[29]

Infection can stem from direct and indirect contact with live poultry, the latter of which includes contact with poultry shipping crates, food/water dishes, soil, and consumption of food or drink where poultry have been. Poultry routinely have fecal contamination on their feathers and feet, so acquisition of Salmonella from live poultry is not restricted to solely handling poultry feces. It is not recommended to keep poultry, even those considered pets, indoors where food is prepared or consumed, or to wash poultry food/water containers in kitchen sinks.[3,31,32] The best way to prevent salmonellosis is to always wash your hands with soap and water immediately after handling live poultry or anything/anywhere poultry have been (**Fig. 1**). In addition, the Centers for Disease Control (CDC) does not recommend that children aged less than 5 years have any direct interaction with backyard poultry, as they are not yet immunocompetent at that age.[29] Extensive recommendations for owners of backyard poultry including coup design, biosecurity protocols, cleaning, and quarantine recommendations are available on the CDC Web page (https://www.cdc.gov/healthy-pets/about/backyard-poultry.html).

Rodents

Of all reported zoonotic illnesses associated with pet small mammals (rodents, rabbits, hedgehogs, sugar gliders, and ferrets) from 1996 to 2017, Salmonella was the most common pathogen, and rodents were associated with over half of those reported cases.[3] S enterica serovars Enteritidis (*Salmonella enteritidis*) and Typhimurium are the most common isolates from rodents.[33] The vast majority of infected rodents, both wild and domestic, are asymptomatic, with the notable exception of guinea pigs. Clinical signs of salmonellosis in infected guinea pigs can include lethargy, anorexia, and hemorrhagic diarrhea in some cases, with a reported incubation period of 5 to 7 days.[1,33] Similar to other species, treatment of Salmonella-infected guinea pigs does not guarantee elimination of a carrier state.[34] The first reported outbreak of salmonellosis associated with exposure to pet guinea pigs in the United States occurred in

HEALTHY FAMILIES AND FLOCKS

Live poultry, such as chickens, ducks, geese, and turkeys, often carry harmful germs such as *Salmonella*. While it usually doesn't make the birds sick, *Salmonella* can cause serious illness when it is passed to people.

HANDWASHING PROTECTS YOU FROM GERMS

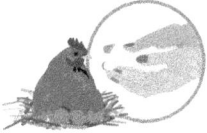

- Always wash your hands with soap and water right after touching live poultry or anything in the area where they live and roam.
- Adults should supervise hand washing for young children.
- Use hand sanitizer if soap and water are not readily available.

HANDLE BIRDS SAFELY

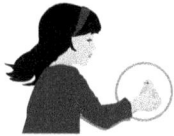

- Children younger than 5 years, adults older than 65 years, and people with weakened immune systems should not handle or touch chicks, ducklings, or other live poultry.
- Do not bring chicks, ducklings and other live poultry to schools, childcare centers, or nursing homes.
- Do not snuggle or kiss the birds, touch your mouth, or eat or drink around live poultry.

SAFELY CLEAN COOPS

- Clean any equipment used to care for live poultry outside, such as cages or feed or water containers.
- Set aside a pair of shoes to wear while taking care of poultry and keep those shoes outside of the house.

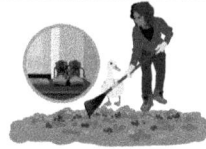

POULTRY BELONG OUTSIDE

- Do not let live poultry inside the house, especially in kitchens.
- Do not let live poultry in areas where food or drink is prepared, served, or stored.

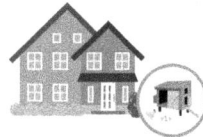

CDC
U.S. Department of
Health and Human Services
Centers for Disease
Control and Prevention

Have a Backyard Flock? Don't Wing it.
Visit www.cdc.gov/features/salmonellapoultry
for more information

Fig. 1. This poster entitled "Healthy Families and Flocks" from the Centers for Disease Control (CDC) describes ways that owners can help prevent zoonoses (*Salmonella* spp. and others) from backyard chickens and their eggs. (Healthy families and flocks, CDC STACKS: https://stacks.cdc.gov/view/cdc/44796.)

2010, and 10 patients were infected, 60% of which were aged less than 12 years.[34] An additional outbreak of salmonellosis linked to infected pet guinea pigs was reported in the United States from 2015 to 2017, with 9 human cases in 8 states.[35]

Twenty-eight cases of rodent-associated multidrug-resistant Salmonella infections (*S enterica* serovar Typhimurium) were documented in the United States from December 2003 to September 2004.[36] Among these cases, 59% reported exposure to pet hamsters, mice, or rats. The median age of affected persons was at the age of

16 years and 40% of patients required hospitalization. In addition, there have been several reported outbreaks of salmonellosis in people linked to contact with live and deceased feeder rodents, mainly mice, both nationally and internationally.[37–39] A global systematic review published in 2023 found 62 publications on zoonotic pathogens associated with pet and feeder murid rodents; *Leptospira* spp. and *Salmonella* spp. were the most prevalent zoonoses, and pet rodents accounted for 71% of the articles with only 26% from feeder rodents.[40] While not the focus of this article, it is important to recognize that at least 8 species of wild rodents serve as reservoirs for *Salmonella* spp., and these infected wild rodents can transmit this bacterium to mammalian livestock and poultry leading to foodborne illnesses in humans.[41,42] Only 15 *Salmonella* Enteritidis cells are needed to successfully infect a mouse (*Mus musculus*), and that same mouse will shed approximately 230,000 Salmonella in a single fecal pellet—and that same mouse will produce up to 100 fecal pellets in 24 hours. Therefore, a single mouse can introduce 23 million *Salmonella* bacteria into an environment (enclosure, house, barn, etc.) in 1 day.[41] Pet rodents are likely an under-recognized source of human salmonella infections; veterinary staff and owners should be aware of this risk from not only live pet rodents, but also wild and deceased feeder rodents.

Hedgehogs

The African pygmy hedgehog (*Atelerix albiventris*) is the most commonly kept species of hedgehog in the United States and is considered a reservoir host for Salmonella.[43] The most common species of Salmonella isolated from hedgehogs are *S enterica* serovar Typhimurium, *S enterica* serovar Stanley, and *Salmonella tilene*.[44] Salmonella is found in both wild and companion hedgehogs, and although human cases are uncommon, there have been 3 separate documented Salmonella outbreaks within the United States.[45] The longest outbreak spanned multiple states from 2011 to 2013, with isolation of *S enterica* serovar Typhimurium that was linked to contact with pet hedgehogs.[45] Additional outbreaks occurred in both 2018 to 2019 and 2020, with the most recent outbreak resulting in 49 cases and 11 hospitalizations.[6] A study investigating the 2018 to 2019 outbreak used whole genome sequencing to determine that isolates were highly related to the isolates from the 2011 to 2013 outbreak.[46] Therefore, although these outbreaks occur in clusters, it is likely that similar strains continue to spread even during non-outbreak periods.[46] This article also highlighted the role of breeders in prevention, citing CDC recommendations to test and remove positive hedgehogs from breeding colonies in order to mitigate the ongoing sale of known Salmonella-positive animals.[46]

Hedgehogs can be asymptomatic carriers of Salmonella or can develop associated clinical signs including diarrhea, with the most classic form being green and mucoid.[44] Other signs include weight loss, anorexia, lethargy, and sudden death.[43] Treatment of Salmonella in pet hedgehogs is controversial given the risk of zoonosis and development of antimicrobial resistance but can include fluid therapy, probiotics, analgesia, and, in severe cases, systemic antibiotics.[44] Routine testing is not recommended in healthy animals, but fecal culture is considered the gold standard diagnostic and should be performed if the hedgehog is showing clinical signs or if a suspected zoonotic transmission has occurred. Subclinical carriers may shed intermittently, with comorbidities or stress increasing the likelihood of shedding.[44] Therefore, additional hygienic precautions or possible isolation should be considered in any ill hedgehog.

Primates

Nonhuman primates, while less commonly kept as household pets, are also considered to be a possible source of Salmonella infection in humans.[47,48] Reports of Salmonella linked to primates are rare, and most commonly occur in children.[47] Findings from the National Research Council suggest that pathogenic Salmonella strains in primates are most often contracted from exposure to infected humans and are less likely to be transmitted back to humans.[49] However, any primate with diarrhea or other gastrointestinal signs should be considered a possible Salmonella risk and should be treated with appropriate caution.

Campylobacteriosis

Campylobacter spp. are Gram-negative, curved bacilli that are transmitted via the fecal-oral route and are responsible for up to 9% of foodborne illness in the United States.[50] The *Campylobacter* genus consists of 32 species and 9 subspecies, with the vast majority of cases of campylobacteriosis in humans being caused by *Campylobacter jejuni* subs. *jejuni*, and a smaller proportion being caused by *Campylobacter coli* and other species.[50] Some species, such as *Campylobacter upsaliensis*, have been frequently isolated from animals but have not yet been reported to cause disease in humans.[51] Most commonly, campylobacteriosis presents as self-limiting gastroenteritis, fever, and weakness, though in a small percentage of cases complications can occur including peripheral neuropathies, reactive arthritis, and chronic intestinal disorders such as irritable bowel syndrome.[50]

Consumption of contaminated meat and eggs from poultry accounts for 50% to 80% of foodborne cases of human campylobacteriosis, though close contact with a variety of species can result in infection as well if proper hygiene is not observed.[51,52] Backyard chickens in particular are a known source of campylobacteriosis, particularly when eggs are consumed without being properly decontaminated.[51] Outbreaks are rarely reported and infections occur sporadically.[3] It has also been suggested that human infections are likely under-reported, as it is not a reportable disease, and cases may be higher than current data suggest.[3] A meta-analysis evaluating the prevalence of Campylobacter in petting zoos and household pets found that pets had a higher prevalence of pathogenic *Campylobacter* sp. than petting zoos, with 34% of fecal samples being positive.[51] Although *C jejuni* does not readily replicate outside of the gastrointestinal (GI) tract, it can survive for several weeks in the environment, including at lower temperatures, meaning that transmission can occur through indirect as well as direct contact with shedding animals.[50] Campylobacter is a common commensal in a variety of animal species and can be shed by clinically healthy animals, though shedding is typically more common in animals with diarrhea.[53]

Although Campylobacter has been well described in mammals and birds, transmission from reptile species is also possible and may be underreported.[52] Species such as *C jejuni* have been isolated from reptile species but are more commonly found in endotherms.[52] In reptiles, the most commonly isolated species of Campylobacter are *C. fetus* subsp *testudinum* and *C fetus* subsp *fetus* both of which have been isolated from clinically healthy as well as symptomatic reptiles. These species are considered to be less pathogenic than *C jejuni* and related species but have been shown to cause disease in immunocompromised humans.[52] A closely related species, *Campylobacter iguaniorum*, has also been identified in reptiles though this species has yet to be linked to human disease.[52] As the number of household reptiles continues to grow, further research is needed to determine the prevalence and zoonotic risk associated with these less common species of Campylobacter.

PARASITIC ZOONOSES

A variety of endoparasites with a tropism for the gastrointestinal tract are capable of being passed from exotic pets to humans. This section is not meant to be a comprehensive list but will cover a few of the more clinically relevant parasites known to cause zoonotic disease in humans.

Giardiasis

Giardia duodenalis, sometimes also referred to as *Giardia intestinalis* and *Giardia lamblia*, is a protozoan enteric parasite commonly found in a variety of mammalian hosts.[54] Infection occurs by swallowing cysts, the infectious stage of that parasite, either indirectly through contaminated food or water, or directly through ingestion of feces.[55] Both humans and animals can be asymptomatic carriers or can develop clinical disease, typically presenting as acute or chronic diarrhea.[55] The exotic pet most often associated with transmission of Giardia is the chinchilla (*Chinchilla chinchilla*), with this species being known to carry zoonotic assemblages of Giardia, as well as multiple documented cases of human disease originating from contact with pet chinchillas.[54–56] Assemblages A and B are considered to have the widest host range, with assemblages C through H being most host-specific and less likely to cause zoonotic disease.[54] One study out of the Czech Republic found that all samples of chinchilla *G duodenalis* (n = 18) were characterized as assemblage B, indicating a higher likelihood of infection from chinchillas than from species shedding Giardia with different assemblages.[54] A 2021 meta-analysis reinforced these findings, stating that many domestic species shed primarily host-adapted assemblages, with zoonotic assemblages being less common than previously thought, and primarily coming from a small number species including chinchillas, guinea pigs, rabbits, and nonhuman primates.[57] Therefore, although caution and good hygiene practices should be implemented with species known to cause giardiasis, this disease is not considered high risk in all mammalian species that likely carry it.

Cryptosporidiosis

Cryptosporidium spp. is an apicomplexan parasite that is known to cause diarrheal disease in humans.[58] Infection happens through ingestion of oocysts and can occur through ingestion of infected water, or close contact with an infected animal.[58] *Cryptosporidium parvum* is the primary species associated with clinical disease in humans and most often originates from domestic ruminants, though it can be passed from a variety of mammalian species including rabbits.[58] Several other Cryptosporidium species have been identified in exotic pet species, including *Cryptosporidium muris* in rodents, *Cryptosporidium wrairi* in guinea pigs, *Cryptosporidium serpentis* in snakes, and *Cryptosporidium molnari* in fish, though none of these have been confirmed to be zoonotic.

Tapeworms

Tapeworms, such as *Echinococcus spp.*, can be found in exotic pet species such as rabbits, but their zoonotic potential relies on the consumption of undercooked meat and is unlikely to occur in the context of pet ownership.[58] One tapeworm of note is *Hymenolepis nana*, a zoonotic parasite that is most often associated with fecal transmission in rodents.[59] Although more common in Europe than the United States, *Hymenolepis* has a worldwide distribution and is the most common cestode infecting humans, particularly children.[59] Multiple surveys studies have been performed in European pet rodent populations, with presence of *H nana* eggs found in a variety of species including Chinchillas, mice, rats, gerbils, squirrels, and hamsters, with prevalences up to 42% in some species.[59–61] One of these surveys also found a significantly higher prevalence of eggs in pet store rodents compared to those in breeder colonies.[59] As with other enteric parasites, hygiene and appropriate disposal of pet fecal material is paramount to disease prevention. A variety of enteric parasites with known zoonotic potential have also been found in reptile and amphibian parasite surveys, but reports of transmission to humans are sparse to nonexistent.[62,63] Pets housed in appropriate conditions with a known acquisition history and proper husbandry are overall low risk for zoonotic parasitism. In most cases, standard hygiene is sufficient for preventing parasite transmission from exotic pets.

General preventative measures

Zoonotic diseases are transmitted by 3 main routes: vector-borne, aerosol, and contact. Contact transmission is the most applicable for gastroenteric diseases and this includes ingestion, cutaneous, percutaneous, or mucous membrane exposure.[64] The single most important preventative measure to prevent zoonotic diseases is consistent and thorough hand hygiene.[3,64,65] Hand hygiene includes standard handwashing with some form of soap and water, use of alcohol-based hand rubs, and appropriate use of gloves. Handwashing should be performed after handling an animal or any surface that an animal has contacted, after contact with feces and bodily fluids, and after removing gloves, if used.[64] Water temperature actually has little impact on the efficacy of handwashing, but warm water, if available, has been shown to increase compliance for most people.[66] Disposable towels are recommended over community or shared towels.[67] Alcohol-based hand sanitizers should contain at least 60% alcohol and are a reasonable alternative for fast disinfection, as they take approximately one-third the time required for appropriate hand disinfection compared with the use of soap and water.[64] However, these products are not effective against all types of pathogens.[3] The use of disposable gloves is also highly encouraged to prevent pathogen transmission especially when handling feces, exudates, bodily fluids, and deceased animals. However, gloves can easily become ripped when handling certain species due to claws and/or scales. Therefore, the use of disposable gloves is never a complete substitute for handwashing.

In addition to handwashing, there are other precautions one can take to prevent zoonotic disease from exotic pets, which may be more challenging to implement due to the strong bonds that can be present between exotic pets and their owners. These include not kissing or holding these animals close to your face and preventing them to roam free within the household, especially areas of food preparation.[3] In some cases, contact with and ownership of certain exotic pets are not recommended at all due to high risk of contracting a zoonotic disease; these include children younger than 5 years, adults aged 65 years or older, pregnant women, and people with weakened immune systems due to disease and/or immunosuppressive drugs.[3] The Compendium of Veterinary Standard Precautions for Zoonotic Prevention in Veterinary Personnel is a good resource for additional methods to prevent these diseases among veterinary hospital personnel.[65]

CLINICS CARE POINTS

- All reptiles should be considered possible shedders of Salmonella. Factors including husbandry, diet, reptile source, and stressors should all be evaluated if clinical salmonellosis is suspected in a reptile or human who has had contact with a reptile. The use of antibiotics is controversial and should be used judiciously in cases of reptile salmonellosis.

- Both Salmonella and Campylobacter should be considered zoonotic risks for backyard poultry owners, particularly as their popularity increases. Clients owning a backyard flock should be educated on proper egg (and meat, if applicable) decontamination to reduce risk of gastrointestinal disease transmission.

- Frozen, thawed feeder rodents still pose a zoonotic risk of salmonellosis, and the same precautions should be followed when handling deceased rodents as live rodents, including handwashing and appropriate disinfection of any surfaces the rodents came into contact with.
- The single most important preventative measure to prevent zoonotic diseases is consistent and thorough hand hygiene that includes standard handwashing with some form of soap and water, use of alcohol-based hand rubs, and appropriate use of disposable gloves.

DISCLOSURE

The authors have nothing to disclose.

REFERENCES

1. Dróźdż M, Małaszczuk M, Paluch E, et al. Zoonotic potential and prevalence of Salmonella serovars isolated from pets. Infect Ecol Epidemiol 2021;11:1975530.
2. Mitchell MA, Shane SM. Salmonella in reptiles. Seminars Avian Exot Pet Med 2001;25–35.
3. Varela K, Brown JA, Lipton B, et al. A review of zoonotic disease threats to pet owners: a compendium of measures to prevent zoonotic diseases associated with non-traditional pets such as rodents and other small mammals, reptiles, amphibians, backyard poultry, and other selected animals. Vector Borne Zoonotic Dis 2022;22:303–60.
4. Galán-Relaño Á, Valero Díaz A, Huerta Lorenzo B, et al. Salmonella and salmonellosis: an update on public health implications and control strategies. Animals 2023;13:3666.
5. Pees M, Brockmann M, Steiner N, et al. Salmonella in reptiles: a review of occurrence, interactions, shedding and risk factors for human infections. Front Cell Dev Biol 2023;11:1251036.
6. Outbreaks linked to animals and animal products. 2024. Available at: https://www.cdc.gov/healthy-pets/outbreaks/index.html. Accessed August 20, 2024.
7. Michael G, Schwarz S. Antimicrobial resistance in zoonotic nontyphoidal Salmonella: an alarming trend? Clin Microbiol Infect 2016;22:968–74.
8. Merkevičienė L, Butrimaitė-Ambrozevičienė Č, Paškevičius G, et al. Serological variety and antimicrobial resistance in Salmonella isolated from reptiles. Biology 2022;11:836.
9. Clancy MM, Davis M, Valitutto MT, et al. Salmonella infection and carriage in reptiles in a zoological collection. J Am Vet Med Assoc 2016;248:1050–9.
10. Jiang H-Y, Ma J-E, Li J, et al. Diets alter the gut microbiome of crocodile lizards. Front Microbiol 2017;8:2073.
11. Williams S, Patel M, Markey P, et al. Salmonella in the tropical household environment–everyday, everywhere. J Infect 2015;71:642–8.
12. Gast RK, Porter JrRE. Salmonella infections. In: Swayne DE, Boulianne M, Logue CM, et al, editors. Diseases of poultry. 2020. p. 717–53.
13. Cox N, Richardson L, Buhr R, et al. Recovery of Campylobacter and Salmonella serovars from the spleen, liver and gallbladder, and ceca of six-and eight-week-old commercial broilers. J Appl Poultry Res 2007;16:477–80.
14. Le Bouquin S, Allain V, Rouxel S, et al. Prevalence and risk factors for Salmonella spp. contamination in French broiler-chicken flocks at the end of the rearing period. Prev Vet Med 2010;97:245–51.

15. Pitesky M, Charlton B, Bland M, et al. Surveillance of Salmonella enteritidis in layer houses: a retrospective comparison of the Food and Drug Administration's egg safety rule (2010–2011) and the California Egg Quality Assurance Program (2007–2011). Avian Dis 2013;57:51–6.
16. Sivaramalingam T, McEwen SA, Pearl DL, et al. A temporal study of Salmonella serovars from environmental samples from poultry breeder flocks in Ontario between 1998 and 2008. Can J Vet Res 2013;77:1–11.
17. Larsen KM, DeCicco M, Hood K, et al. Salmonella enterica frequency in backyard chickens in Vermont and biosecurity knowledge and practices of owners. Front Vet Sci 2022;9:979548.
18. Waltman WD, Gast R. Salmonella enterica. In: Williams SMW, editor. A laboratory manual for the isolation and identification of avian pathogens. 6th edition. Jacksonville, FL: American Association of Avian Pathologists; 2016. p. 103–9.
19. Gast RK, Stone HD, Holt PS, et al. Evaluation of the efficacy of an oil-emulsion bacterin for protecting chickens against Salmonella enteritidis. Avian Dis 1992;992–9.
20. Arnold ME, Gosling RJ, La Ragione RM, et al. Estimation of the impact of vaccination on faecal shedding and organ and egg contamination for Salmonella Enteritidis, Salmonella Typhiumurium and monophasic Salmonella Typhimurium. Avian Pathol 2014;43:155–63.
21. McIlroy S, McCracken R, Neill S, et al. Control, prevention and eradication of Salmonella enteritidis infection in broiler and broiler breeder flocks. Vet Rec 1989;125:545–8.
22. Seo KH, Holt P, Gast R, et al. Combined effect of antibiotic and competitive exclusion treatment on Salmonella Enteritidis fecal shedding in molted laying hens. J Food Protect 2000;63:545–8.
23. Iwabuchi E, Maruyama N, Hara A, et al. Nationwide survey of Salmonella prevalence in environmental dust from layer farms in Japan. J Food Protect 2010;73:1993–2000.
24. Parveen S, Taabodi M, Schwarz JG, et al. Prevalence and antimicrobial resistance of Salmonella recovered from processed poultry. J Food Protect 2007;70:2466–72.
25. Shah DH, Paul NC, Sischo WC, et al. Population dynamics and antimicrobial resistance of the most prevalent poultry-associated Salmonella serotypes. Poultry Sci 2017;96:687–702.
26. Manning J, Hargis B, Hinton Jr A, et al. Effect of selected antibiotics and anticoccidials on Salmonella enteritidis cecal colonization and organ invasion in Leghorn chicks. Avian Dis 1994;256–61.
27. Davies R, Wray C. Persistence of Salmonella enteritidis in poultry units and poultry food. Br Poultry Sci 1996;37:589–96.
28. Guo C, Hoekstra RM, Schroeder CM, et al. Application of Bayesian techniques to model the burden of human salmonellosis attributable to US food commodities at the point of processing: adaptation of a Danish model. Foodb Pathog Dis 2011;8:509–16.
29. Stapleton GS, Habrun C, Nemechek K, et al. Multistate outbreaks of salmonellosis linked to contact with backyard poultry—United States, 2015–2022. Zoonoses Public Health 2024;71:708–22.
30. Waltenburg MA, Perez A, Salah Z, et al. Multistate reptile-and amphibian-associated salmonellosis outbreaks in humans, United States, 2009–2018. Zoonoses Public Health 2022;69:925–37.

31. Behravesh CB, Brinson D, Hopkins BA, et al. Backyard poultry flocks and salmonellosis: a recurring, yet preventable public health challenge. Clin Infect Dis 2014;58:1432–8.

32. Souza MJ. Zoonotic diseases. In: Greenacre C, Morishita T, editors. Backyard poultry medicine and surgery. 2nd ed. Hoboken, NJ: Wiley Blackwell; 2021. p. 195–205.

33. Mitchell M, Tully TN Jr. In: Quesenberry K, Orcutt CJ, Mans C, et al, editors. Ferrets, rabbits, and rodents clinical medicine and surgery. 4th ed. St. Louis, MO: Elsevier; 2021. p. 609–19. Zoonotic Diseases Associated with Small Mammals.

34. Bartholomew ML, Heffernan RT, Wright JG, et al. Multistate outbreak of Salmonella enterica serotype enteritidis infection associated with pet Guinea pigs. Vector Borne Zoonotic Dis 2014;14:414–21.

35. Robertson S, Burakoff A, Stevenson L, et al. Recurrence of a multistate outbreak of Salmonella enteritidis infections linked to contact with Guinea pigs-eight states, 2015-2017. MMWR (Morb Mortal Wkly Rep) 2018;67(42):1195–6.

36. Swanson SJ, Snider C, Braden CR, et al. Multidrug-resistant Salmonella enterica serotype Typhimurium associated with pet rodents. NEJM 2007;356:21–8.

37. Plotogea A, Taylor M, Parayno A, et al. Human Salmonella enteritidis illness outbreak associated with exposure to live mice in British Columbia, Canada, 2018–2019. Zoonoses Public Health 2022;69:856–63.

38. Cartwright E, Nguyen T, Melluso C, et al. A multistate investigation of antibiotic-resistant Salmonella enterica serotype I 4,[5], 12: i:-infections as part of an international outbreak associated with frozen feeder rodents. Zoonoses Public Health 2016;63:62–71.

39. Vrbova L, Sivanantharajah S, Walton R, et al. Outbreak of Salmonella Typhimurium associated with feeder rodents. Zoonoses Public Health 2018;65:386–94.

40. Shivambu N, Shivambu TC, Chimimba CT. Zoonotic pathogens associated with pet and feeder murid rodent species: a global systematic review. Vector Borne Zoonotic Dis 2023;23:551–60.

41. Jahan NA, Lindsey LL, Larsen PA. The role of peridomestic rodents as reservoirs for zoonotic foodborne pathogens. Vector Borne Zoonotic Dis 2021;21:133–48.

42. Lapuz RRSP, Umali DV, Suzuki T, et al. Comparison of the prevalence of Salmonella infection in layer hens from commercial layer farms with high and low rodent densities. Avian Dis 2012;56:29–34.

43. Ruszkowski JJ, Hetman M, Turlewicz-Podbielska H, et al. Hedgehogs as a potential source of zoonotic pathogens—a review and an update of knowledge. Animals 2021;11:1754.

44. Keeble E, Koterwas B. Salmonellosis in hedgehogs. Vet Clin North Am Exot Anim Pract 2020;23:459–70.

45. Anderson T, Marsden-Haug N, Morris J, et al. Multistate outbreak of human Salmonella Typhimurium infections linked to pet hedgehogs–United States, 2011–2013. Zoonoses Public Health 2017;64:290–8.

46. Hoff C, Nichols M, Gollarza L, et al. Multistate outbreak of Salmonella Typhimurium linked to pet hedgehogs, United States, 2018–2019. Zoonoses Public Health 2022;69:167–74.

47. Renquist DM, Whitney Jr RA. Zoonoses acquired from pet primates. Vet Clin North Am Sm Ani Pract 1987;17:219–40.

48. Burgos-Rodriguez AG. Zoonotic diseases of primates. Vet Clin North Am Exot Anim Pract 2011;14:557–75.

49. Murphy F, Roberts J, Bayne K. Occupational health and safety in the care and use of nonhuman primates. Washington, DC: National Academies Press; 2003.

50. Chlebicz A, Śliżewska K. Campylobacteriosis, salmonellosis, yersiniosis, and listeriosis as zoonotic foodborne diseases: a review. Int J Environ Res Publ Health 2018;15:863.
51. Pintar KD, Christidis T, Thomas MK, et al. A systematic review and meta-analysis of the Campylobacter spp. prevalence and concentration in household pets and petting zoo animals for use in exposure assessments. PLoS One 2015;10:e0144976.
52. Masila NM, Ross KE, Gardner MG, et al. Zoonotic and public health implications of Campylobacter species and squamates (lizards, snakes and amphisbaenians). Pathogens 2020;9:799.
53. Burnens AP, Angéloz-Wick B, Nicolet J. Comparison of Campylobacter carriage rates in diarrheic and healthy pet animals. J Vet Med Ser B 1992;39:175–80.
54. Lecová L, Hammerbauerová I, Tůmová P, et al. Companion animals as a potential source of Giardia intestinalis infection in humans in the Czech Republic–A pilot study. Vet Parasitol Reg Stud Reports 2020;21:100431.
55. Tůmová P, Mazánek L, Lecová L, et al. A natural zoonotic giardiasis: infection of a child via Giardia cysts in pet chinchilla droppings. Parasitol Int 2018;67:759–62.
56. Martel A, Donnelly T, Mans C. Update on diseases in chinchillas: 2013–2019. Vet Clin North Am Exot Anim Pract 2020;23:321–35.
57. Cai W, Ryan U, Xiao L, et al. Zoonotic giardiasis: an update. Parasitol Res 2021;1–20.
58. Souza MJ. Bacterial and parasitic zoonoses of exotic pets. Vet Clin North Am Exot Anim Pract 2009;12:401–15.
59. Jarošová J, Antolová D, Šnábel V, et al. The dwarf tapeworm Hymenolepis nana in pet rodents in Slovakia—epidemiological survey and genetic analysis. Parasitol Res 2020;119:519–27.
60. Brustenga L, Morganti G, Baldoni E, et al. High prevalence of hymenolepis (rodentolepis) nana in amateur breeding facilities of Chinchillas (Chinchilla lanigera) and sugar gliders (Petaurus breviceps) from Italy. Acta Parasitol 2023;68:913–5.
61. d'Ovidio D, Noviello E, Pepe P, et al. Survey of Hymenolepis spp. in pet rodents in Italy. Parasitol Res 2015;114:4381–4.
62. Leung TL. Zoonotic parasites in reptiles, with particular emphasis on potential zoonoses in Australian reptiles. Curr Clin Microbiol Rep 2024;11:88–98.
63. Hallinger MJ, Taubert A, Hermosilla C. Endoparasites infecting exotic captive amphibian pet and zoo animals (Anura, Caudata) in Germany. Parasitol Res 2020;119:3659–73.
64. Williams CJ, Scheftel JM, Elchos BL, et al. Compendium of veterinary standard precautions for zoonotic disease prevention in veterinary personnel: national association of state public health veterinarians: veterinary infection control committee 2015. J Am Vet Med Assoc 2015;247:1252–77.
65. Compendium of measures to prevent disease associated with animals in public settings, 2023: national association of state public health veterinarians animal contact compendium committee. J Am Vet Med Assoc 2023;261:1887–94.
66. Michaels B, Gangar V, Schultz A, et al. Water temperature as a factor in hand-washing efficacy. Food Serv Technol 2002;2:139–49.
67. Boyce J, Pittet D. Guideline for hand hygiene in health-care settings: recommendations of the healthcare infection control practices advisory committee and the HICPAC/SHEA/APIC/IDSA hand hygiene task force. Infect Control Hosp Epidemiol 2002;23:S3–40.

Application of Diagnostic Imaging in Exotic Animal Gastroenterology

Robert J.T. Doneley, BVSc, FANZCVS (Avian Medicine)

KEYWORDS

- Radiology • Ultrasound • Fluoroscopy • Contrast imaging • Computed tomography
- MRI

KEY POINTS

- Good quality imaging is a key element in the diagnosis of gastroenteric diseases of exotic pets.
- Available modalities include plain radiography, contrast radiography, fluoroscopy, computed tomography, ultrasound, and MRI.
- Understanding which modality to use, how to use it, and when, is essential for its effective use.
- Knowledge of the required restraint and positioning of the patient are essential in obtaining a high-quality image.
- Once a high-quality image has been obtained, knowledge of anatomy and expected normal can assist the clinician in making a diagnosis.

INTRODUCTION

Diagnostic imaging is an important component of the clinical examination of the gastrointestinal tract of birds, reptiles, and small mammals. From assessing motility to looking for neoplasia or foreign bodies, diagnostic imaging has both supplemented and largely replaced exploratory surgery as a primary diagnostic tool.

Imaging modalities can be broadly divided into 2 groups; those using ionizing radiation (eg, radiology, computed tomography [CT], and fluoroscopy); and those that do not use radiation, such as ultrasound and MRI. Each has its own indications, advantages, disadvantages, safety concerns, and expenses.

Regardless of the chosen modality, there are 2 facets to the optimal utilization of diagnostic imaging—obtaining a high-quality image, and then interpreting it. This

Avian and Exotic Pet Service, UQ Veterinary Medical Centre, Building 8156, Main Drive, University of Qld, Gatton, Queensland 4343, Australia
E-mail address: r.doneley@uq.edu.au

Vet Clin Exot Anim 28 (2025) 381–411
https://doi.org/10.1016/j.cvex.2024.11.008
1094-9194/25/© 2024 Elsevier Inc. All rights are reserved, including those for text and data mining, AI training, and similar technologies.

Abbreviations	
CBCT	cone-beam computed tomography
CT	computed tomography
D	dimensional
IV	intravenous
PDW	proton–density-weighted
T	tesla

article will discuss how to obtain high-quality images of the gastrointestinal tract using the modalities commonly used in clinical practice, and how to interpret them.

OBTAINING HIGH-QUALITY IMAGES WITH RADIOLOGY, FLUOROSCOPY, AND COMPUTED TOMOGRAPHY

The goal in diagnostic imaging is to obtain high-quality images, which are suitable for the clinical purpose, using the minimum radiation dose to the patient and veterinary staff. Image quality is difficult to define because it is subjective in its nature, but a high-quality image enables the observer to extract information from the image that assists in making an accurate diagnosis.

To obtain a high-quality image requires:

1. Equipment and techniques are used to provide:
   a. Good contrast, that is, the difference in density between 2 adjacent structures. High-radiographic contrast is obtained where density differences are distinct (black to white). Low-radiographic contrast occurs where adjacent regions have a low-density difference (dark gray to light gray). The greater the contrast, the more visible features become.
   b. Appropriate exposure, which is determined by the amount of radiation energy used relative to the patient's body size. When insufficient energy is used, most of the radiation is absorbed by the patient and does not reach the receiver, producing an under-exposed (white) image. Conversely, excessively high-energy radiation produces an over-exposed image, that is, too dark to provide details.
2. The patient is positioned so that the relevant part of the body is the center of the image focus.
3. The patient must not move during the imaging. Movement—even rapid breathing—blurs the imaging and reduces the sharpness of the image. Scatter of the radiation beam at the periphery of the film will also reduce the image sharpness if the beam is not collimated.

Equipment and Technique

Radiology
Most modern small animal X-ray machines, especially digital units, can produce quality images of birds and exotic patients. The X-ray generator should be capable of 5.0 to 7.5 mAs exposures, have a range of 40 to 100 kVp, and be adjustable in small increments. Rapid exposure times (ie, 0.02 of a second and faster) should be possible to minimize patient movement artifact. If using film, high-definition mammography or extremity films can be used for small patients, and dental radiographs can be used for very small patients.[1] Radiography of small patients scatters fewer X-rays and therefore anti-scatter techniques such as grids are not required.

Fluoroscopy

Fluoroscopy is an imaging modality that uses the continuous emission of X-rays, captured on a screen, to produce a dynamic image that provides real-time visualization of body structures and function. In contrast to radiographic gastrointestinal contrast studies (which require multiple episodes of handling, sedation, or anesthesia, often over several hours), fluoroscopy is usually performed with the patient in a container, reducing the need for manual or chemical restraint and allowing the diagnosis of gastrointestinal motility functional disorders, as well as an assessment of organ position and size, and the specific locations of strictures or foreign bodies. Fluoroscopy lacks the sharpness and contrast of digital radiographs but can be paired with digital imaging (eg, via a horizontal beam through the restraint box) if more detailed is required (**Fig. 1**). Because of their slow gastrointestinal times, fluoroscopy is rarely used in reptiles, as the same result can be obtained with contrast radiography.

By using minimal restraint during fluoroscopy, the masking effects on gastrointestinal motility caused by repetitive handling and anesthesia are avoided, as is exposure of staff to excessive radiation.[2,3] Although low doses of radiation are used, repeated exposure may result in a relatively high cumulative dose to the patient. Therefore, precautions, such as performing the study at paced intervals for only short bursts of time, should be used.[4]

Computed tomography

CT uses an X-ray tube rotating around the patient's body and opposite rows of detectors, to measure X-ray attenuations by different tissues. X-ray attenuation, and therefore contrast, can be enhanced by the use of intravenous (IV) contrast media. Each rotation of the X-ray tube (housed in the gantry) takes approximately 1 second; the data collected by the receptors are processed by computer software to produce 2 dimensional (2D) cross-sectional (tomographic) images of the body (slices), which are then reconstructed by computer software into either transverse, coronal, or sagittal planes (**Fig. 2**) multiplanar reconstructions which, in turn, can then be assembled into a 3D reconstruction of part or whole of the patient's body.

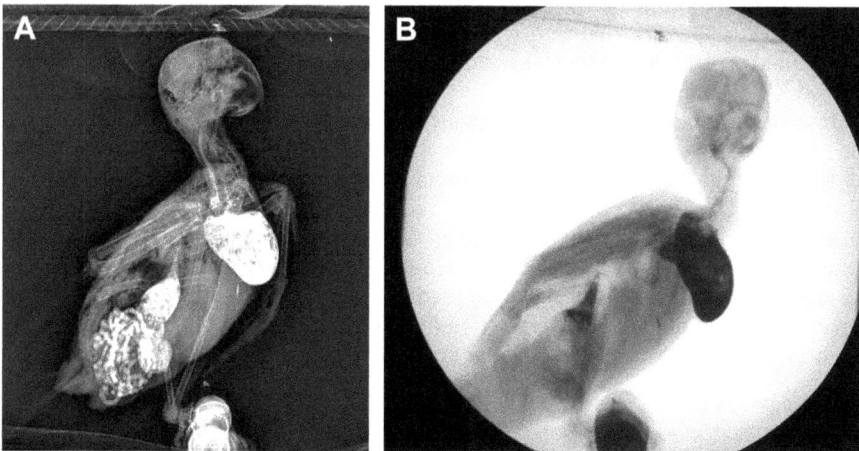

Fig. 1. A comparison of (*A*) fluoroscopy and (*B*) radiology of the same patient only minutes apart. It can be seen how fluoroscopy lacks resolution and contrast when compared to radiology.

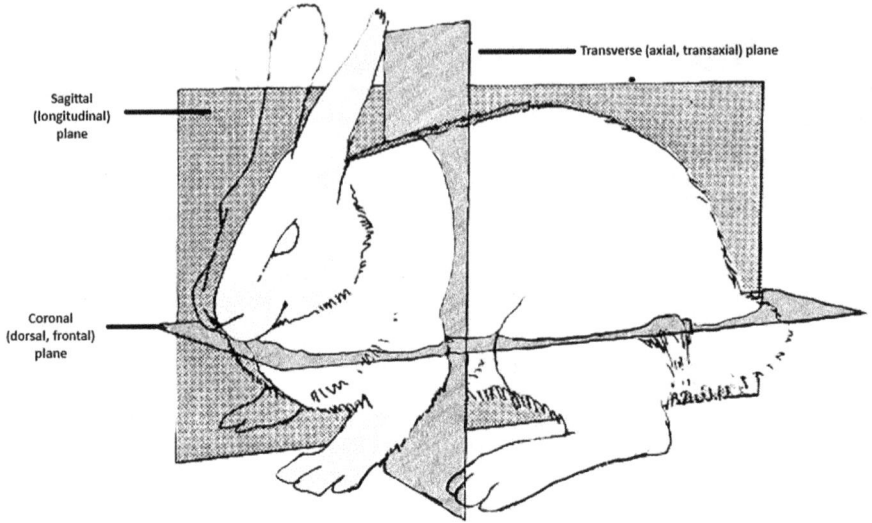

Fig. 2. The anatomic planes used in computed tomography and MRI scanning.

This modality overcomes the interference from superimposition of one tissue over another, allowing examination of tissues/structures that would have otherwise remained undetected with conventional radiographs. However, the resolution of the individual slices is less than that of conventional radiographs. Resolution can be increased by taking more and thinner slices—the thinner the slice, the greater the resolution. Slice thickness is controlled by (1) the speed with which the patient passes through the gantry (a rapid transit produces fewer and thicker slices), and (2) the number of detectors opposite the X-ray tube. Current technology can now take 16, 32, 40, 64, or 128 slices in a single rotation, producing thinner slices (higher resolution) in a short time (reduced radiation exposure and increased patient safety).

An emerging technology is Cone-Beam Computed Tomography (CBCT), widely used in medicine for head and neck imaging (such as dentistry) and has increasingly been used in veterinary medicine. It involves the use of a C-arm rotating around a patient placed on a small imaging platform (40 cm), taking capturing slices using a cone-shaped X-ray beam.

Most CBCT systems have internal shielding and therefore do not require special room buildout. The units are reasonably mobile, allowing their use in several locations within a hospital and compared to more conventional CT units, they are less expensive.[5]

However, this technology has 2 major drawbacks: firstly, it is very slow when compared to conventional CT (1 rotation around the patient can take 15–30 sec), making movement artifacts highly likely; and secondly, while it has high spatial resolution, it also has poor contrast resolution. This makes CBCT ideal for hard tissue imaging (eg, bones and teeth), but less suitable for abdominal imaging.

Contrast imaging

Oral contrast studies are sometimes necessary to distinguish one tissue or structure from its surroundings, or to provide greater detail of that tissue/structure, but they are also useful for assessing.

- The anatomy and motility of the gastrointestinal tract

- The presence of a perforation in the tract causing leakage of contrast into the peritoneal cavity
- The presence of an obstruction
- To outline the tract in an other lowcontrast image of the coelom / abdomen
- IV contrast can also be used to enhance imaging of the vascular supply and perfusion of the gastrointestinal tract.

Gastrointestinal studies use contrast media, a group of chemical agents developed to aid in the characterization of pathology by improving the contrast resolution of an imaging modality. These agents absorb X-rays, and thus appear white on a radiograph, providing contrast to an image. Contrast media are comparatively inexpensive and well-tolerated by most patients; complications from their use are rare.

Commonly used contrast media can be used orally or intravenously, and sometimes both. The 2 types most often used in oral studies of the gastrointestinal tract are:

a. Water-soluble iodinated contrast agents for example, Iohexol (Omnipague, GE Healthcare) and diatrizoate (Urograffin, Bayer; Gastrogaffin, Bayer)
b. Barium sulfate

A contraindication for a barium study is when gastrointestinal tract rupture is suspected, as barium leakage into the peritoneum can have catastrophic consequences including peritonitis, granuloma formation, and adhesions.[6] If this is suspected, an oral study using iodinated media is preferred. However, a disadvantage of the water-soluble contrast media is their hypertonicity; by drawing fluid into the gastrointestinal lumen, these agents may cause diarrhea and dehydration. They should be avoided in dehydrated patients or those with known renal disease. Iohexol is less hypertonic than diatrizoate and has minimal pulmonary complications if aspirated. If necessary, these contrast media can be diluted 1:1 with water.[7]

Care must be taken with barium contrast studies in reptiles as large volumes in a patient with reduced gastrointestinal motility can dry out and obstruct the tract. This situation is not common but should be considered in patients with pre-existing ileus or dehydration. If, at the completion of a study, any remaining barium should be removed through soaking in warm water, the use of warm water enemas, or massage.[8]

Oral contrast studies are generally restricted to radiographic and fluoroscopic examinations, although occasionally, they are also used for CT studies. Recommended techniques for contrast studies are shown in **Table 1**.

The 3 most common mistakes made when using contrast media[5] are:

1. *Failing to take plain survey images immediately before contrast administration.* This can rule out other disease processes, to adjust the unit's settings and the patient's positioning, to confirm adequate preparation of the abdomen/caudal coelom (colon and bladder), and to use as a pre-contrast comparison.
2. *Using an insufficient volume of contrast medium.* Too small a volume does not distend the lumen sufficiently to appreciate detail.
3. *Taking too few images after oral contrast medium is given.*

If detailed imaging of the gastrointestinal mucosal lining is required, a double contrast study can be performed. The required volume of contrast is calculated, but half of this is administered as contrast media and the other half as air, using a feeding tube. The contrast coats the mucosal surface while the air distends the gastrointestinal lumen, enhancing the contrast.

Table 1
Recommended techniques for orally administered gastrointestinal contrast studies in birds, reptiles, and small mammals

Species	Preparation	Volume of Contrast Media to Be Administered	Radiology	Fluoroscopy
Birds	Fast the bird for 1–4 h. If fasting fails to empty the crop, the contents should be removed with a large bore feeding tube before administering the contrast media.	20 mLs/kg via rubber or metal feeding tube. Alternatively, a feeding tube passed through the crop into the proventriculus in the anesthetized patient allows a smaller volume of contrast media (5–10 mLs/kg) to be used[9]	Take at 5, 15, and 30 min, then hourly afterward till the study is complete	• Still fluoroscopic images are performed at 5, 15, 30, 60, 120, 180, 240, and 300-min time points after barium administration. • 60 s video exposures are taken at the 30, 60, 120, and 240-min time points to assess contractility.[2,3,10]
Lizards	Ensure the patient is well-hydrated and warmed so it can reach and maintain its preferred body temperature. Fasting for several days (up to a week in snakes) may be needed to empty the gastrointestinal tract.	10–15 mLs/kg via stomach tube[11]	Take at 5, 15, 30, and 45 min, and then 1, 2, 3, 4, 5, 6, 8, 10, 12, 24, 30, and 36 h[12]	There are very limited reports on the use of fluoroscopy in reptiles, presumably because the slow gastrointestinal transit time renders this modality less useful. It can be used to assess localized contractility after localizing an area of interest.
Chelonians			Take initial images at 5 min then at 30, 60, 90, 120, and 150 min, and then at 3, 4, 6, 8, 12, 24, 48, 72, and 96 h[13]	
Snakes		25 mLs/kg via stomach tube[14]	Take initial images at 5 min, then at 1, 2, 3, 6, 9, 12, 48, and 72 h[14]	
Rabbits and rodents	Usually not fasted	20 mLs/kg by esophageal or stomach tube[15]	Take images at 5, 15, 30, 60 min, then hourly for 2–4 h	
Ferrets	Fast up to 8 h	8–13 mL/kg administered by a curve-tipped dosing syringe	Take images at 5, 10, 20, 40, 60, 90, and 120 min after barium administration. If the stomach is not empty at 120 min, a further image can be taken at 150 min[16]	Fluoroscopy may be useful in selected cases for imaging of the intrathoracic tract of the esophagus, when used in conjunction with contrast medium. This can allow assessment of megaesophagus or facilitate the removal of a foreign body.

Care must be taken to minimize spillage of the media onto the patient's feathers, skin, or fur, as it may complicate the interpretation of the image.

An oral study may not produce sufficient distention for a large intestinal or cloacal examination. The large intestine can be examined with a retrograde infusion of contrast into the colon (ie, barium enema) with 1 to 2 mL/kg of contrast media.[1] A cloacagram is taken under anesthesia. The cloaca is gently irrigated with warm sterile saline (to remove fecal material), and a temporary ventoplasty is performed. With the ventoplasty sutures loosely tightened, an iodinated contrast media is introduced through the vent into the cloaca using a soft, primed catheter (to avoid air bubbles). When it begins to reflux, the sutures are tightened, and the first image taken. A small volume of contrast media is reintroduced prior to each radiographic exposure to allow for leakage.[17]

IV contrast is often ideal for viewing vasculature and organ systems.[18] The transit and accumulation of this contrast media in different organs (enhancement) improves the differentiation of internal structures.[19] Using media with an iodine concentration of 250 to 300 mg/mL at the dose of 1 to 2 mLs/kg (250 – 600 mg/kg) is given as a rapid bolus. However, their short duration of effect requires the use of a rapid bolus or continuous bolus infusions in conjunction with rapid sequence scanning techniques. This requirement can be hampered by the viscosity of the media. While many have a low viscosity that can easily pass through the small gauge IV catheters, some may require dilution with sterile normal saline.[18,19] Images are taken almost immediately because of the rapid clearance from the blood.

Caution must be observed in using IV contrast in small patients. One retrospective study of 134 contrast-enhanced CT scans in 120 birds demonstrated a mortality rate of 45.4% in small birds (<150g) compared with a mortality rate of 0.8% (1/120) for large birds (>150 g). Although the relationship between contrast media and death could not be confirmed, this study justifies caution when using contrast IV media.[20]

Restraint

Regardless of the species, positioning of the patient is vital for the accurate interpretation of a diagnostic image. Taking time to properly position the patient will reduce the number of repeat exposures needed to get a diagnostic image.[21] The best way to properly position a patient is with sedation or anesthesia; only very tame (or very sick) patients can be positioned conscious with minimal or no restraint. This is often less stressful for the patient (and therefore safer) than manual restraint. Not only does sedation/anesthesia facilitate positioning, but it also helps to avoid movement artifacts associated with sudden, unexpected movements or a rapid, panting respiratory rate. General anesthesia is strongly recommended for radiographic studies of snakes. The relaxed state of the patient makes positioning of the patient easier, and it eliminates spinal curvatures associated with normal muscular contractions.[8]

The use of sedation/anesthesia will also minimize staff exposure to radiation. An adequately restrained patient can be positioned using radiolucent tape, foam wedges, and sandbags rather than manually holding them (**Fig. 3**).

For fluoroscopic studies, the patient is usually restrained by placing it in a suitable container (a cardboard box or a purpose-made Perspex cage). If possible, the patient should be placed in the container until it has acclimatized to the confinement.

Birds may require fasting for a few hours before the procedure. The purpose of fasting is to allow gastric emptying and minimize the risk of regurgitation and aspiration but reptiles and small mammals rarely require this.

Positioning

Radiology
Good radiographic technique requires that a minimum of 2 orthogonal views (at 90° from each other) be taken for every study. By capturing the same region from different

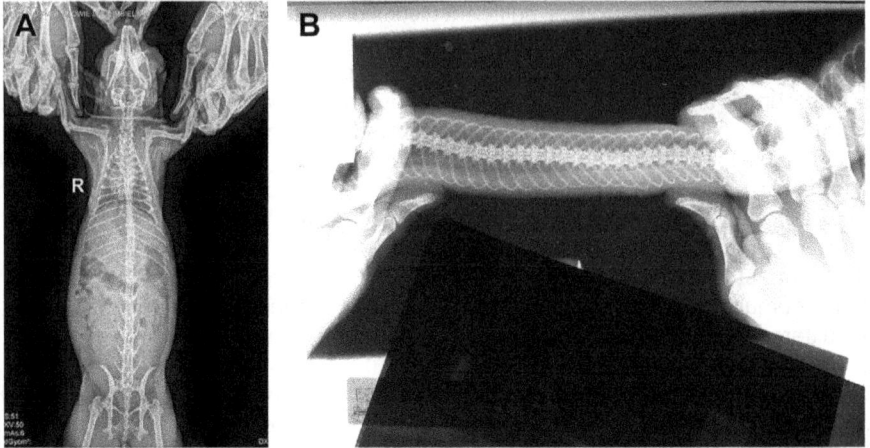

Fig. 3. The images show good positioning of the patient (*A*) a rabbit and (*B*) a snake, but an unacceptably high risk to the holder.

angles, orthogonal views help minimize the effect of tissue superimposition and allow for better visualization of anatomic details and potential pathology. Recommended positioning for these orthogonal views is described in **Table 2** (**Figs. 4–7**).

Fluoroscopy
As the patient is usually not chemically restrained during a fluoroscopic study, it is important to minimize acute stressors such as loud voices, unexpected movement of the box, and so forth that may result in the patient moving. If the patient is a bird, a single perch can be placed in the container so that the bird can sit comfortably with its tail off the ground (**Fig. 8**).

Computed Tomography

Although the CT computer software can correct asymmetry of the patient positioning, better results are obtained if the patient is positioned in ventral recumbency and is symmetric. This may require placing the patient (especially birds) in a V-shaped trough made of radiolucent material, for example, cardboard (**Figs. 9–11**). Limbs can be extended slightly, but superimposition is not a major issue with CT (an advantage over radiology).

OBTAINING HIGH-QUALITY IMAGES WITH ULTRASOUND AND MRI
Ultrasonography

Ultrasonography provides the best images of organs that are largely composed of fluid and soft tissue. The abdomen is ideally suited to this.[22] Ultrasonography allows real-time evaluation of physiologic processes (eg, gastrointestinal motility) and organ perfusion. It is also used to detect the presence of free fluid in the body or contained fluid within structures such as ovarian follicles, gall bladders, and urinary bladders. Ultrasound-guided aspirates allow safer and more accurate sampling of masses and cysts.[5] It is considered a safe imaging modality as is relatively non-invasive, does not use ionizing radiation, and can be used without general anesthesia.

The most common uses of ultrasound as an imaging technique for gastrointestinal disease include evaluation of the internal organs for shape, size, and architecture, the

Table 2
Standard positioning for birds, reptiles and small mammals while been radiographed

Position	Technique	Image
Birds		
Lateral	Lateral recumbency, with the wings extended dorsally and the legs pulled caudally. The limbs can be held in position with adhesive tape, sandbags, or ties.	On the image the acetabulae should be superimposed, as should the coracoids.
Ventrodorsal	Dorsal recumbency with the wings extended laterally and the legs caudally alongside the tail, with the femurs ideally parallel to the spine and each other.	The carina of the keel (seen as a thin air space in the carina) should be superimposed over the vertebrae.
Position	**Technique**	
Reptiles		
Lateral	Taken with a horizontal beam to prevent organ displacement and subsequent difficulty interpreting the images. Snakes should be anesthetized or restrained in a translucent plastic tube to keep the body straight. Lizards and chelonians should have their legs extended rostrally and caudally, and restrained.	The ribs should be superimposed, and the spine not rotated.
Ventrodorsal/ dorsoventral	If necessary, use sedation and/or plastic tubes to keep the spine as straight as possible. The legs should be extended rostrally and caudally and restrained.	The ribs and spine should be symmetric.
Craniocaudal (for chelonians)	The head and limbs should be extended out of the shell, which can be achieved by placing the patient on an elevated stand that touches the plastron only.	Left and right lung fields should be visible and symmetric
Small mammals		
Right lateral	The thoracic limbs must be extended cranially to prevent superimposition of the brachial muscles over the mediastinal portion cranial to the heart. The pelvic limbs should be extended caudally.	The ribs should be superimposed, and the spine and pelvis not rotated. The cranial thorax and caudal abdomen should be visible.
Dorsoventral	This is preferred for whole body radiographs, including thorax and abdomen. V troughs (foam or Perspex), radiolucent foam, tape, and cotton wool can be used to optimize positioning, which is performed in a similar manner to small animal radiology.	The sternum should be superimposed on the spine.

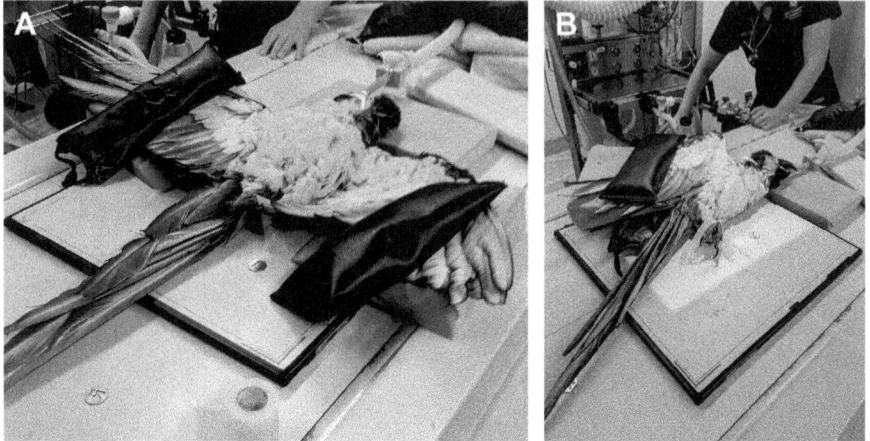

Fig. 4. The standard (A) lateral and (B) VD positioning of a bird been radiographed, using sandbags, foam wedges, and adhesive tape to position the patient.

detection of free fluid, and a guide for cystocentesis and fine needle aspirate biopsies. As pregnancy in some ways mimic gastrointestinal disease, pregnancy testing via ultrasound is useful as an exclusion technique.

Sonogram

The sonogram, an image produced by the reflection of high frequency sound waves generated by a transducer (probe), is based on the unique echoes produced by different tissues and their compressibility. The appearance of tissue on the sonogram represents its echogenicity compared with surrounding structures (**Fig. 12**).

- Structures that return minimal echo, such as serous fluids, blood, and urine, will appear black on the sonogram and are *anechoic*.
- Tissue that reflects more waves than neighboring tissues (eg, air, bone) will appear whiter, or *hyperechoic*, on the sonogram.
- Tissue that reflects ultrasound beams less than the adjacent tissues (eg, muscle vs bone) appear darker, or *hypoechoic*, on the screen.

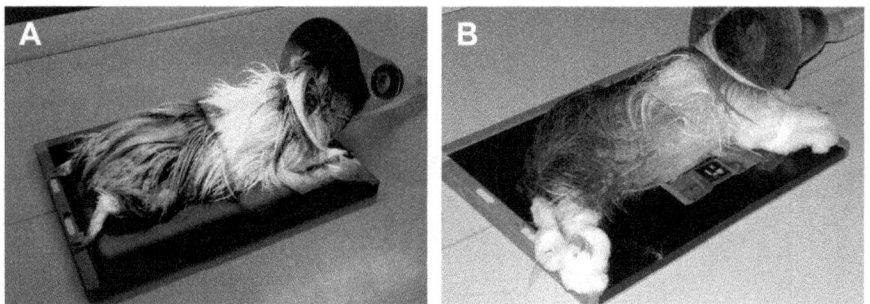

Fig. 5. The standard (A) lateral and (B) DV positioning of a guinea pig been radiographed, using sandbags, foam wedges, and adhesive tape for positioning. Note the cotton wool placed between the front and black legs to prevent rolling the body when securing the upper legs.

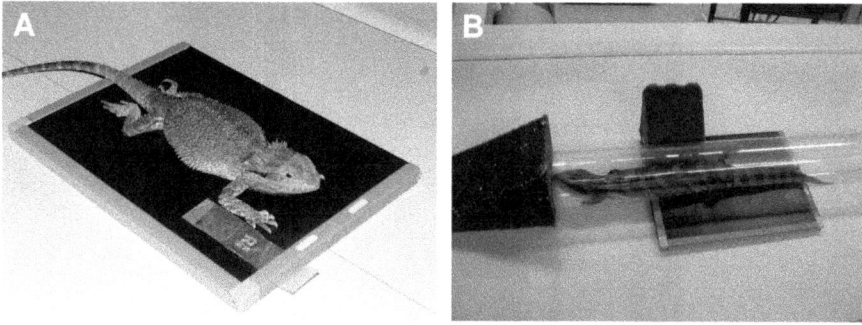

Fig. 6. Dorsoventral positioning for lizards (A) is usually simple, although acrylic tubes (B) can assist with both restraint and positioning.

- Tissues of the same density are *isoechoic*, that is, difficult to distinguish between.[23]

Ultrasonography therefore cannot be used to scan gas-filled structures (eg, avian air sacs, mammalian lungs) or bony tissues, as the sound beam is totally reflected at soft tissue/gas interfaces and absorbed at soft tissue/bone interfaces. Intestinal gas, air sacs, and bone also *shadow* any other organs beyond them.

Sonographic lesions are sometimes quite characteristic of a given disease process, but more often the changes are nonspecific. Although ultrasonography can be quite sensitive to detect disease, the changes are not specific for a given disease in most cases unless a characteristic change in anatomic presentation and echogenicity are detected.

Transducers

The focal range (depth) of the transducer is inversely related to its frequency as the result of attenuation (the loss of acoustic energy as the wave travels). High frequency transducers provide a more detailed picture, but the field of imaging is reduced.[23]

As a rule, the smaller the patient, the higher the frequency that will be required. For very small patients (<50g), a frequency of between 7 MHz and 12 MHz is often suitable—note that 10 to 15-mHz linear array hockey stick probes are now becoming available. Larger patients may require a transducer with a frequency of 3.5 to 7 MHz. Lower frequencies can be used to localize an area of interest, and then a higher frequency transducer can be used to examine it in detail.

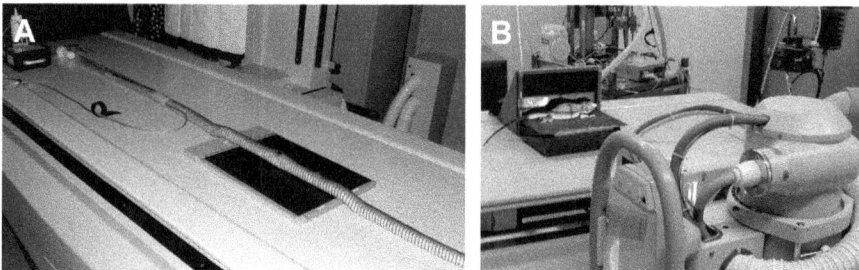

Fig. 7. A lateral view of a snake using a vertical beam (A) can give a distorted appearance due to organ displacement. A horizontal beam (B) gives better results.

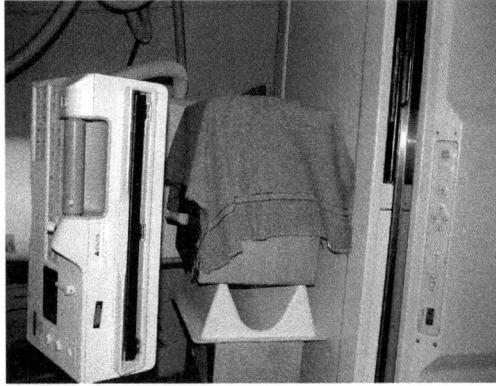

Fig. 8. Fluoroscopic study. The bird is enclosed in the cardboard box, sitting on a perch (the end of which can be seen on the left side). The towel is to keep the bird calm during the study.

Three types of transducers are commonly used in practice.

- *Linear* - higher frequency transducers with an often-large rectangular footprint (surface that touches the patient's skin), which may be impractical on very small patients.
- *Curvilinear* - lower frequency transducers with a convex footprint.
- *Phased-array* (also known as *sector*) – low frequency transducers that generate an image from a point and are good for getting between ribs.

Both curvilinear and phased-array probes generate sector images, narrow in the near field and wide in the far field. Because of their smaller footprint, available frequencies, and the sector image, curvilinear probes are often preferred.[24] Further

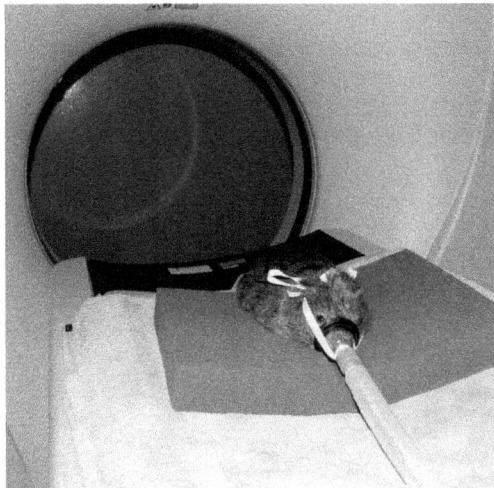

Fig. 9. Guinea pig positioned on a foam pad for computed tomography (CT). Good liaison between the radiographer and anesthetist is needed to ensure equipment does not become tangled when the CT gurney moves into the gantry.

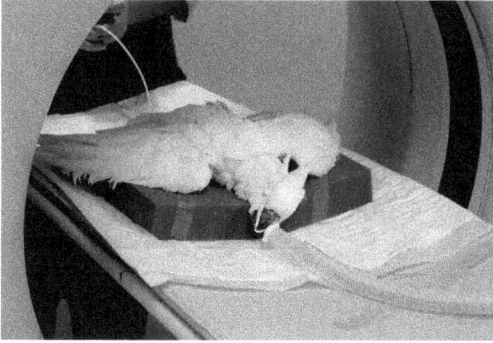

Fig. 10. Cockatoo positioned on a foam pad for a computed tomography.

reports evaluating the hockey stick transducers are currently lacking, but they could offer another option for the sonographer.

Technique

Any air between the patient's skin and the transducer will produce artifacts that make interpretation difficult, if not impossible. It is therefore vital to prepare the skin appropriately.

1. Birds: Preferably use an apteryla as the coupling point. In species where this is not possible, feathers may have to be plucked. Acoustic coupling gel is then applied to the bare skin. If possible, avoid alcohol as it can accelerate loss of body heat. The standard approaches used in birds are illustrated in **Fig. 13**
2. Reptiles: Air trapped between the scales can be particularly challenging to the sonographer. Patients undergoing ecdysis are poor candidates because of air between the layers of the skin. In some species, for example, the blue tongue skink (*Tiliqua* spp), osteoderms may make ultrasound an unsuitable imaging modality.[25] Methods used to improve transducer contact in other reptiles include rubbing gel between the scales and immersing the animal in warm water.

While snakes and lizards are relatively easy to ultrasound, using the heart (in snakes) or the liver and gallbladder (in lizards) as starting points for the examination,

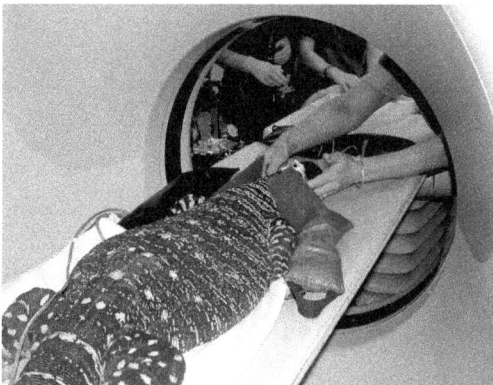

Fig. 11. A large lace monitor during a computed tomography scan of its head.

Hyperechoic	Isoechoic	Hypoechoic	Anechoic
Bone Air Diaphragm Collagen Fat	Renal cortex compared to liver	Muscle Liver compared to spleen	Serous fluid Blood Urine

Fig. 12. The scales of echogenicity in sonograms.

chelonians can be more challenging. The carapace and plastron severely limit the examination of internal organs but there are 3 suitable contact points along each side: the cranial mediastinal approach provides good access to the heart and liver; the axillary window allows visualization of the lateral liver and kidneys; and the pre-femoral window will provide access to the intestinal tract.[26] (**Fig. 14**)

3. Small mammals: The ventral and ventrolateral surfaces of the abdomen are clipped of hair, and a combination of alcohol and ultrasound-specific coupling gel is applied to the skin, eliminating any air between the probe's surface and surface of the skin. Fur must be clipped to achieve adequate skin contact but not so much as to allow excessive loss of body heat.

In some cases, the use of stand-offs should be considered. These are gel-filled or water-filled pads, such as fingers of a disposable glove. They act as an acoustic interface, allowing better sound wave penetration and enhancing contact with irregularly shaped anatomic structures such as reptilian skin. After placing coupling gel on the skin, a stand-off is placed over the area of interest and the operator scans through the stand-off.

It is recommended that a systematic approach to imaging be used to ensure that the Location, Echotexture, Measurements, Outline, Number and Size of any findings are

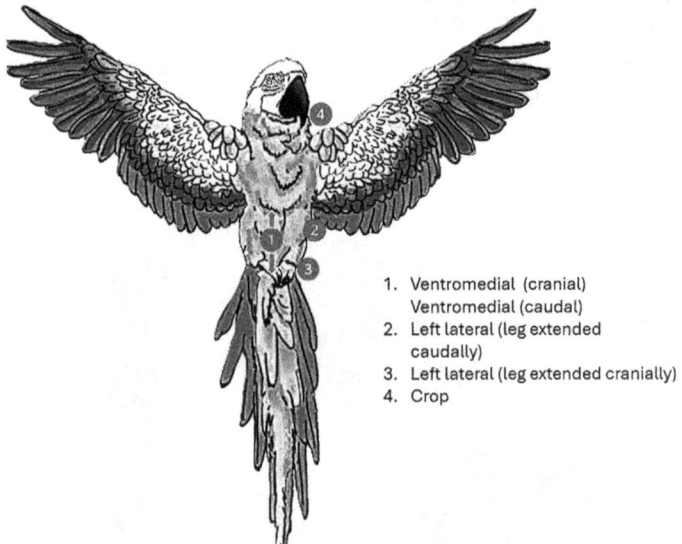

1. Ventromedial (cranial)
Ventromedial (caudal)
2. Left lateral (leg extended caudally)
3. Left lateral (leg extended cranially)
4. Crop

Fig. 13. Acoustic windows in birds.

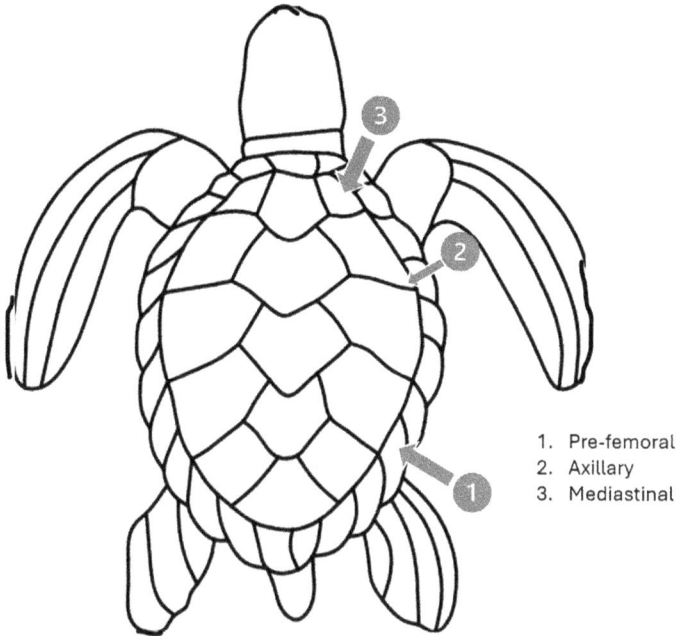

1. Pre-femoral
2. Axillary
3. Mediastinal

Fig. 14. Acoustic windows in chelonians.

considered.[27] Whenever possible each organ should be scanned in 2 planes: transverse and sagittal/longitudinal.[1,27]

During the examination the following should be noted:

- Normal anatomy/variants of abdominal organs and structures in at least 2 planes. This should include assessment of size, outline, and ultrasound characteristics
- Relative echogenicity of abdominal organs
- Pathologic findings including focal and diffuse processes and associated hemodynamic findings (pre-operative and post-operative assessments)
- The presence of any intra-abdominal fluid, focal fluid collections, and peritoneal or retroperitoneal fat or masses
- Where clinically relevant: vascular anatomy including position, course, and lumen of relevant vessels (hemodynamic observations including the presence/absence of flow, its direction, velocity, and Doppler waveform).

Color Doppler

Ultrasonic color Doppler combines anatomic information derived using ultrasound, with velocity information obtained from Doppler technology. It generates a color map depicting movement of blood (Doppler mode) superimposed on grey-scale images of tissue anatomy (B mode). The most common use of the technique is to image the movement of blood through the organs, blood vessels, and the heart. Blood flow toward the probe is colored red, while flow away from the probe is colored blue. Color Doppler can be used to:

a. Identify abnormal vascularity, such as hyperemia or neovascularization, in intestinal diseases such as edema, inflammation, or malignancy.
b. Determine if an abdominal mass is avascular (eg, an abscess) or vascular (eg, neoplasia)

MRI

Like CT, MRI displays objects in slices. Unlike CT, MRI does not utilize radiation, but rather uses a powerful magnetic field in combination with high-frequency radio waves to align and spin protons (nuclei of hydrogen atoms) in the body, and then obtain signals resulting from these protons. Because most hydrogen atoms in the body are trapped in water molecules, the MRI image produced represents the different types, distributions, and volumes of water in various tissues, allowing differentiation of soft tissue types. Images are composed of a series of 2D images or "slices" that may be viewed alone or in 3D reconstructions. The use of IV contrast agents such gadolinium is considered a routine procedure for MRI scans to enhance contrast and compare pre-contrast and post-contrast images.[18]

This ability to differentiate soft tissues and the wide variety of ways in which image contrast (weighting) can by generated for visualizing the body's anatomy and physiology makes MRI a superior imaging tool for soft tissues. However, CT is more useful for imaging bony structures, has better resolution, a much shorter investigation time, and is currently more readily available than MRI.

The strength of the magnetic field used in MRI, the magnetic flux density, is expressed in Tesla (T). In clinical veterinary medicine, MRI units typically range from 0.2 to 3 T.

By changing the settings of the MRI scanner (eg, pulse repetition time and echo time), different tissue weightings are obtained and subsequently used to analyze the tissue composition.[18] The 3 types of weightings commonly used are as follows:

- T1-weighted images (longitudinal relaxation or simply T1) relate to the rate of recovery of the proton spins after each perturbation (called excitation) required to elicit an observable signal. Therefore, tissues with long T1 (eg, water) appear hypo-intense.
- T2-weighted images (transverse relaxation or T2), relate to the rate of decay of the observable signal. Therefore, in contrast to T1, tissues with long T2 appear hyper-intense.
- Proton–density-weighted (spin–density-weighted) images (PDW): Contrast between tissues is primarily dependent on the number of available spins (protons) (ie, brightness is highest in tissues with a high-protein density); these images minimize the T1 and T2 effects, therefore resulting in less contrast than T1 or T2 images; although these images may be useful for depicting normal anatomy, they are used less often.

Because each type of tissue has its own characteristics for T1, T2, and PDW, the images obtained from these 3 weighting types can be combined to identify the origin of the examined tissue.

Limiting factors for the use of MRI use are:

- A full investigation may take at least 45 minutes, requiring extended anesthesia times with limited access to the patient during the procedure.
- The small size of most exotic patients in combination with the low spatial resolution of most systems (less than 0.5 T) limits the diagnostic value of MRI has in small patients, especially since the minimal slice thickness needs to be 1 to 3 mm to achieve a useable signal-to-noise ratio with these machines.
- Imaging may be hindered by the high respiratory and heart rates or by the presence of artifacts caused by the presence of air sacs and/or a transponder.[18]
- The magnetic field of an MRI dictates the use of specialized modifications to metal-containing equipment such as anesthetic machines, patient monitors, etc.

INTERPRETATION OF IMAGES

A systematic approach for image interpretation in exotics, as in small animal imaging, is recommended. The first step is to assess the overall image quality (**Box 1**).

- Is the exposure and contrast suitable for interpretation?
- Are there any artifacts affecting image quality?
- Is the patient positioned appropriately to accurately assess internal structures?

The next step is to interpret the image. This should be done carefully and methodically, on either an organ-based approach or via a rostral to caudal evaluation. Abnormalities can be described in terms of size, shape, location, number, margination, or opacity. The definition and examples of specific uses of each term are shown in **Table 3**.

EVALUATION OF THE GASTROINTESTINAL TRACT USING RADIOLOGY
Plain/Survey Films

Radiographic evaluation of the gastrointestinal tract should begin with plain (noncontrast) films even though, in some cases of coelomic or abdominal disease, these radiographs may be of relatively low yield (eg, loss of serosal detail, ill-defined soft tissue masses, and lack of contrast). Even so, there are sufficient potential findings to warrant survey films.

The preferred projections for examining the gastrointestinal tract of birds, reptiles, and small mammals, along with notes on expected findings, are contained in **Table 4**.

Birds

Generalized or localized ileus is a common finding in birds with severe systemic illness, heavy metal toxicosis, gastrointestinal disease, the presence of a foreign body, and infectious diseases (eg, *Macrorhabdus ornithogaster* infection or Proventriculus Dilatation Disease). With the loss of normal peristaltic activity, the gastrointestinal tract is often distended with fluid, gas, or ingesta.

- Distention of the crop with fluid or ingesta suggests either generalized ileus or a primary crop problem (eg, foreign body).
- Distention of the proventriculus (with or without gas) may be due to generalized ileus associated with systemic illness or lead toxicosis. It is also seen with lead toxicosis, infectious diseases, or foreign bodies.
- Intestinal loops distended with fluid or gas are abnormal. It can be associated with:
  a. generalized ileus for example, lead toxicosis, pancreatic disease

---

Box 1
Errors in interpretation

Everyone who interprets diagnostic images makes errors, regardless of their level of expertise. Two specific errors in interpretation that all clinicians make deserve particular consideration:

- *Bias* results from expecting to find something and then making the imaging findings fit that expectation.
- *Satisfaction of search* pertains to finding an obvious radiographic abnormality and then stopping the search for more lesions, regardless of whether the finding explains the clinical signs.

Avoiding these errors is a gradual transition that comes with experience.

Table 3
Standard radiographic terms used to describe abnormalities seen on radiographs

Term	Definition	Example
Size	Change in size of a structure with the overall shape remaining as expected	• Hepatomegaly • Splenomegaly • Gastric dilation
Shape	Change in the shape of a structure such that the overall expected shape has been altered	• Volvulus • Proventricular dilation
Location	Change in the expected location of a structure	• Displacement of the ventriculus by an enlarged liver • Cranial displacement of the intestines by ovarian follicles in a lizard
Number	Change in the expected number of structures	
Margination	Change in the expected outline of a structure	• Thickening of the stomach or intestinal wall
Opacity	Change in the expected opacity of a structure	• Increased radiopacity of the celom in cases of ascites
Contrast enhancement	Contrast agents work by altering the way imaging modalities interact with body tissues.	• Differentiating structures • Highlighting lesions
Mass effect	The effect of masses on normal tissues is that of displacement	• Organomegaly in birds, displacing the liver laterally & giving the appearance of hepatomegaly.

    b. intraluminal obstruction due to inflammation, foreign bodies,[30] parasites, intussusception, stricture, granuloma, or neoplasia

Gastrointestinal obstruction with foreign bodies such as knotted cotton fiber, ingluvioliths, coins, plastic, and so forth usually will produce a generalized ileus (if the obstruction is complete) or a localized ileus (if the obstruction is partial) (**Fig. 15**). It is normal to see radiopaque particulate matter (grit) in the ventriculus. Distension of the ventriculus with this material, often with it moving rostrally into the proventriculus or caudally into the intestines, is abnormal and indicates gastric impaction.

The proventriculus can be displaced dorsally by hepatomegaly or in any direction by other extraluminal masses. The ventriculus can be displaced caudodorsally by hepatomegaly and cranially by a mass effect in the mid or caudal coelom. Extraluminal coelomic masses such as eggs, ovarian disease, splenomegaly, gonadal enlargement, and nephromegaly, can displace the intestines ventrally.

Metallic densities in the gastrointestinal tract should be viewed with caution. Not all metallic densities are made of or contain lead, and not all lead particles can be seen radiographically. Lead toxicosis cannot be diagnosed based on the presence of metallic densities in the gastrointestinal tract; radiographs should be used to assess the presence, quantity, and size of metallic particles in the gastrointestinal tract after the diagnosis has been made.

Absolute hepatomegaly (ie, the liver is physically enlarged) may be due to hepatic diseases such as lipidosis, neoplasia, or chlamydiosis, and can cause dorsal displacement of the proventriculus, caudodorsal displacement of the ventriculus, and compression of the intestines ventrally, dorsally, cranially or caudally. Relative liver

Table 4
Recommended views for gastrointestinal imaging in birds, reptile, and small mammals

Species	Recommended Views to Examine the Gastrointestinal Tract	Comments
Birds	Lateral Ventrodorsal	The air-filled coelom of birds lends itself to good contrast and differentiation of internal organs. This contrast can be lost; however, if the air sacs are compressed from the outside for example, by fluid, fat, organomegaly, reproductive activity, or neoplasia.
Lizards	Dorsoventral (highest value) Lateral-horizontal beam	Reptiles usually have poor coelomic radiographic contrast due to the close anatomic proximity of the internal organs, the lack of internal fat, the absence of a diaphragm to clearly demarcate the thorax and
Snakes	Lateral (highest value)-horizontal beam Dorsoventral	abdomen, and effect of a shell or osteoderms on the image.[8] The stomach is often not identifiable in lizards and snakes unless it is gas-filled or radiopaque material was recently ingested. The chelonian stomach can sometimes be identified in the left mid portion of the coelom.
Chelonians	Dorsoventral (highest value) Lateral-horizontal beam Craniocaudal-horizontal beam	The intestinal serosal detail is usually indistinct. Relatively more gas is found in the digestive tract in lizards than in snakes or chelonians, but even so it is usually present in only small amounts. Sometimes the presence of ingesta or fecal material can highlight the intestinal tract.
Small mammals	Lateral Dorsoventral	Contrast is provided by the presence of intra-abdominal and retroperitoneal fat. In young and cachexic animals, which have little intra-abdominal fat, radiographic images of the abdomen are low in contrast.[28] The stomach, located on the left and within the costal arch, usually contains ingesta and small amounts of gas. In rabbits, the stomach can extend below the costal arch and almost to the right body wall. Radiographically, the stomach appears oval to pear-shaped in both guinea pigs and rats. In rats and mice, the stomach also sits within the costal arch. The cecum in hindgut fermenters (rabbit and guinea pig) is normally full of ingesta and small amounts of gas. The rabbit cecum lies mainly on the right of the ventral abdominal wall and extends caudally over to the left side. In the lateral projection, the cecum is typically situated in the middle of the ventral abdomen. In guinea pigs, the cecum lies equally in both halves of the abdomen and extends in a more dorsal direction.[1,28] This large cecal size, combined with the proximity of other organs, often results in poor contrast and poor serosal detail.[20,29] The liver can be seen in the cranial abdomen but, in rabbits, the caudal border is not clearly visible on a lateral view (it can be seen in guinea pigs). The rest of the gastrointestinal tract is usually filled with non-homogeneous ingesta[28]
Ferrets	Dorsoventral Lateral	The stomach should not contain gas, although small amounts may be seen in the small intestine. The gastrointestinal contents are frequently homogenous with low contrast, making it difficult to identify separate areas of the tract. The small intestines in the ferret form a major part of the gut length and approximately two-thirds of their length are situated in the right half of the abdomen and a third in the left caudal abdomen caudal to the stomach.[28]

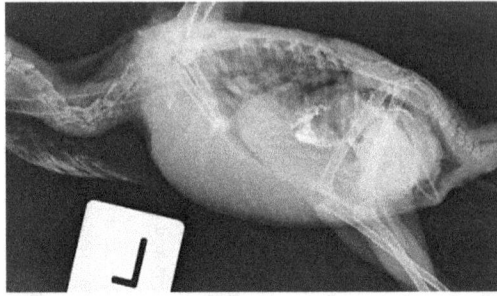

Fig. 15. A fibrous foreign body in the proventriculus causing localized ileus. It has been out-lined by contrast media and subsequently surgically removed.

enlargement (ie, the liver is normal-sized but appears enlarged) can be due to a cranial coelomic mass (eg, an egg, pyometra, ascites, or organomegaly) displacing the liver lobes laterally. On a ventrodorsal view, a distended proventriculus can appear as left-sided hepatomegaly.

Loss of serosal detail is common, often associated with obesity or, more commonly, ascites (eg, yolk peritonitis, congestive heart failure, intestinal dilation with fluid, and severe oviductal disease). The entire coelom becomes distended and radiopaque with little or no contrast. The air sac space is lost, and the liver appears compressed tightly against the body wall.

Other findings in the coelom can include an egg, collapsed eggs (or their remnants), or metastatic/dystrophic tissue mineralization. While these findings may be incidental, their presence should be a consideration in the diagnostic process.

Reptiles

It is important to note that gastrointestinal motility of reptiles is slow when compared with mammals, making an incorrect diagnosis of ileus possible.[31] Ileus has been asso-ciated with the presence of ovarian follicles, extra-luminal masses (eg, neoplasia[32]), hypocalcemia, dehydration,[33] hypothermia, and constipation.[31] Gaseous tympany of the intestinal tract is occasionally visualized in reptiles, but is not a consistent finding.[31]

Intestinal obstruction is characterized by enlargement of the diameter of the diges-tive tract, but a prominent obstructive gas pattern is not always seen.[31–33] **(Fig. 16)** The accumulation of luminal contents in a dilated segment of intestines is commonly seen with a focal intestinal obstruction.[8]

The presence of rocks, gravel, or sand is not uncommon in the gastrointestinal tract, although large quantities may indicate constipation or an obstruction **(Fig. 17)**. In some species, intestinal foreign material may have to be distinguished from uroliths—the latter usually have a lamellated appearance.

Rabbits and rodents

Gastrointestinal stasis and ileus in rabbits and guinea pigs are acquired disorders associated with decreased motility resulting from either mechanical obstruction, reduced peristalsis, or both.[28] It should be noted that, even in healthy animals, the contents of the diet may affect the transit time. Low-fiber concentrated feeds are associated with quicker transit times (8 – 10 hours), while high-fiber diets with a low-energy concentration have longer transit times (up to 30 hours).[34]

Diagnosing gastrointestinal obstructions is challenging in rabbits (and, to a lesser extent, in guinea pigs), as reduced peristalsis may be hard to differentiate from an

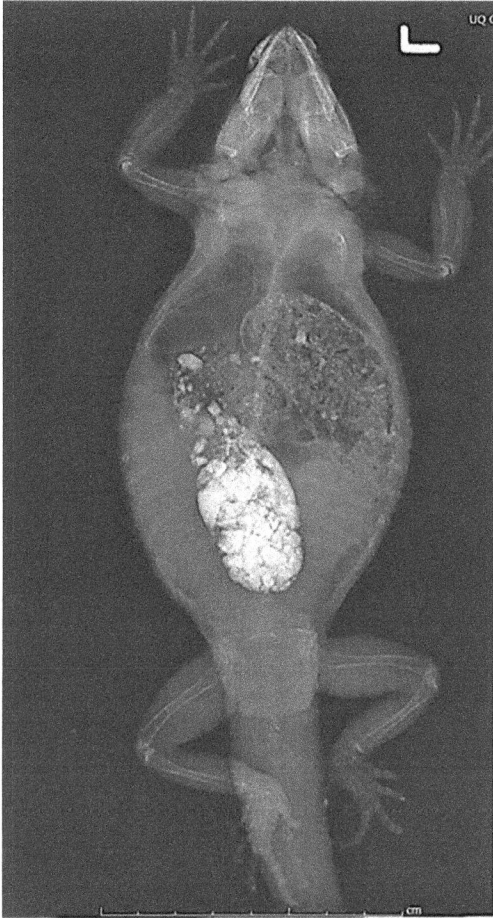

Fig. 16. Gastrointestinal impaction in a bearded dragon following ingestion of soil, probably in response to metabolic bone disease.

obstructive ileus. Careful evaluation of the stomach size and the relative amounts of ingesta, fluid, and gas is a key part of the radiographic interpretation (**Fig. 18**). A stomach distended with fluid density and gas often has a 'halo' appearance, indicating an obstructive pattern. This clinical suspicion can be strengthened with the presence of gaseous distension of the intestines and cecum.[28,35] The intestinal tract can be examined for luminal size, position within the abdomen, wall thickness, and pattern. If dilation or plication is noticed within the intestinal tract, the clinician should consider obstructive disease as a possible diagnosis.[36] Serial plain radiographs may help to determine if an obstruction is moving through the gastrointestinal tract or is lodged firmly.[36,37]

Ferrets

Radiographic signs of gastroenteric diseases in ferrets are like those seen in dogs and cats. With a rapid gastrointestinal time (less than 3 hours), generalized ileus appears to be rare in ferrets, although localized ileus is often seen with obstructive disease.

Doneley

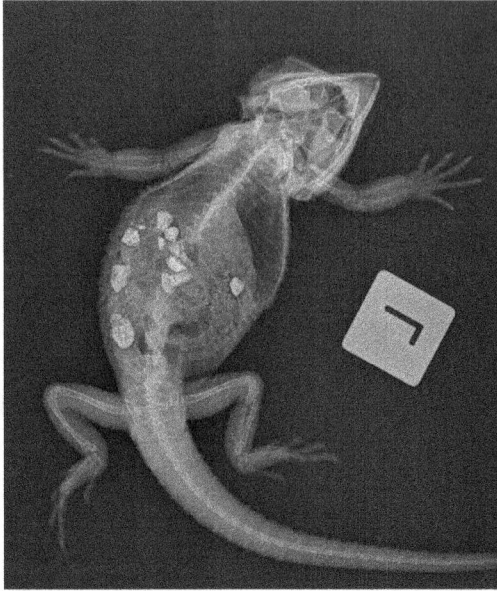

Fig. 17. Constipation in a bearded dragon.

Obstructive disorders such as foreign bodies are common, especially in young ferrets, and are often located in the pylorus, duodenum, or small intestine. Cranial to the obstruction the intestine will be markedly dilated, but beyond the obstruction the intestine will often appear normal.

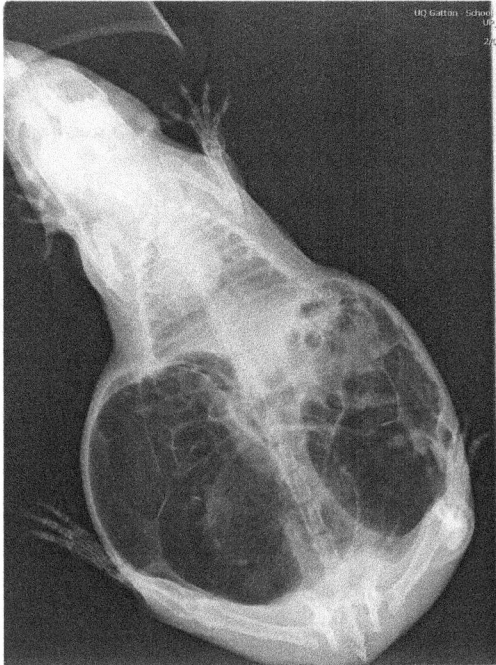

Fig. 18. Gastric stasis and ileus in a guinea pig.

Contrast Radiography

If good quality survey radiographs are not diagnostic, further imaging should be considered. In most veterinary practices, a contrast study using radiology is very achievable and will provide much needed information. Fluoroscopy has some advantages (mainly through been able to observe contractility) but for most clinical cases, a well-performed radiographic contrast study is a good diagnostic modality.

When interpreting a contrast study,[38] the clinician needs to examine:

- The transit times
- Lesions or anatomic alterations that persist throughout the study
- Intraluminal filling defects or foreign bodies
- Changes in luminal size, either constrictions or dilation
- Mucosal thickening or defects

These requirements are demonstrated in **Figs. 19–21**—radiographs of an eclectus parrot (*Eclectus roratus*) with a proventricular foreign body.

Gastrointestinal motility may be altered by the anatomy of the tract[3] (absence/presence of a crop or caecum), the species[39] (transit times are faster in birds of prey than in psittacine species), its age, its size, its diet, and its health. Stress and medications (including sedatives and anesthetics)[40] can have significant effects. It can also be affected by the contrast media used, with water-soluble iodinated contrast media having significantly shorter transit times than barium.[8]

Fluoroscopy

The main indication for fluoroscopy in birds is to observe gastrointestinal motility. After contrast, media is placed directly into the crop—obvious contractions of the crop can be seen, usually passing a bolus of media into the distal esophagus and proventriculus. The movement of these esophageal boluses can seem quite random, sometimes remaining in the esophagus until the next bolus, other times been regurgitated back to the crop. Once in the proventriculus, the bolus may be regurgitated back into the esophagus (but not to the crop).

Proventricular contractions, moving media into the ventriculus, occur when the proventriculus is sufficiently filled. Just after a proventriculus contraction occurs, a ventricular contraction begins. These are easily seen on fluoroscopy, occurring 3 to 4 times each minute. Toward the end of the contraction, media can be seen entering the duodenum. Reflux from the ventriculus into the proventriculus, and from the duodenum into the ventriculus is seldom seen.

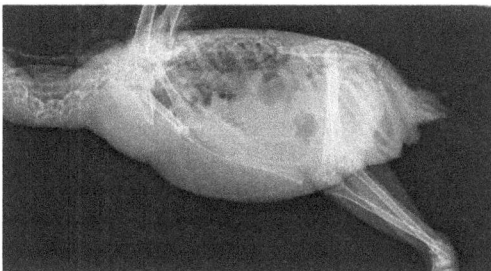

Fig. 19. Plain survey radiograph of an Eclectus parrot presented for intermittent vomiting. Some gas can be seen in the proventricular region, but it is difficult to assess due to loss of serosal detail.

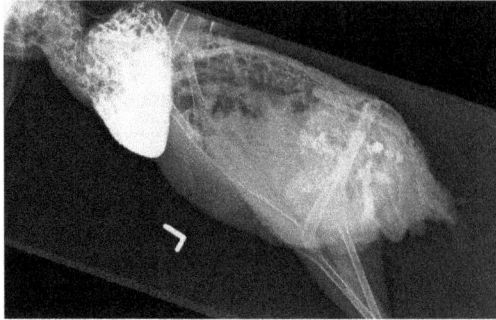

Fig. 20. Radiograph taken 1 hour after the administration of 20 mLs/kg barium sulfate. Most of the barium is still in the crop, although small amounts have passed through to the small intestine (delayed transit time). A possible radiopaque linear object is in the proventriculus.

Peristaltic waves in the duodenum and small intestine are rapid and can move in either direction, or as segmental contractions (producing a *string of pearls* appearance). The colon is slightly wider and less convoluted than the small intestines. Only occasional slow segmental contractions are observed in the colon.[40]

Ultrasound

The exotic animal clinician must appreciate the wide variation in anatomy between the various species that may be encountered. Care must be taken not to overinterpret normal structures in an unfamiliar species, and whenever possible, known standards should be consulted.

The inability of ultrasound waves to pass through air-filled structures (such as lungs or avian air sacs) limits its use in some gastrointestinal conditions in birds. It is difficult to successfully ultrasound the gastrointestinal tract of a healthy bird, although water given by gavage 10 to 15 minutes to sonography can act as a negative contrast, enhancing visualization of the tract.[29] When the air sacs are compressed by enlarged organs (such as the liver), fat, or fluid, ultrasound becomes an invaluable tool where plain radiographs may be of little assistance.

The ventriculus is usually easily identifiable due to the presence of hyperechoic grit with shadowing behind it. There is usually a hypoechoic around the grit (ingesta) and

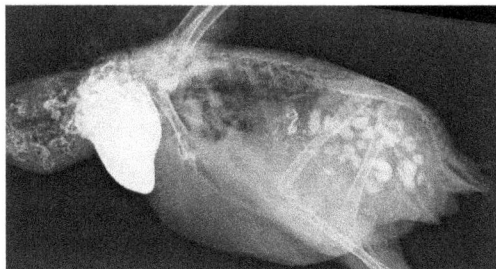

Fig. 21. Radiograph taken at 2 hours. While more contrast has passed into the intestine, the majority is still in the crop (delayed transit). The intestinal tract is not filling as expected (intraluminal filling deficits), and the radiopaque linear object is identified in the proventriculus (lesion that is persisting). A partial obstruction by a fibrous foreign body was successively removed endoscopically.

then the hypoechoic muscle wall. Directing the transducer cranially from the ventriculus may reveal the proventriculus, but it is often difficult to see if it is not enlarged. Caudal to the ventriculus, the intestines can be identified by their peristaltic waves. The pancreas may be visible as a hyperechoic area with the duodenal loop on the ventral body wall (a spacer may be required to visualize the pancreas).[34,41] Reference intervals for intestinal wall thickness and stratification are gradually becoming available.

The ability to sonographically image the reptile gastrointestinal tract is greatly dependent on the degree and type of filling within its lumen. Gaseous and stony or sandy contents hamper the imaging, while fluid contents enhance the quality. The structure of both the stomach and the intestinal wall can be assessed. In lizards and chelonians, the stomach has a thin wall and lies in the left part of the body cavity. In herbivorous reptiles, the stomach is often quite large and, when both stomach and ceca are filled with ingesta, they can be difficult to differentiate.[9]

The ultrasonographic anatomy of the reptilian small intestine is like that of mammals, with 5 wall layers visible. The stomach wall of inappetent (or fasted) snakes is readily imaged but when it is distended with ingesta, only one side of the stomach (that closest to the transducer) can be assessed. The wall of the large intestine is thinner and has indistinguishable layers.[9]

Many lizards have 2 intracoelomic fat bodies that extend from the pelvic region to the lateral body wall on both sides. Their echogenicity is much greater than that of the liver and this disparity can be used when assessing the liver parenchyma. The size of the fat body can also be used as a measure of the nutritional status of the animal.[9]

Ultrasound examination of the reptilian gastrointestinal tract also allows the detection of linear (and other) foreign bodies, intestinal lacerations, intussusceptions, and free coelomic fluid.

Herbivorous small mammals will always have some gas in the gastrointestinal tract, which can often be overcome by using different planes and applying pressure on the abdomen as needed. The presence of large amounts of gas in the intestine (eg, as seen with ileus) may limit the application of ultrasound.[10]

Unlike most animals that have a 5-layered intestinal wall, ultrasonographic layering of the gastrointestinal wall in guinea pigs and rabbits only shows 3 layers: an outer line of reflection (corresponding to the serosa); an anechoic middle layer (muscularis); and a hyperechoic inner interface (mucosa and submucosa). This may be because the mucosa and submucosa are too thin to be differentiated in the ultrasonographic examination. A small volume of anechoic free fluid in the abdomen is considered normal.[10]

Computed Tomography

Radiolucent tissues, such as air-filled structures, attenuate fewer X-rays and appear darker, while more radiodense tissues, for example, bone or metal, attenuate more X-rays and appear whiter. A CT image includes more shades of gray (greater contrast resolution) than a radiograph. Whereas radiography provides 5 shades of gray (ie, gas, fat, fluid/soft tissue, bone, and metal), CT can distinguish between thousands of shades of gray, including a distinction between soft tissue and fluid. Contrast resolution is further improved with the addition of an IV contrast medium, increasing the conspicuity of lesions with greater blood flow or capillary permeability.[11,12,21,42] (**Fig. 22**) The dynamically acquired images can then be visualized as variably sized slices or summed to provide reconstructions in various planes.

CT facilitates the detection and examination of intracoelomic organs (liver, kidney, and spleen), especially when contrast medium is used. The gastrointestinal tract

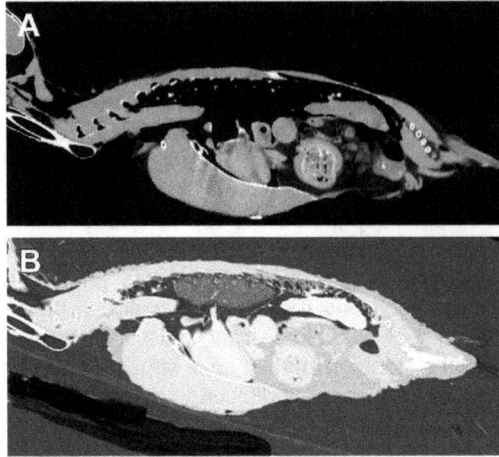

Fig. 22. The use of intravenous contrast in the computed tomography of a blue and gold maw. (*A*) pre-contrast, (*B*) post-contrast.

can also be visualized, but recognizing pathology in the intestinal tract may require the administration of orally-administered contrast media.[13–16,43] It is also useful in determining the size and extent of tumors and other abnormalities, as well as the effect of disease on surrounding normal anatomy, helping to develop a more appropriate treatment plan.[22,42,44]

Interpretation of MRI images

When scanning exotic patients, confirm with the radiologist about the resolution of the image that can be obtained with the available magnets (**Box 2**). An MRI scanner equipped with a magnet of 1.3 T field strength appears to be suitable to image small mammals such as small rabbits or ferrets. Very small patients may require field strength greater than 7 T. However, *weaker* magnets with field strength of only 0.2 to 0.4 T will have significantly less resolution and produce images that may not have enough resolution to be diagnostically useful.[18,22,42]

Because the MRI imaging is based on the responses of tissues and/or circulatory characteristics (eg, flow rates), this imaging modality is good for understanding the forms and positions of soft tissues, tracking changes, and identifying pathologic conditions.[18]

Box 2
Terminology

Three planes are commonly generated (veterinary terminology is in bold type and medical terminology is in parentheses):
- *Sagittal plane* (sagittal)
- *Transverse plane* (transaxial)
- *Dorsal plane* (coronal). **Fig. 2**

The intensity of the tissue density is described as:
- *Hyperintense* - bright (white)
- *Hypointense* - dark (black)
- *Isointense* - gray

- On a T1-weighted image, fat, gadolinium, methemoglobin, and melanin are hyperintense. Tissues such as brain parenchyma appear isointense, and tissues such as free water hypointense.
- On a T2-weighted image, tissues with the strongest signal are hyperintense. These include free water or watery tissues such as tumors, edema, and inflammation. Brain has an intermediate signal (isointense), while fat appears darker than on a T1 sequence.
- PDW-weighted images can be used to differentiate cystic from solid structures but exhibit less tissue contrast resolution than T1 and T2 sequences.[42]

Tissues with small amounts of hydrogen protons are hypointense on spin echo sequences; dense cortical bone, calcification, fibrous tissue, gas, and implanted materials are good examples of tissue with void hypointense signals. Flowing blood may also show as a hypointense (void) signal in some sequences.

As a rule, pathophysiological processes associated with inflammation, edema, or tumoral infiltrations show increased water content. This increases the relaxation time of the affected tissue, which translates in a hyperintense lesion on a T2 spin echo sequence. Exceptions to this rule include lesions with short relaxation time, and those that are composed of fat, hemorrhage, melanin, or contrast-enhancing characteristics. The presence of abnormalities should always be confirmed in more than 1 plane to avoid overinterpretation of various artifacts.

MRI is useful for detecting abscesses and metastatic disease. It can provide sufficient resolution to assess detailed diagnosis and prognosis, and the potential for surgical treatment. The presence of abnormalities should always be confirmed in more than 1 plane (dorsal or coronal, lateral or sagittal, and transverse or axial [see **Fig. 2**]) to avoid overinterpretation of various artifacts.

MRI has a potential value in visualizing the gastrointestinal tract, liver, spleen, and urogenital tract. In birds, it is less useful for imaging the heart and lungs of birds due to blurring produced by the normal heart and respiratory rates of small mammals and birds. The pancreas and adrenal glands may not be visible in some patients.

THE FUTURE OF DIAGNOSTIC IMAGING

Other advanced imaging modalities, already in use in human medicine, may eventually prove beneficial in exotic mammal medicine. While fluoroscopy, CT and MRI are not new to human or small animal medicine, their use in exotic or non-traditional pets is vastly underutilized. This may be related to the cost or the availability of the necessary equipment, even with some universities finding it difficult to justify updating their available equipment. However, with increased expectations of clients and their financial willingness, it is now not uncommon for private practices to utilize *entry level* CT scanners and fluoroscopes.

On the horizon for exotic pet medicine are other modalities, already in use in medicine. Nuclear diagnostic imaging, involving injection of radioactive isotopes, includes PET and scintigraphy. This technology provides functional information, rather than morphologic information, and can be used in addition to other standard modalities.

PET scans, utilizing CT and MRI technologies, can detect and trace radioactive material as it is injected into the patient, particularly radioactive-labelled glucose. This glucose isotope will concentrate in tissues with a high-energy consumption (such as neoplasms), allowing not only the detection of these masses but also their metabolic activity.

Scintigraphy, similarly to PET scans, generates images by detecting the emission of gamma rays from the patient. It has been used to detect conditions such as hyperthyroidism and muscle tears. The disadvantages of nuclear diagnostic imaging at this time include the higher radiation dose administered to the patient, the persistent radioactivity of the patient for several days, the availability of facilities offering this modality; the regulatory oversight required for the use of radioactive materials, and its cost. This current limited use means that their diagnostic value in exotic pet medicine has still to be assessed.

Without a doubt, it is in the best interest of the patient, the client, and the veterinarian to be aware of these different modalities, to recognize their applications (and limitations), and then to successfully integrate them into exotic pet medicine.

SUMMARY

For many veterinarians, the presentation of a bird, reptile, or small mammal for evaluation of a gastrointestinal problem poses an almost existential crisis. In any situation, by going back to first principles the veterinarian can work through a case and then reflect on how to apply them to their patient. This article reviews how a high-quality image of diagnostic value can be obtained using the more common imaging modalities (the principles), thus providing the clinician with the information needed to select the most appropriate modality and interpret the results (the application).

CLINICS CARE POINTS

- Sedation and/or anesthesia are often much safer and less stressful for exotic pets than manual restraint.
- Remember the old computer motto: Garbage In = Garbage Out. Poor quality, non-diagnostic images provide little information but take away the client's ability to pay for an accurate diagnosis and treatment.
- Invest in good quality imaging equipment.
- Always keep in mind those errors in interpretation - bias and satisfaction of search.

DISCLOSURE

The author has nothing to disclose.

REFERENCES

1. Guzman D. Ferret, rabbit, and rodent diagnostic imaging. In: Wild West veterinary conference. 2015. Available at: https://www.vin.com/doc/?id=7432394. Accessed August 26, 2024.
2. Vink-Nooteboom M, Lumeij JT, Wolvekamp WTC. Radiography and image-intensified fluoroscopy of barium passage through the gastrointestinal tract in six healthy Amazon parrots (*Amazona aestiva*). Vet Radiol Ultrasound 2003; 44(1):43–8.
3. Doss GA, Williams JM, Mans C. Determination of gastrointestinal transit times in Barred Owls (Strix Varia) by contrast fluoroscopy. J Avian Med Surg 2017;31(2): 123–7.
4. Coke RL, Lennox AM, Speer BS. Advanced imaging for diagnosing surgical conditions. In: Am board vet practitioners conference proceedings. 2017. Available at: https://www.vin.com/members/cms/project/defaultadv1.aspx?pid=19449&catId= &id=8207835&said=&meta=&authorid=&preview=. Accessed August 21, 2024.

5. Quesenberry K. Applications of advanced diagnostic imaging in birds. In: Pacific veterinary conference proceedings. 2018. Available at: https://www.vin.com/members/cms/project/defaultadv1.aspx?pid=20885&catId=&id=8550755&said=&meta=&authorid=&preview=. Accessed August 22, 2024.

6. Karanikas I, Kakoulidis DD, Gouvas ZT, et al. Barium peritonitis: a rare complication of upper gastrointestinal contrast investigation. Postgrad Med 1997;73(859): 297–8.

7. Williams J, Biller DS, Myer CW, et al. The use of iohexal as a gastrointestinal contrast agent in three dogs, five cats, and one bird. JAVMA (J Am Vet Med Assoc) 1993;202(4):625–7.

8. Silverman S. Diagnostic imaging. In: Mader DR, editor. Reptile medicine and surgery. 2nd edition. Philadelphia, PA: W.B. Saunders; 2006. p. 471–89. ISBN 9780721693279.

9. Pees M. Ultrasonography. In: Krautwald-Junghanns ME, et al, editors. Diagnostic imaging of exotic pets: birds, small mammals, reptiles, schluetersche. Germany: ProQuest Ebook Central; 2010. Available at: https://ebookcentral.proquest.com/lib/uql/detail.action?docID=616948. Accessed September 12, 2024.

10. Gómez MN, Domínguez Miño E, García de Carellán A, et al. Abdominal ultrasound features and reference values in healthy Guinea pigs (Cavia porcellus). Vet Rec 2024;194(2):e3668. Available at: https://doi.org/10.1002/vetr.3668. Accessed September 12, 2024.

11. Langan JN. Radiographic positioning and interpretation. In: American Association of zoo veterinarians conference. 2013. Available at: https://www.vin.com/doc/?id=6046976. Accessed August 26, 2024.

12. Monks D. A quick method for contrast radiography of the proximal gastrointestinal tract of the anesthetized avian patient. Exot Dvm 2003;5(5):17–8.

13. Schumacker J, Toal RL. Advanced radiography and ultrasonography in reptiles. Seminars Avian Exot Pet Med 2001;10(4):162–8.

14. Mathes KA, Radelof K, Engelke E, et al. Specific anatomy and radiographic illustration of the digestive tract and transit time of two orally administered contrast media in inland bearded dragons (Pogona vitticeps). PLoS One 2019;14(8): e0221050.

15. Meyer J. Gastrografin as a gastrointestinal contrast agent in the Greek tortoise (Testudo hermanni). J Zoo Wildl Med 1998;29(2):183–9.

16. Banzato T, Russo E, Finotti L, et al. Development of a technique for contrast radiographic examination of the gastrointestinal tract in ball pythons (Python regius). Am J Vet Res 2012;73(7):996–1001.

17. Doneley B. Diagnostic imaging. In: Avian medicine and surgery in practice: companion and aviary birds. 2nd edition. Boca Raton, FL: CRC Press; 2018. p. 95–107.

18. Wyneken J. Computed tomography and magnetic resonance imaging. In: Mader DR, Divers SJ, editors. Current therapy in reptile medicine and surgery. Philadelphia: Saunders; 2013. p. 93–106.

19. Pietsch H., CT contrast agents, In: Kiessling F. and Pichler B., Small animal imaging, 2011, Springer; Berlin, Heidelberg. 141-149. Available at: https://doi.org/10.1007/978-3-642-12945-2_11 (Accessed 21 August 2024).

20. McCready JE, Gardhouse SM, Appleby R, et al. Mortality rate of birds following intravenous administration of iodinated contrast medium for computed tomography. J Am Vet Med Assoc 2021;259(1):77–83.

21. Chen S. Diagnostic imaging of exotic companion small Mammals. In: Southwest veterinary symposium. 2019. Available at: https://www.vin.com/doc/?id=9222355. Accessed August 26, 2024.

22. Tarbell AL, Fischetti AJ. Diagnostic imaging. In: Quesenberry K, Orcutt CJ, Mans C, Carpenter JW, editors. Ferrets, rabbits, and rodents. 4th edition. Philadelphia, PA: W.B. Saunders; 2020. p. 559–68. ISBN 9780323484350.

23. Thorsen AJ, Lakin GE. Basic physics of ultrasonography. Semin Colon Rectal Surg 2010;21(4):186–90.

24. Fulton RF. Focused basic ultrasound principles and artifacts. In: Lisciandro GR, editor. Focused ultrasound techniques for the small animal practitioner. 1st edition. Hoboken, NJ: Wiley; 2014. p. 1–16.

25. Hochleithner C, Holland M. Ultrasonography. In: Mader DR, Divers SJ, editors. Current therapy in reptile medicine and surgery. Philadelphia, PA: W.B. Saunders; 2014. p. 107–27. ISBN 9781455708932.

26. Penninck DG, Stewart JS, Paul-Murphy J, et al. Ultrasonography of the California desert tortoise (Xerobates agassizi): anatomy and application. Vet Radiol 1991; 32(3):112–6.

27. British Medical Ultrasound Society. Small animal veterinary guidelines for professional ultrasound practice. (6th edition) Available at: https://www.bmus.org/mediacentre/news/small-animal-veterinary-guidelines-for-professional-ultrasound-practice/ (Accessed 22 August 2024).

28. Reusch B. Rabbit gastroenterology. Vet Clin North Am Exot Anim Pract 2005;8(2): 351–75.

29. Krautwald-Junghanns M-E, Stahl A, Pees M, et al. Sonographic investigation of the gastrointestinal tract of granivorous birds. Vet Radiol Ultras 2024;3(6):576–82.

30. Molazem M, Soroori S, Soflaei R, et al. Radiologic features of radiolucent foreign bodies ingestion in common Mynah (Acridotheres tristis). Vet Med Sci 2023;9(3): 1163–71.

31. Mans C. Clinical update on diagnosis and management of disorders of the digestive system of reptiles. J Exot Pet Med 2013;22(2):141–62.

32. Helmick KE, Bennett RA, Ginn P, et al. Intestinal volvulus and stricture associated with a leiomyoma in a green turtle (Chelonia mydas). J Zoo Wild Med 2000;31(2): 221–7.

33. Benson KG. Reptilian gastrointestinal diseases. Seminars Avian Exot Pet Med 1999;8(2):90–7.

34. Krautwald-Junghanns M-E, Pees M, Reese S, et al. Diagnostic imaging of exotic pets: birds, small mammals, reptiles. 1st edition. Germany: Schluetersche: ProQuest Ebook Central; 2010. Available at: http://ebookcentral.proquest.com/lib/uql/detail.action?docID=616948. Accessed August 22, 2024.

35. Beaufrère H. Medical management of gastrointestinal stasis in rabbits. In: Proceedings Pacific veterinary conference. 2022. Available at: https://www.vin.com/doc/?id=10876786&pid=28856. Accessed September 5, 2025.

36. Ritzman TK. Diagnosis and clinical management of gastrointestinal conditions. Vet Clin North Am Exot Anim Pract 2014;17(2):179–94. ISSN 1094-9194, ISBN 9780323297271.

37. Debenham JJ, Brinchmann T, Sheen J, et al. Radiographic diagnosis of small intestinal obstruction in pet rabbits (Oryctolagus cuniculus): 63 cases. J Small Anim Pract 2019;60(11):691–6.

38. Sander J. Using contrast radiography to diagnose gastrointestinal diseases in birds. Vet Med 1996;9(7):652–5.

39. Doss GA, Williams JM, Mans C. Contrast fluoroscopic evaluation of gastrointestinal transit times with and without the use of falconry hoods in red-tailed hawks (Buteo jamaicensis). J Am Vet Med Assoc 2017;251(9):1064–9.

40. Martel A, Mans C, Doss GA, et al. Effects of midazolam and midazolam-butorphanol on gastrointestinal transit time and motility in cockatiels (Nymphicus hollandicus). J Avian Med Surg 2018;32(4):286–93.
41. Le Roux AB, Quesenberry K, Donnelly KA, et al. Disseminated pancreatic adeno-carcinoma in an Eclectus parrot (Eclectus roratus). J Am Vet Med Assoc 2020; 257(6):635–41.
42. van Zeeland YRA, Schoemaker NJ, Hsu EW. Advances in diagnostic imaging. In: Speer BL, editor. Current therapy in avian medicine and surgery. Philadelphia, PA: W.B. Saunders; 2016. p. 531–49.
43. Silverman S, Tell LA. Radiology equipment and positioning techniques. In: Silverman S, Tell L, Nugent-Deal J, Palmer-Holtry KL, editors. Radiology of ro-dents, rabbits, and ferrets. Phildelphia, PA: W.B. Saunders; 2005. p. 1–8. ISBN 9780721697895.
44. Schwarz LA, Solano M, Manning A, et al. The normal upper gastrointestinal exam-ination in the ferret. Vet Radiol Ultras 2003;44(2):165–72.

Avian Gastroenterology
Anatomy and Assessment

Ashton Hollwarth, BSc, BVMS, CertAVP (Zoo Med), ANZCVS (Avian Medicine & Surgery), DipECZM (Avian), MRCVS*, Lucia Gomez Prieto, DVM, MRCVS

KEYWORDS

- Gastroenterology • Anatomy • Physiology • Cytology • Fecal examination

KEY POINTS

- The anatomy of the avian gastrointestinal tract differs vastly between different species, based on environment, diet, feeding strategy, and evolutionary adaptations.
- Species-specific adaptations to diet and environment shape the external and internal anatomy of different families of birds.
- Distinct lymph nodes are absent across the alimentary tract of birds, but gut-associated lymphatic tissue is present.
- The gastrointestinal tract of avian patients is difficult to examine physically, so to investigate gastrointestinal concerns, clinicians must use diagnostic testing.

INTRODUCTION

Avian patients commonly present for gastrointestinal complaints as the symptoms of digestive disorders, such as abnormal droppings or vomiting, are readily observable by owners. The avian gastrointestinal system varies enormously between different species, based on diet, feeding habits, food availability, and environment. Because of these differences, nutrition and gastrointestinal diseases can differ greatly between species. It is important for practitioners to be aware of and understand these species differences and how they relate to functional anatomy and species predispositions for gastrointestinal diseases. The objectives of this article are to review the anatomy and physiology of the avian gastrointestinal tract, describe the anatomic differences between different orders of birds, and to discuss diagnostic tools that practitioners can use to investigate gastrointestinal disease in their avian patients in clinical practice.

Great Western Exotics, Unit 10 Berkshire House, County Park, Shrivenham Road, Swindon, Wiltshire SN1 2NR, UK
* Corresponding author.
E-mail address: ashton.hollwarth@vets-now.com

Vet Clin Exot Anim 28 (2025) 413–424
https://doi.org/10.1016/j.cvex.2024.11.009
1094-9194/25/© 2024 Elsevier Inc. All rights are reserved, including those for text and data mining, AI training, and similar technologies.

Abbreviations	
CT	computed tomography
DPG	deep proventricular glands
GALT	gut-associated lymphatic tissue
GLDH	glutamate dehydrogenase
SPG	superficial proventricular glands

ANATOMY AND PHYSIOLOGY

The digestive system of avian species is adapted to its specific feeding habits and diet. The beak or bill is formed by the bones of the jaw and its keratin cover, known as rhamphotheca. The cutting edge of the keratin of both the maxillary beak (rhinotheca) and the mandibular beak (gnathotheca) is known as tomium. The culmen and gonys are the median longitudinal lines of the rhinotheca and gnathotheca respectively.[1] The bill-tip organ, a sensory organ situated at the tip of the upper and lower beaks in most birds, can be found only on the gnathotheca of the chicken (*Gallus gallus domesticus*).[2,3] This organ intervenes in food selection and prehension.

The beak is species-specific with Psittaciformes having a wide and curved rhinotheca, Galliformes having a triangular beak with hooked rhinotheca, Anseriformes having a beak with a flattened and rounded tip, and birds of prey possessing a hooked rhinotheca (**Fig. 1**). The shape and size of the gnathotheca depends on the characteristic of the upper beak. Birds with a straighter beak tend to have a lower length ratio of lower-to-upper beak, for example, waterfowl. Psittacines, on the other hand, have a curved rhinotheca, and therefore this ratio tends to be the highest.[4]

The oral cavity and pharynx, often called oropharynx, differs from those of mammals in lacking a soft palate and consequently, the nasopharynx. The oropharynx is connected to the nasal cavity by a small fissure in the palate called the choana. Caudal to the choana, the infundibular cleft connects the oropharynx to the avian tuba auditiva.[1,5] The palate is often covered by a keratinized mucosa, making transverse ridges and shallow grooves, and in some species, papillae are present (**Figs. 2** and **3**).[5] Especially well-developed ridges are present in seed-eating passerines, to help in cutting and removing the shells of seeds.[1,6]

The tongue is adapted to facilitate prehension, manipulation, and swallowing of food. A protrusible tongue is observed in nectar and pollen feeding birds, such as hummingbirds.[7,8] Woodpeckers have a brush-like tip enabling them to capture small insects and extract tree sap.[9] A thick and muscular tongue is present in nut-eaters and shell-eaters, including psittacines and passerines. Many fish-eating species have

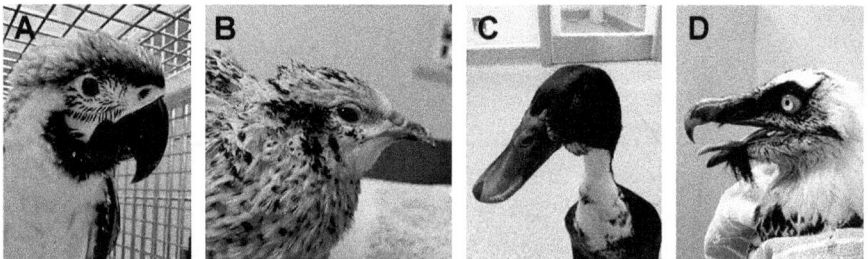

Fig. 1. Beaks of different avian species. (*A*) Blue-and-yellow macaw (*Ara ararauna*), (*B*) Japanese quail (*Coturnix japonica*), (*C*) Indian runner duck (*Anas platyrhynchos domesticus*), (*D*) Bearded vulture (*Gypaetus barbatus*).

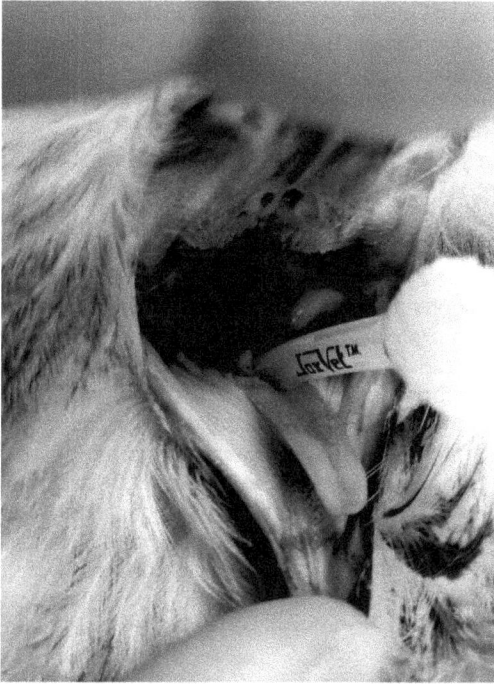

Fig. 2. Oropharynx with palate papillae of a Eurasian eagle-owl (*Bubo bubo*).

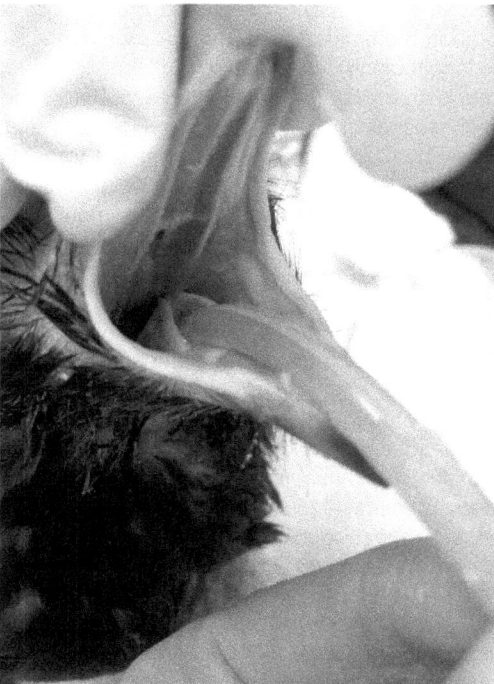

Fig. 3. Oropharynx, laryngeal mound, and choana of a Harris hawk (*Parabuteo unicinctus*).

strong tongue papillae to hold slippery food. In waterfowl, the tongue is adapted to filter water particles through lateral bristles and tooth-like processes that interlock with the lamellae of the maxillary beak. This process occurs after a groove on the dorsal surface of the tongue is filled with water.[1] Other adaptations of waterfowl include using the previously described bristles and processes to tear grass or break hard pieces of food, for example, in the Egyptian goose (*Alopochen aegyptiaca*).[10] Some Galliformes have caudally directed lingual papillae that helps prevent regurgitation of food bolus.[11,12] At the base of the tongue, the laryngeal mound presents the opening of the glottis into the larynx.

Upon grasping the food, the tongue presses it toward the palate. Reflexive closure of the choana, infundibular cleft, and glottis occurs to prevent food from entering the nasal cavity or respiratory system. A coordinated sequence of movements of the tongue facilitates the transfer of the food bolus from the oral cavity to the pharynx and ultimately to the esophagus.[1,5]

The avian sense of taste differs from mammals by having tastebuds mainly on the palate, base of the tongue and pharynx, and around salivary glands instead of on the dorsal surface of the tongue.[13] Salivary glands are distributed throughout the oropharynx and may vary between species. These include the maxillary salivary gland, palatine glands, rostral and intermediate mandibular glands, and lingual glands. It has been hypothesized that dry diet birds, such as granivores, would have more developed salivary glands to help swallowing. Recent studies have proven the presence of well-developed salivary glands also in fish-eating birds like the cattle egret (*Bubulcus ibis*).[14]

The alimentary canal differs from that in mammals, with distinctions including the presence of the crop in some species, a stomach divided into proventriculus and ventriculus, the presence of 2 ceca, and the replacement of the anus by a cloaca.[5]

The esophagus is thin-walled and generally lies on the right side of the neck, in contrast to the course in mammals.[5,15] The esophagus is divided into cervical and thoracic regions. It is longitudinally folded allowing a great distension for food passage. The crop (or ingluvies) is an esophageal dilation present before the esophagus enters the coelomic cavity whose main function is food storage.[1] Other functions include the production of crop milk by Columbiformes, which is fed to nestlings, composed of proliferated epithelial cells filled with lipids that have desquamated from the crop mucosa.[16] The crop is absent in many bird species, for example, owls, gulls, ratites and, penguins.[17–20] Crop size and shape varies across species, being large in Galliformes, bilobed in pigeons, with a lateral sac-like diverticulum that lies transverse across the neck in some psittacine species, and a simple widening of the distal crop in some ducks and geese (**Figs. 4** and **5**).[1,15,21] The distribution of secretory glands across the mucosa of the esophagus and crop varies among species, and they contribute to enhance the food passage.[1,22]

The avian stomach, situated on the left side of the coelomic cavity, is divided into the proventriculus or glandular stomach (*pars glandularis*) cranially, and the ventriculus or muscular stomach (*pars muscularis*), caudally. The proventriculus and ventriculus generally consists of mucosal, submucosal, muscular, and serosal layers. The proventricular mucosa, in most species, presents longitudinal folds increasing the surface. These folds are more numerous in nectarivores passerines, in which food volume present in the proventriculus is greater, compared to granivore or omnivore passerines.[5,6,23–25]

The superficial proventricular glands (SPG) are involved in mucus production, while the deep proventricular glands (DPG) are associated with the production of stomach enzymes including pepsinogen and hydrochloric acid. DPG have been described in

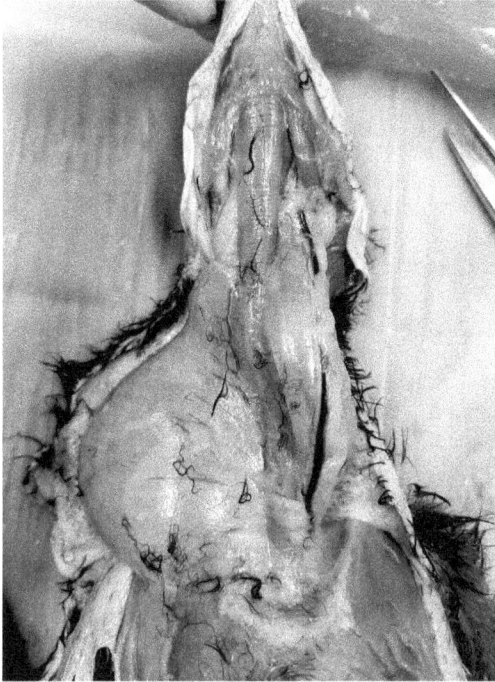

Fig. 4. Esophagus and crop of a juvenile hooded vulture (*Necrosyrtes monachus*).

many avian species with inconsistent distribution.[23–27] The majority of the proventricular wall in omnivores and carnivores, such as the common moorhen (*Gallinula chloropus*), domestic fowl (*Gallus gallus*), hooded crow (*Corvus cornix*), pallid scops-owl (*Otus brucei*), and common kestrel (*Falco tinnunculus*), is occupied by DPG. In carnivores, the proventriculus tends to be large and these glands produce an acidic secretion suggesting a strong glandular digestion.[23,25–28]

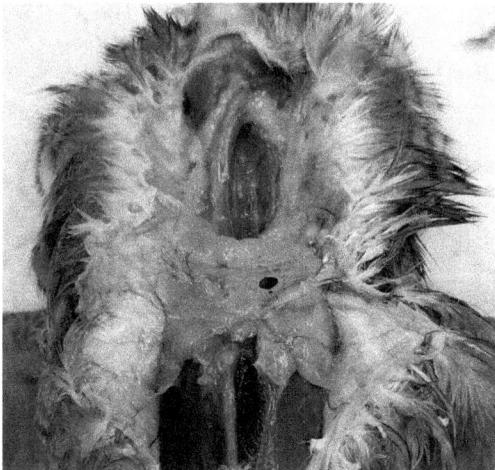

Fig. 5. Crop of a budgerigar (*Melopsittacus undulatus*).

An intermediate area (ie, the isthmus) separates the proventriculus and ventriculus, which usually lacks DPG but may still have SPG.[26] A robust ventriculus, or gizzard, grinds down seeds and fibrous material. This structure is well developed in birds with a granivorous, omnivorous, and herbivorous diet in contrast to carnivores in which it is less developed.[5,9,29] This is achieved by having a well-developed muscular layer, a thicker noncellular keratin layer that covers the mucosa, called the koilin or cuticle, and the presence of grit (**Fig. 6**).[6,26,30] A pellet or casting formed of nondigestible residuals of food material, such as feathers, is formed in the gizzard and later regurgitated in raptors and crows.[31] This pellet may also contain bones in owls, due to a higher stomach pH compared to other raptors.[32–34]

The intestines run from the pylorus to the cloaca and the length, size, and shape varies among species. Macroscopic differentiation between small intestinal segments is challenging due to its uniform diameter but can be achieved by visualization of the opening of the bile and pancreatic ducts in the distal duodenum and the presence of the Meckel's diverticulum, residual of the yolk sac, at the end of the jejunum.[23,30] The duodenum is U-shaped and the pancreas is present between the duodenal loops, holding together descending and ascending duodenums.[6,23,30,35,36] The jejuno-ileum, arranged in loops or coiled, is the intestinal segment where digestion, conducted by the pancreatic enzymes and bile, and absorption occurs.[6,20,23] Small intestines vary in length across species, generally being longer in granivores.[9,31] Microscopically, the avian intestines are characterized by villi formation of the epithelial mucosa. These villi vary in size between species and between intestinal segments within the same species.[6,23,30,37,38]

The colorectum is short and tubular, ending in the gastrointestinal section of the cloaca, the coprodeum. Bilateral ceca, if present, arise from the cranial part of the colon at the ileo-cecal-colic junction and run cranially along the small intestine. Ceca are usually blind-ended and tubular in shape; however, in the common barn owl (*Tyto alba*) they are very thin at the caudal portion adjacent to the insertion to the colorectum with a large blind end, which gives an appearance of a microphone.[23,30,35,36] Ceca are absent in psittacines.[29,39]

The avian large intestine enters the cloaca into the coprodeum, which is the largest of the 3 parts of the cloaca. In some species, such as the great horned owl (*Bubo virginianus*), American kestrel (*Falco sparverius*), and domestic duck, there is a recto-

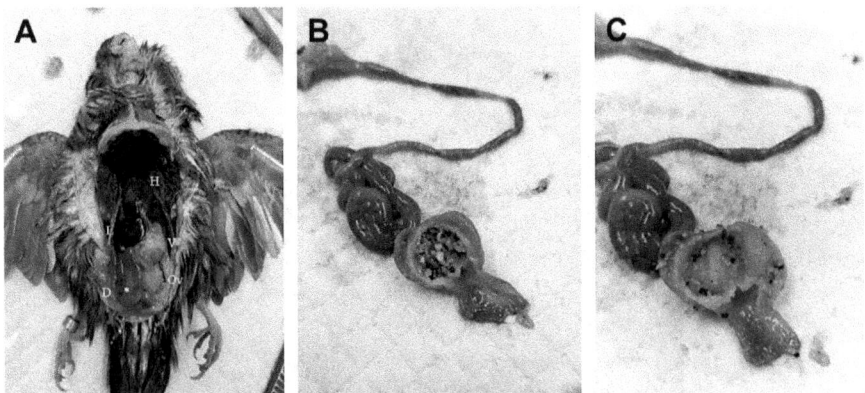

Fig. 6. (*A*) Celomic cavity and celomic organs of a budgerigar during *postmortem* examination. (*B*) Proventriculus and ventriculus opened before removing food and grit. (*C*) Proventriculus and ventriculus after removing food and grit, with visible ventricular cuticle. *, Pancreas; D, Duodenum; H, Heart; L, Liver; Ov, Oviduct; V, Ventriculus.

coprodeal sphincter.[37,40] The coprodeum connects to the urodeum where the urinary and reproductive tracts open. The coprodeum and the urodeum are separated by the coprourodeal fold. The last chamber of the cloaca is the proctodeum, which has a role in avian immune system, as it opens to the *Bursa of Fabricius.*[37]

The coprodeum is a vascular and glandular organ and lacks villi in Psittaciformes, Falconiformes, and Columbiformes.[37,41] Feces stored in the coprodeum mix with the urine and urates from the urodeum to form the urofeces that are excreted together. The function of the coprodeum and colorectum includes regulation of the osmotic balance by reabsorption of sodium from intestinal loses, and by postrenal modification of the urine with water absorption after retroperistaltism of the urine into the large intestine.[38,42,43] In some species, retroperistaltism of urine may reach the cecum, in which bacterial decomposition of uric acid occurs.[44] Urofeces are excreted directly from the coprodeum through the vent, the external horizontal opening of the cloaca formed by ventral and dorsal lips. These urofeces do not contact the urodeum or the proctodeum during evacuation.[37] In the common ostrich, the coprodeum acts similar to a mammalian bladder, storing only urine and not participating in osmotic balance regulation. In this species, feces are stored in the distal large intestine rather than in the coprodeum and are excreted separately from the urine.[45]

Distinct lymph nodes are absent across the alimentary tract of birds, but gut-associated lymphatic tissue (GALT) is present.[23,30,46]

The liver is the main organ for de novo lipogenesis in avian species.[47] It is dark red-brown in color and relatively large in birds with right and left lobes, the left one being subdivided into caudo-dorsal and caudo-ventral parts.[30,48] The visceral surface of the right lobe is in contact with the duodenum, and the left lobe with the proventriculus, ventriculus, and spleen.[28] Cranially both lobes are in contact with the heart leaving a characteristic cardiac impression.[36] The gall bladder is thin-walled, positioned on the visceral surface of the right liver lobe and its duct drains to it.[30] The gall bladder is absent in most psittacines.[48]

The pancreas is pale pink to yellow in color and is situated in the mesoduodenum.[6,23,30,35,36] The pancreas varies in length and structure between species, having from 2 to 4 pancreatic lobes named dorsal, ventral, third, and splenic pancreatic lobes. Three ducts from the exocrine pancreas, dorsal, ventral, and the third lobes respectively, drain into the duodenum.[5,30] The avian exocrine pancreas is composed of pyramidal acinar cells with zymogen granules, and the endocrine part is distributed in Islets of Langerhans. Five types of endocrine cells have been found in the avian pancreas: alpha cells secreting glucagon, beta cells secreting insulin, delta cells secreting somatostatin, pancreatic polypeptide secreting cells, and neuropeptide Y secreting cells.[49–51]

EXAMINATION AND DIAGNOSTIC INVESTIGATION

Examination of the gastrointestinal tract in its entirety is difficult with physical examination alone. The oral cavity and cloaca can be physically examined, and the crop, when present, as well as the ventriculus and intestines can often be palpated on physical examination. However, a thorough examination of the gastrointestinal tract requires diagnostic modalities.

When examining the oral cavity, normal anatomy for the species being examined needs to be considered, including beak shape, form and texture, normal tongue anatomy and mobility, appearance of the glottis and choana, and normal appearance of the oral mucosa. External examination of the vent lips is possible, but full cloacal examination is likely to require the use of endoscopy.

Examination of feces can provide practitioners with a vast amount of information. Droppings should be assessed for size, color, consistency, urine, and uric acid to fecal volumes, and presence of any foreign material or hemorrhage, considering what is normal for the species (**Fig. 7**). Feces can also be further examined for the presence of parasites, or cytologically to assess bacterial, fungal, or yeast organisms. Culture and sensitivity testing can be considered if abnormal organisms are identified in cytology. In a similar manner to visual examination of the droppings, castings from birds who naturally cast pellets can also be examined for consistency and presence of any foreign materials. Crop or proventricular washes can be performed using warmed saline in an attempt to identify infectious organisms such as *Trichomonas* spp. or *Macrorhabdus ornithogaster*.

Diagnostic imaging is immensely useful for the investigation of gastrointestinal disease. Both plain and contrast radiographs can be used to assess the gastrointestinal tract and are useful for determining organomegaly, mass effects, filling defects, or gas or fluid distension. Computed tomography (CT) can also be used to assess the gastrointestinal tract and has the advantage of avoiding superimposition of organs. The use of intravenous contrast agents in conjunction with CT can be used to assess the liver and pancreas. Fluoroscopic studies can be performed to assess the passage of contrast material to determine gastrointestinal transit time, filling defects, and gastric contractility.

Endoscopy is a useful tool to evaluate the gastrointestinal tract, both internally and externally. Its benefits include a minimally invasive examination of the gastrointestinal tract and surrounding structures, and the ability to take biopsies or remove foreign bodies without requiring celiotomy. Both rigid and flexible endoscopy can be employed in assessment of the gastrointestinal tract, dependent on patient size. Rigid endoscopy is usually employed in smaller birds less than 400g to evaluate

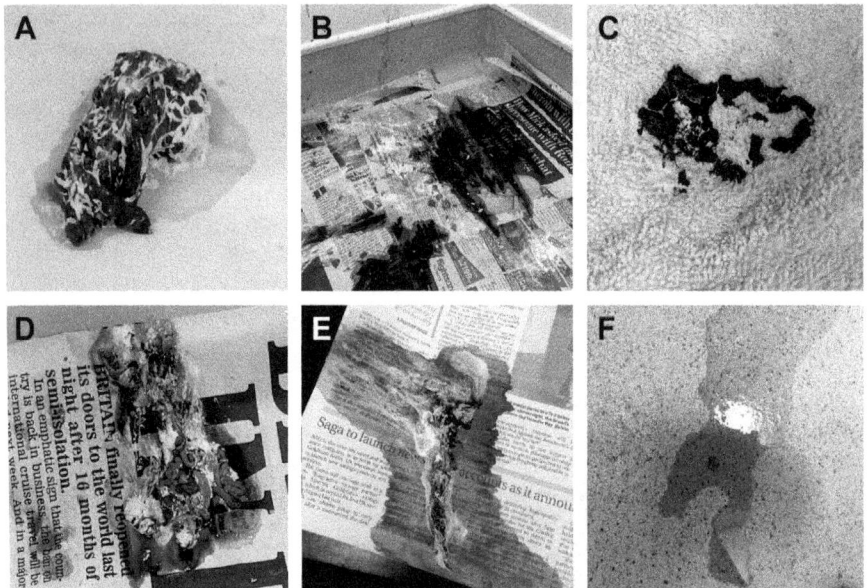

Fig. 7. Examples of different fecal presentations that a practitioner may encounter. (*A*) Normal dropping from a parrot. (*B*) Diarrhea. (*C*) Melena. (*D*) Hemorrhage. (*E*) Polyuria. (*F*) Biliverdinuria.

the upper gastrointestinal tract, with flexible endoscopy being required in birds of larger sizes.[52] Cloacoscopy can be achieved with a rigid endoscope and instrument sheath in order to provide warmed saline insufflation. If assessment of the liver, pancreas, or coelom is required, celioscopy with the use of a rigid endoscope can be used. A standard left-sided approach is useful to assess the gastrointestinal tract and the left liver lobe. A right-sided approach can be used to assess the pancreas and right liver lobe. A ventral approach can be used to assess both the liver lobes without requiring patient repositioning.[52]

Hematology and biochemistry can be useful in patients with systemic disease that manifests with gastrointestinal symptoms and can help discriminate primary gastrointestinal pathology from secondary gastrointestinal signs. When attempting to identify hepatic disease, there are several markers to consider. In the racing pigeon, plasma aspartate aminotransferase and bile acids have been found to be the most sensitive indicators of hepatic disease, and glutamate dehydrogenase (GLDH) was determined to be the most liver-specific enzyme.[53] As a general rule when comparing enzyme activity and attempting to determine between hepatic and musculoskeletal disease, plasma creatinine kinase activity does not increase in response to hepatic disease, and GLDH, gamma-glutamyl transferase, and bile acids do not increase following muscle damage. In addition, biochemistry can assist in diagnosing pancreatic disease, as activity of both amylase and lipase have been reported to increase in cases of active pancreatitis.[53]

SUMMARY

The avian gastrointestinal system is highly diverse between different avian families, reflecting the ecological niches that each species inhabits in the wild. These differences reflect the varied feeding strategies, diets, and habitats of these birds. It is important for practitioners to understand the species anatomic and physiologic differences to ensure the best treatment of patients under their care.

CLINICS CARE POINTS

- Avian gastrointestinal anatomy is closely related to feeding strategies. Clinicians can often gleen deduce the feeding strategy and diet of an avian patient based on the anatomy of their beak, oral cavity and gastrointestinal tract.

- The gastrointestinal tract of avians is vastly different between speices, and to that of mammals. In particular, most birds have an outpouching of the oesophagus - the crop - and have stomachs divided between the glandular (proventriculus) and muscular (ventriulus) areas. The feeding stratefy of each species defines the presence or absence of a crop, and its anatomy, as well as the length and size of the proventriculus, ventriculus, small intestine and caea, if present.

- Diagnostic testing of the gastrointestinal tract can be very minimally invasive. Samples of faeces can be used for staining, such as Gram staining or new methylene blue staining which can be performed quickly and at a low cost in clinic. Faecal samples can also be submitted for culture and sensitivity, PCR testing or faecal occult blood testing.

- Other diagnostic testing, such as blood sampling and endoscopy, can be more invasive, but can yield important diagnostic information about underlying conditions. Clinicians should not avoid more invasive testing if it is indicated, as pathology external to the gastrointestinal tract can result in gastrointestinal symptoms.

DISCLOSURE

The authors have nothing to disclose.

REFERENCES

1. King AS, McLelland J. External anatomy. In: King AS, McLelland J, editors. Birds, their structure and function. 2nd edition. Bath: Bailliere Tindall; 1984. p. 9–22.
2. Gentle MJ, Breward J. The bill tip organ of the chicken (Gallus gallus var. Domesticus). J Anat 1986;145:79–85.
3. Avilova KV. Spatial organization of the epithelial structures in the bill tip organ of waterfowl (Anseriformes, Aves). Biol Bull Rev 2018;8:234–44.
4. Cheng Y, Lei F. Avian lower beak is always overlooked: its coordinate role in shaping species-specific beak should not be underestimated. Integr Zool 2023;19(2): 339–42.
5. Konig HE, Liebich HG, Korbel R, et al. Digestive system (apparatus digestorius). In: Konig HE, Rudiger K, Liebich HG, editors. Avian anatomy, textbook and colour atlas. 2nd edition. Sheffield: 5M Publishing Ltd; 2009. p. 92–117.
6. Taha AM, Al-Duleemy AS. Morphological description of the digestive canal in Taeniopygia guttata (zebra finch) and Sturnus vulgaris (starling). J Basic Appl Zool 2020;81(1):1–10.
7. Rico-Guevara A, Hurme KJ, Rubega MA, et al. Nectar feeding beyond the tongue: hummingbirds drink using phase-shifted bill opening, flexible tongue flaps and wringing at the tips. J Exp Biol 2023;226(1):1–11.
8. Gartell BD, Jones SM, Brereton RN, et al. Morphological adaptations to nectarivory of the alimentary tract of the swift parrot Lathamus discolor. EMU 2000;100(4): 274–9.
9. Jung J, Naleway SE, Yaraghi NA, et al. Structural analysis of the tongue and hyoid apparatus in a woodpecker. Acta Biomater 2016;37:1–13.
10. Hassan SM, Moussa EA, Cartwright AL. Variations by sex in anatomical and morphological features of the tongue of Egyptian Goose (Alopochen aegyptiacus). Cells Tissues Organs 2009;191(2):161–5.
11. Parchami A, Dehkordi RAF, Bahadoran S. Fine structure of the dorsal lingual epithelium of the common quail (Coturnix coturnix). World Appl Sci J 2010;10(10):1185–9.
12. Erdogan S, Sagsoz H, Akbalik ME. Anatomical and histological structure of the tongue and histochemical characteristics of the lingual salivary glands in the Chukar partridge (Alectoris chukar, Gray 1830). Br Poult Sci 2012;53(3):307–15.
13. Kudo K, Nishisimura S, Tabata S. Distribution of taste buds in layer-type chickens: scanning electron microscopic observations. J Anim Sci 2008;79(6):680–5.
14. El-Bakry AM, Iwasaki S. Ultrastructure and histochemical study of the lingual salivary glands of some bird species. Pak J Zool 2014;46(2):553–9.
15. Klingler JJ. On the morphological description of tracheal and esophageal displacement and its phylogenetic distribution in Avialae. PLoS One 2016;11(9):1–37.
16. Jin C, He Y, Jiang S, et al. Chemical composition of pigeon crop milk and factors affecting its production: a review. Poult Sci J 2023;102(6):1–14.
17. Shawki NA, Mahmoud FA, Mohamed MY. Seasonal variations in the digestive tract of the little owl, Athene noctua: anatomical, histological and scanning electron microscopical studies. Microsc Microanal 2022;28(3):844–57.
18. Ince NG, Pazvant G, Kahvecioglu KO. Macro anatomic investigations on digestive system of Marmara region sea gulls. J Anim Vet Adv 2010;9(12):1757–60.

19. Umar Z, Qureshi AS, Shahid R, et al. Histological and histomorphometric study of the cranial digestive tract of ostriches (Struthio camelus) with advancing age. Vet Med 2021;66(04):127–39.
20. Kline S, Kottyan J, Phillips J, et al. The radiographic and endoscopic anatomy and digestive mechanisms of captive African penguins (Spheniscus demersus). J Zoo Wildl Med 2020;51(2):371–8.
21. Hallsworth EG, Coates JI. The growth of the alimentary tract of the fowl and the goose. J Agric Sci 1962;58(2):153–63.
22. Rajabi E, Nabipour A. Histological study on the esophagus and crop in various species of wild bird. Avian Biol Res 2009;2(3):161–4.
23. Abdellatif A, Farag A, Metwally E. Anatomical, histochemical and immunohisto-chemical observations on the gastrointestinal tract of Gallinula chloropus (Aves: Rallidae). BCM Zool 2022;7(1):61.
24. Ogunkoya YO, Cook RD. Histomorphology of the proventriculus of three species of Australian passerines: lichmera indistincta, Zosterops lateralis and Poephila guttata. Anat Histol Embryol 2009;38(4):246–53.
25. Beheiry RR. Histochemical and scanning electron microscopy of proventriculus in Turkey. J Adv Vet Anim Res 2018;5(3):290–8.
26. Alsanosy AA, Noreldin AE, Elewa YHA, et al. Comparative features of the upper alimentary tract in the domestic fowl (Gallus gallus domesticus) and kestrel (Falco tinnunculus): a morphological, histochemical and scanning electron micro-scopy study. Microsc Microanal 2021;27(1):201–14.
27. Maksoud MKMA, Ibrahim AAH, Nabil TM, et al. Histomorphological, histochemi-cal and scanning electron microscopic investigation of the proventriculus (Ventriculus glandularis) of the hooded crow (Corvus cornix). Anat Histol Embryol 2022;51(3):380–9.
28. Al-Saffar FJ, Al-Samawy ERM. Microscopic and morphometric study of the pro-ventriculus and ventriculus of the striated scope owl (Otus scors brucei) in Iraq. Kufa J Vet Med Sci 2014;5(2):9–23.
29. Aizawa J, Tivane C, Rodrigues MN, et al. Gross anatomical features of the gastro-intestinal tract (GIT) of Blue-and-yellow macaws (Ara ararauna) - oesophagus to cloaca. Anat Histol Embryol 2013;42(6):432–7.
30. Zaher M, El-Ghareeb AW, Hamdi H, et al. Anatomical, histological and histo-chemical adaptations of the avian alimentary canal to their food habits: I-Coturnix coturnix. J Life Sci 2012;9(3):253–75.
31. Hirschberg RM. Anatomy and physiology. In: Chitty J, Lierz M, editors. BSAVA Manual of raptors, pigeons and passerine birds. 1st edition. Quedgeley: British Small Animal Veterinary Association; 2008. p. 25–41.
32. Smith CR, Richmond ME. Factors influencing pellet egestion and gastric pH in the barn owl. Wilson Bull 1972;84(2):179–86.
33. Graves GR. Field measurements of gastrointestinal pH of new world vultures in Guyana. J Raptor Res 2017;51(4):465–9.
34. Duke GE, Jegers AA, Loff G, et al. Gastric digestion in some raptors. Comp Bio-chem Physiol Part A Physiol 1975;50(4):649–56.
35. Oyelowo F, Usende I, Abiyere E, et al. Comparative gross morphology and morpho-metric investigations on the alimentary tract of three age groups of Barn owl (Tyto alba) found in North-Central Nigeria. Int J Vet Sci 2017;6(1):7–12.
36. Morales Espino A, Deniz S, Fumero-Hernandez F, et al. A cadaveric study using anatomical cross-section and computed tomography for the coelomic cavity in juvenile cory's shearwater (Aves, Procellariidae, Calonectris borealis). Animals 2024;14(6):858.

37. Taylor WM. Clinical significance of the avian cloaca: interrelationships with the kidneys and the hindgut. In: Speer BL, editor. Current therapy in avian medicine and surgery. 1st edition. St. Louis: Elsevier; 2016. p. 329–44.

38. Arnason SS, Elbrond VS, Lavert G. Transport characteristics and morphology of the colon and coprodeum in two wild birds of different habitats, the rock ptarmigan (Lagopus mutus) and the (Uria aalge). Comp Biochem Physiol, Part A: Mol Integr Physiol 2015;185:86–96.

39. Wanmi N, Sulaiman MH, Gosomji I, et al. Study on the macrometry of gastrointestinal tract of wild west African Senegal parrot (Poicephalus senegalus versteri). Anat J Afr 2017;6(3):1065–70.

40. Mahdi AH. The structure and innervation of the sphincters in the large intestine of the domestic duck (Anas platyrhynchos) [PhD thesis]. Edinburgh: Royal (Dick) School of Veterinary Studies, University of Edinburgh; 1989.

41. Johnson OW, Skadhauge E. Structural-functional correlations in the kidneys and observations of colon and cloacal morphology in certain Australian birds. J Anat 1975;120(3):495–505.

42. Elbrond VS, Jones CJP, Skadhauge E. Localization, morphology and function of the mitochondria-rich cells in relation to transepithelial Na+-transport in chicken lower intestine (coprodeum). Comp Biochem Physiol, Part A: Mol Integr Physiol 2004;137(4):683–96.

43. Elbrond VS, Laverty G, Dantzer V, et al. Ultrastructure and electrolyte transport of the epithelium of coprodeum, colon and the proctodeal diverticulum of Rhea Americana. Comp Biochem Physiol, Part A: Mol Integr Physiol 2009;152(3):357–65.

44. Barnes EM, Impey CS. The occurrence and properties of uric acid decomposing anaerobic bacteria in the avian caecum. J Appl Bacteriol 1974;37(3):393–409.

45. Skadhauge E, Erlwanger KH, Ruziwa SD, et al. Does the ostrich (Struthio camelus) coprodeum have the electrophysiological properties and microstructure of other birds? Comp Biochem Physiol Part A. Mol Integr Physiol 2003;134(4):749–55.

46. Ruan Y, Wang Y, Guo Y, et al. T cell subset profile and inflammatory cytokine properties in the gut associated lymphoid tissues of chickens during infectious bursal disease virus (IBDV) infection. Arch Virol 2020;165:2249–58.

47. Laveille GA, Romsos DR, Yeh Y, et al. Lipid biosynthesis in the chick. A consideration of site of synthesis, influence of diet and possible regulatory mechanisms. Poult Sci J 1975;54(4):1075–93.

48. Veladiano IA, Banzato T, Bellini L, et al. Normal computed tomographic features and reference values for the coelomic cavity in pet parrots. BMC Vet Res 2016; 12:182.

49. Goodarzi N, Bashiri A. Histology and immunofluorescent study of the pancreas in lovebird (Agapornis personatus). Vet Med Sci 2024;10(2):e1394.

50. Palmieri C, Shivaprasad HL. An immunohistochemical study of the endocrine pancreas in raptors. Res Vet Sci 2014;97(3):587–91.

51. Mohammadi A, Goodarzi N. Immunofluorescence study of the endocrine pancreas in the common pheasant (Phasianus colchicus). Zoomorphology 2024;143:249–54.

52. Divers SJ. Avian diagnostic endoscopy. Vet Clin North Am Exot Anim Pract 2010; 13(2):187–202.

53. Lumeij JT. Avian clinical biochemistry. In: Kaneko JJ, Harvey JW, Bruss ML, editors. Clinical biochemistry of domestic animals. 6th edition. London: Elsevier; 2008. p. 839–72.

Avian Gastroenterology
Noninfectious and Infectious Disease

Ashton Hollwarth, BSc, BVMS, CertAVP (Zoo Med), ANZCVS (Avian Medicine &
Surgery), DipECZM (Avian), MRCVS*, Lucia Gomez Prieto, DVM, MRCVS

KEYWORDS

- Gastroenterology • Crop burn • Foreign body • Bacterial gastroenteritis
- Herpesvirus • *Macrorhabdus ornithogaster*

KEY POINTS

- Foreign bodies of the crop, proventriculus, and ventriculus are a common presentation in birds, usually accompanied by clinical signs of lethargy, weight loss, hyporexia or anorexia, regurgitation, and coelomic distension.
- Clinicians must consider normal anatomy and physiology in avian patients when attempting to investigate the cause of gastrointestinal signs.
- Bornavirus and avian influenza are key viral differential diagnoses for birds presenting with gastrointestinal and neurologic signs.
- *Macrorhabdus ornithogaster* is a common fungal pathogen of captive birds, and most commonly seen in budgerigars (*Melopsittacus undulatus*). Treatment is difficult and has not been widely studied.

INTRODUCTION

Once gastrointestinal signs have been identified, practitioners can use diagnostic investigations to discover the cause. Gastrointestinal disease in birds presents with varying signs, and there are many infectious and noninfectious causes of gastrointestinal illness. Some of these are the result of physical complications, such as thermal burns, foreign bodies, or intussusception. Other causes are acquired by contact with other birds or contact with contaminated materials, resulting in development of infectious diseases. The objectives of this article are to discuss the most commonly encountered noninfectious diseases, and discuss best management and prevention of these syndromes, as well as to outline commonly encountered infectious diseases in avian practice and discuss how best practitioners can manage these cases when infectious disease is suspected.

Great Western Exotics, Unit 10 Berkshire House, County Park, Shrivenham Road, Swindon, Wiltshire SN1 2NR, UK
* Corresponding author.
E-mail address: ashton.hollwarth@vets-now.com

Vet Clin Exot Anim 28 (2025) 425–451
https://doi.org/10.1016/j.cvex.2024.11.010   **vetexotic.theclinics.com**

Abbreviations	
ABV	avian bornavirus
DM	diabetes mellitus
PCR	polymerase chain reaction
PDD	proventricular dilation disease

NONINFECTIOUS DISEASE
Crop Burns

Crop burns are observed in juvenile birds, usually psittacines, following gavage feeding of improperly warmed formula that causes thermal injury to the crop mucosa. Overheated formula or formula that is poorly stirred can result in hot areas within the mixture, resulting in thermal burns and subsequent mucosal and skin necrosis (**Fig. 1**).[1] Occasionally, this is also seen in adult birds following ingestion of a caustic substance. A scab is formed over the affected area which eventually lifts away and results in a fistula over the crop. Often, the first indication of this type of injury is evidence of formula on the skin around the thoracic inlet, which some owners may mistake as regurgitation. Treatment of these injuries requires surgery to debride the necrotic tissue, after waiting 3 to 5 days for the damaged tissue to declare itself.[2] The skin and crop wall are often adhered following formation of the fistula; therefore, while under general anesthesia, the crop wall and skin need to be separated, debrided, and closed in separate layers. The crop wall should be closed with a continuous suture pattern but does not require inversion.[2]

Crop Impaction

Crop impaction is diagnosed with some frequence. Small psittacines have been reported to ingest small volumes of fibrous material over time, which result in formation of an ingluvolith within the crop.[3] Formation of ingluvoliths is a common presentation in cockatiels (*Nymphicus hollandicus*), who ingest fibrous material, resulting in clinical signs of vomiting, lethargy, and weight loss.[4,5] These are often diagnosed by palpation of the crop, which reveals a firm, mobile mass. Investigation into a population of cockatiels with fibrous ingluvoliths showed that affected birds were significantly more likely to be male and under 3 years of age.[5] A mortality rate of 33% in this population has led

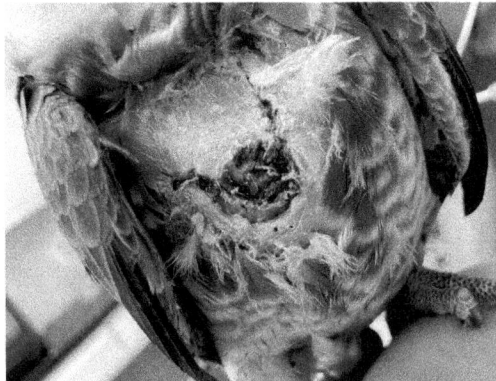

Fig. 1. Necrotic material over the thoracic inlet following a crop burn in a juvenile gray parrot (*Psittacus erithacus*).

to the recommendation that fibrous materials should not be offered to cockatiels as cage accessories.[5] In addition, crop impaction has been reported in nestlings whose parents were fed inappropriate diets high in grit and in individuals fed large volumes of peanuts that became imbibed within the crop.[6,7]

Crop impactions are also observed in chickens, acutely as a result of ingestion of bulky fibrous material such as plant matter, feathers, bedding material, water-absorbent feed, or indigestible materials such as plastics or metals.[8,9] They can also result from underlying diseases that affect normal peristalsis, such as obstructions further distal in the digestive tract, heavy metal toxicity, endoparasitism, and pathology of the vagus nerve.[9,10]

Foreign Bodies

Foreign bodies in the crop have also been reported in several species, including ingestion of feeding tubes in neonates, an elastic hair band, and fish bones.[11–15] In addition, inappropriate diets in juveniles undergoing the weaning process can result in ingestion of whole food items that are unable to be emptied from the crop, for example, large whole nuts. Tracheal obstruction has also been reported in a peahen following lingual entrapment with a string foreign body.[16] Removal of crop impaction or foreign bodies depends on the size of the foreign material and the patient's condition. Manual removal with forceps may be possible, if the foreign material is small enough to pass through the oral cavity, which can be the case for single items. In the case of ingluvoliths that cannot be milked orad (**Fig. 2**), an ingluviotomy is often required. When making the incision, a site should be chosen over the left lateral crop wall, close to the thoracic inlet.[2] Stay sutures should be placed within the crop wall and the crop should be entered over an avascular area. Ingluviotomy to remove foreign bodies has been reported under general anesthesia or standing using local anesthesia infiltration, resulting in favorable outcomes in all cases reported.[5,7,14,17]

In addition to the crop, foreign bodies elsewhere in the gastrointestinal tract are also often diagnosed. The proventriculus or ventriculus are common areas for foreign bodies to be identified, including wood, metal wire, plant fibers, synthetic fibers,

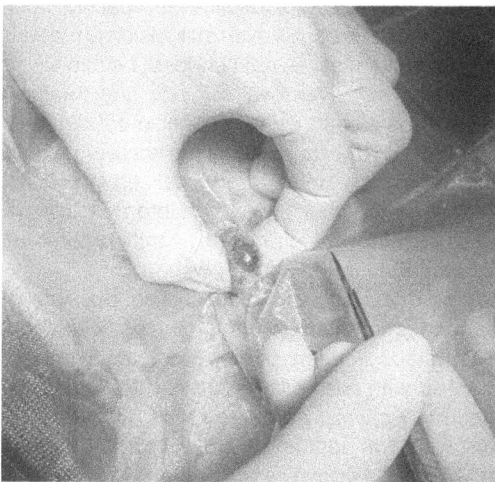

Fig. 2. Dissection through the skin and exposure of the crop wall in a blue-fronted Amazon parrot (*Amazona aestiva*) to retrieve a foreign body within the crop that could not be milked orad.

stones, rubber, plastic, artificial turf, paper and grass, and polyacrylamide gel.[18–28] Clinical signs of gastrointestinal foreign body are often vague, but when present include lethargy, weight loss, hyporexia or anorexia, regurgitation, and coelomic distension.[22] Radiopaque foreign bodies can be identified with plain radiographs or fluoroscopy, and nonradiopaque foreign bodies can be identified following administration of oral contract agents.[10,20,23,26,29] Endoscopy can be utilized for both diagnosis and treatment.[21,22,25–27] Computed tomography can also aid in diagnosis and is of particular use when there are concerns for secondary celomitis.

Perforating foreign bodies with subsequent granulomatous inflammation or peritonitis have been described following ingestion of wire.[19,25,30–33] A case of vegetative endocarditis has also been reported in a Toco toucan (*Ramphastos toco*) following perforation of a sharp foreign body of vegetal origin.[34] Other complications of foreign body ingestion have also been reported. Ingestion of stones in 2 parakeet auklets (*Aethia psittacula*) resulted in formation of ventricular diverticula of varying sizes, identified during surgery and necropsy.[24] Erosive enteritis was identified in a flock of lesser flamingos (*Phoeniconiasis minor*) who ingested decomposed granite, resulting in several mortalities.[29]

Treatment of gastrointestinal foreign bodies is influenced by the nature of the foreign body, the size and stability of the patient, and availability of treatment options. Endoscopy is a common modality for treatment and has been utilized in a number of species.[21,22,25–27] Endoscopy is recommended for the removal of foreign objects in the upper gastrointestinal tract if possible, as it is a less invasive procedure associated with lower patient morbidity compared with surgery.[22] Endoscopic-assisted removal of feeding tubes from the proventriculus in 2 blue-and-yellow macaws and a Triton cockatoo (*Cacatua galerita Triton*) reported that the most suitable patient positioning appeared to be ventral recumbency.[35] To facilitate entry within the gastrointestinal tract, the endoscope can be inserted via the oral cavity, or via an ingluvotomy to facilitate passage deeper aborad within the gastrointestinal tract when the length of the endoscope is insufficient in larger birds.[22]

In cases where a foreign body cannot be removed endoscopically, proventriculotomy is the surgery of choice for gastric foreign bodies and has been used successfully to remove proventricular (**Fig. 3**) or ventricular foreign bodies in a number of species.[5,30,32,33] Left lateral, transverse, or midline approaches to the ventriculus can be used to expose the isthmus, through which an incision is made to access the lumen of the proventriculus and ventriculus.[2] A rigid endoscope can also be inserted into this incision to facilitate foreign body removal.[36] Once any foreign material has been removed, the incision can be closed using monofilament suture material in a simple continuous pattern, over which the caudal tip of the left liver lobe can be tacked.[2] Concerns around leakage of gastric contents and localized infection exist; however, the application of an adipose patch over proventriculotomy incisions in Japanese quail (*Coturnix japonica*) was shown to result in significantly greater inflammation in birds with placement of a patch than in those birds without.[37]

In cases where surgical or endoscopic removal is not possible, several reports exist of successful medical management of gastric foreign bodies. A comparison of medical protocols to remove metallic foreign bodies from the ventriculus of budgerigars showed that birds treated with fine or large grit had the quickest expulsion times of 36 days and 47 days, respectively, compared with 63 days in the control group.[38] Medical management with oral sodium chloride and psyllium successfully resulted in expulsion of a metallic foreign body in a North Island brown kiwi (*Apteryx mantelli*).[19] Ventricular impaction with plant fibers in a Guam kingfisher (*Todiramphus cinnamominus*) was successfully medically managed with the use of natural peanut butter, which facilitated the casting of the impacted material.[20]

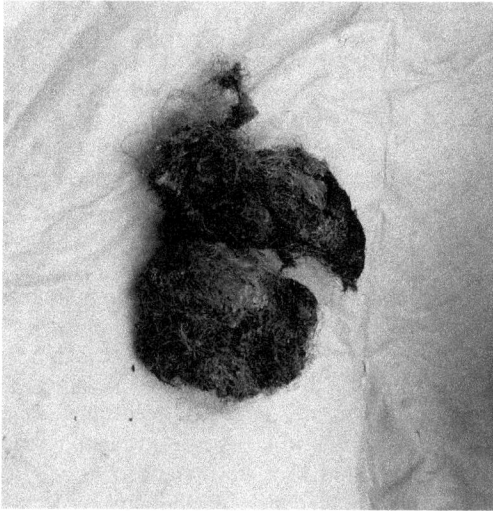

Fig. 3. A trichobezoar of synthetic fibers removed from the proventriculus of a little owl (*Athene noctua*) via a proventriculotomy.

Intussusception

Intussusception is a rare but serious condition in avian patients that often carries a grave prognosis. Clinical signs are often vague, but can include depression, hemorrhagic diarrhea, regurgitation, anorexia, coelomic pain, palpable coelomic mass, cloacal prolapse, and tenesmus.[39] Intestinal intussusception has been reported in juvenile Amazon parrots (*Amazona* spp), tawny eagle owls (*Aquila rapax*), white-cheeked turacos (*Touraco leuotis*), and in greater rheas (*Rhea americana*) following ingestion of large volumes of sand.[39–42] Proventricular intussusceptions have been reported in chickens and a blue-and-yellow macaw.[43,44] Antemortem diagnosis is difficult, usually involving either plain radiographs or contrast radiographs following oral barium administration or contrast enema.[45–47] Successful surgical outcomes have been reported for intestinal intussusceptions in macaws and a tawny eagle; however, generally the prognosis for this condition is grave.[39,40,46]

Cloacal Prolapses

Prolapse of the cloaca is commonly seen in clinical practice. A report identifying cloacal prolapses in birds of prey reported the colon as the most commonly prolapsed organ (35%).[48] In contrast, in a population of psittacines with cloacal prolapse, only 4.7% of the cases reported colonic prolapse.[49] Prolapsed tissue is susceptible to desiccation, trauma, infection, and ischemia, so immediate surgical correction is required. Cloacal endoscopy can be useful in identifying the prolapsed tissue and determining the extent of the pathology.[45] In cases where the prolapsed tissue is not extensive, replacing the protruding tissue and applying lateral vent sutures at approximately one-third and two-thirds of the vent distance may be adequate.[2] In cases of extensive intussusception, surgical correction of the intussusception or resection and anastomosis of the affected tissue is indicated.[36]

Cloacoliths

Cloacoliths are formed when droppings are unable to be completely voided, usually secondary to an underlying condition, such as spinal disease or prolonged egg incubation.[48] In psittacines, they appear to be prevalent in Amazon parrots and macaws.[50] Most cloacoliths in birds are rough, round aggregates formed of uric acid.[51,52] The recommended treatment for cloacolithiasis is removing the aggregated material under general anesthesia.[51] This may involve breaking down the cloacolith piecemeal, potentially with the use of endoscopy or forceps.[48,50] Following removal, the cloaca should be flushed with warm saline to ensure all portions of the cloacolith have been evacuated.[51] Antiinflammatories, antibiotics, and opioid analgesia should be considered.[52]

Hypovitaminosis A

Hypovitaminosis A is considered to be the most common nutritional disease in psittacines fed a seed-only diet.[53] Vitamin A is essential for mucous membranes and epithelium, including glands. A state of hypovitaminosis A results in squamous metaplasia of epithelium and mucous glands.[54] Mucous glands then fill with keratin which plugs the opening of the gland, resulting in severe distension of the gland and localized swelling. Clinically, this appears as nodules with white-beige, thick material within. Vitamin A deficiency has also been reported to affect keratin growth. Following removal of vitamin A in the diet of grey parrots (Psittacus erithacus), it was reported that ridges developed on the beak, which resolved when vitamin A was supplemented in the diet.[54] Definitive diagnosis can be achieved via liver biopsy and quantification of vitamin A levels, with normal levels of vitamin A ranging between 2 and 5 IU/kg.[53]

Obesity

Obesity is a common problem in captive birds, especially in those housed indoors with minimal exercise. Where their wild counterparts would have to spend hours foraging for food, accounting for anywhere between 56% and 90% of daily activities, captive birds are comparatively sedentary.[55] In addition, well-meaning owners often provide ad libitum inappropriate diets, such as seed-only diets. Seed-only diets have been recorded as being deficient in vitamins A, B2, B3, B5, B12, D, E, K and choline, calcium, phosphate, sodium, manganese, zinc, iron, iodine, and selenium, as well as having excessive amounts of fat.[53,56–58] Obesity has been linked to atherosclerosis, hypercholesterolemia, hepatic lipidosis, lipoma and xanthoma formation, joint disease, and pododermatitis.[59,60] Formulated pelleted diets have been suggested as a way to combat and avoid obesity; however, a calorific deficiency is the only definitive way to treat obesity.[55,56]

Hepatic Lipidosis

Hepatic lipidosis, also known as fatty liver syndrome, is a syndrome of excessive lipid within hepatocytes. In pet birds, this appears to be most common in Amazon parrots, cockatiels, budgerigars, macaws, and rose-breasted cockatoos (Eolophus roseicapilla).[61] This syndrome is commonly associated with diets that are excessive in fats, but a significant increase in hepatic lipogranuloma lesions has also been reported as a result of excessive dietary protein in cockatiels.[62]

Iron Storage Disease

Hemochromatosis, or iron storage disease, has also been associated with inappropriate diets that are excessive in iron, diets rich in protein, and diets with excessive ascorbic acid.[63] Toucans, birds of paradise, mynahs, and starlings are taxa that are particularly susceptible to developing iron storage disease.[64] Hemosiderosis refers to excessive accumulation of iron in tissues, whereas hemochromatosis, or iron storage disease, refers to a disease state that results in organ damage as a consequence of this excessive accumulation. Birds affected with iron storage disease may have acute mortality, or may develop ascites, secondary to hepatic or cardiac failure.[61] Antemortem diagnosis is difficult, as it requires liver biopsy to quantify iron levels within the hepatic tissues.[65] Visually, affected livers are golden brown in appearance, and presence of iron can be confirmed histologically with Prussian blue staining.[61] Comparison of treatment methods in common starlings (*Sturnus vulgaris*) identified regular phlebotomy and subcutaneous deferoxamine as an effective treatment method.[65]

Diabetes Mellitus

Diabetes mellitus (DM) has been reported in several orders of birds. Birds with DM are frequently affected by type I diabetes, which is commonly associated with an underlying disease in avian patients.[66,67] Avian glucose regulation relies significantly more on glucagon than insulin, which is in contrast to glucose regulation in mammals.[68] Insulin facilitates uptake of glucose into the cells in postprandial birds, and glucagon is responsible for maintaining glucose levels in the fasting bird.[69] Common clinical signs of DM in birds include polyuria, polydipsia, weight loss, polyphagia, and lethargy.[67] DM is commonly diagnosed based on clinical signs and the presence of persistent hyperglycemia, alongside glucosuria and response to insulin therapy. Successful treatment has been reported in 5 birds using long-acting insulin therapy, and 1 bird utilizing glipizide and dietary modification.[70–74]

Exocrine Pancreatic Insufficiency

Exocrine pancreatic insufficiency develops due to loss of functional pancreatic tissue. As a result, a syndrome of maldigestion results, particularly of fats and starches.[75] Resulting clinical signs include steatorrhea, seen as voluminous, pale droppings, often described as "popcorn droppings," and weight loss. Diagnosis is via histopathology of a pancreatic biopsy, which can either be performed endoscopically or surgically. Histologically, affected pancreas will have loss of zymogen and atrophy of acinar cells. Management involves correcting the underlying cause, if possible, and transitioning the affected individual onto a formulated diet with vegetables, supplemented with pancreatic enzymes.[75]

Neoplasias

Neoplastic processes affecting the gastrointestinal system are commonly reported. Common tumors of the beak and oral cavity include fibrosarcomas, squamous cell carcinomas, and melanomas. Fibrosarcoma is considered to be the most common neoplasm affecting the beak, and papillomatosis is considered the most common neoplasm of the oral cavity.[54] It is unusual for primary oral cavity melanoma to occur, as this usually occurs secondary to beak melanoma.

Proventricular carcinoma is most common in budgerigars, gray-cheeked parakeets (*Brotogeris pyrrhoptera*), lovebirds (*Agapornis* spp), cockatiels, and Amazon parrots.[76] These usually occur at the isthmus, and infiltrate laterally, rather than protruding into the lumen of the gastrointestinal tract.[54] Common primary neoplasms of the intestine include carcinomas, sarcomas, and papillomas.[54] Fibrosarcoma formation within the cecal wall has been reported as a sequela of *Heterakis* infection.[54,77]

INFECTIOUS DISEASES
Bacterial Diseases

Avian chlamydiosis
Chlamydia psittaci infection is most commonly reported in psittacines, however, it affects many avian groups.[78,79] Cockatiels seem to be overrepresented.[80] It is a

zoonotic disease, known as psittacosis or ornithosis in humans.[80] It is transmitted via the feco-oral route.[81] In birds, *C psittaci* has tissue tropism for the liver, causing multifocal necrotic hepatitis as the main pathology, with reported systemic dissemination.[81,82] Clinical signs are nonspecific and include lethargy, anorexia, depression, oculo-nasal discharge, conjunctivitis, biliverdinuria, and bright green diarrhea.[82–84] Hematology often shows leukocytosis, with associated heterophilia and monocytosis.[85] Biochemistry may show elevation of hepatic enzymes; however, in some birds, biochemistry parameters are within normal range.[85] Diagnosis is established through isolation of the bacteria from oropharyngeal or cloacal swabs, or in feces, as well as by the immunofluorescence identification of *C psittaci* antigen in tissue specimens.[79,83,85] Diagnosis via serology relies on paired serologic titers, taken at least 2 weeks apart, run simultaneously at the same laboratory.[86] Avian chlamydiosis must also be suspected after a positive enzyme-linked immunosorbent assay in clinically ill birds; however, positive results may also be seen in asymptomatic birds.[87] Different antibiotics have been proven to be effective, for example, doxycycline and azithromycin.[84] Balsamo and colleagues (2017) published a detailed compendium of control measures of *C psittaci* among birds and humans.[88]

Mycobacteriosis
Several mycobacterial organisms have been reported in birds. *Mycobacterium avium*, with a feco-oral transmission, has been reported in domestic fowl, raptors, and other captive avian groups, and in wildlife such as the griffon vulture (*Gyps fulvus*).[89,90] The course of infection is slow, with granulomatous formation across different coelomic organs including small and large intestine, liver and spleen, and respiratory tract.[90–92] Clinical signs include chronic weight loss, depression, diarrhea, respiratory signs, and occasionally jaundice, if the liver is affected.[91,93,94] *Mycobacterium genavense* has also been commonly reported in different avian species, including Columbiformes, Sphenisciformes, Psittaciformes, and Passeriformes.[95,96] The course of infection of *M genavense* shows resemblance to *M avium* infection, characterized by granuloma formation and corresponding signs depending on the affected organ.[95,96]

Diagnosis includes imaging and visualization of internal granulomas, visualization of intracellular acid-fast-positive bacteria on Ziehl-Neelsen-stained fecal smears or tissues, and real time polymerase chain reaction (PCR) in feces.[89–91,93,95–97] Fecal culture after decontamination has also been suggested as a possible diagnostic technique.[98] Intradermal tuberculin test and rapid agglutination may be used to diagnose *M avium* in chickens; however, these tests failed to diagnose in meat-breed pigeons.[94,99] Because of its zoonotic risk and poor prognosis despite treatment, euthanasia should be considered.[94,97,100,101]

Necrotic enteritis or clostridial enterotoxemia
Clostridial enterotoxemia is caused by *Clostridium perfringens*, anaerobic commensal bacteria of the gastrointestinal tract of avian species.[102,103] *Clostridium* spp associated enteritis has been reported in commercial poultry, raptors, and psittacines.[102–104] Overgrowth of these bacteria has been associated to different factors such as high-protein fishmeal supplemented starter diet and *Eimeria* spp infections.[105] Clinical signs include lethargy, diarrhea which can be hemorrhagic, dehydration, and death in acute cases.[104,106] Antemortem diagnosis includes fecal cultures and PCR.[102] Postmortem findings include visualization of a diphtheritic pseudomembrane in the small intestine, cecum, and colorectum, with necrotic contents and intestinal ulcers.[104,107] Treatment includes the use of antibiotics; however, due to its fatal outcome, prevention of this disease is the key. Fluid-therapy and treatment of comorbidities is highly recommended.

Antibiotic-free prevention methods have been studied in recent literature, but so far have failed to provide significant protection.[108,109] In the Azure-winged magpie (*Cyanopica cyanus*), supplementation with polyamine putrescine has showed reduced inflammation and colonization of *C perfringens*.[110] Prevention of C perfringens involves maintaining proper hygiene and ensuring the appropriate source and manipulation of food. This is particularly crucial for raptors, with emphasis on slow defrosting of food and the prompt removal of uneaten pieces within a few hours.[103] In chickens, a *Lactobacillus casei* vector vaccine has been proven effective against necrotic enteritis.[111]

Campylobacteriosis
Campylobacter spp, nonpathogenic bacteria in poultry, has an important role in public health due to its zoonotic risk. Commercial poultry can be asymptomatic carriers of *Campylobacter* spp.[112] To reduce the further development of antibiotic resistance, the use of bacteriocins to control Campylobacter spp has been studied and proven effective in chickens.[113,114]

Escherichia coli
Escherichia coli is part of the normal gut flora of avian species and has also a zoonotic risk.[115,116] Only some strains of *E coli*, known as avian pathogenic E coli, may cause colibacillosis in poultry.[117] Due to its high multidrug resistant characteristics, only after pure isolation of *E coli* in feces of clinically sick birds, treatment should be considered.[91,103,117]

Salmonellosis
Salmonella spp have been reported to cause various diseases in many avian species. *Salmonella enteritidis* and *Salmonella typhimurium* are nonpathogenic in poultry; however, special attention must be paid due to their zoonotic risk.[91,118] Both bacteria have also been isolated in wild raptors acting as asymptomatic carriers.[119,120] S *typhimurium* causes diarrhea and rapid death due to septicemia in raptors, pigeons, passerines, and psittacines.[106,121,122]

Fowl typhoid is caused by *Salmonella enterica* subsp, *Gallinarum* (S *Gallinarum*). Clinical signs include watery bright yellow to green diarrhea, fever, tachypnea, and pale and shrunken combs.[123] Gross postmortem findings include hemorrhagic enteritis, presence of hemorrhagic liver with necrotic foci, edematous lungs, and renomegaly, and histology demonstrates septicemia with degeneration and necrosis.[123]

Salmonella pullorum (S *enterica* subsp *enterica* serovar *Gallinarum* biovar *Pullorum*) is the etiologic agent of the disease called bacillary white diarrhea that affects poultry. Clinical signs are usually gastrointestinal-related, with white diarrhea, but neurologic signs were reported in recent outbreak of laying hens.[124,125] Mortality rate may reach a 100% rate in young individuals.[125]

Transmission of *Salmonella* spp is mainly horizontal, but vertical transmission of S *pullorum* has been proven in chickens.[126,127] Diagnosis of *Salmonella* spp is based on fecal or cloacal swab cultures, and treatment includes fluid-therapy and antibiotic based on sensitivity testing due to its multidrug-resistant pattern.[119,121,125] In chickens, there are vaccinations commercially available for S *enteritidis* and S *typhimurium*.[128,129]

Pseudotuberculosis
Pseudotuberculosis, caused by *Yersinia pseudotuberculosis*, is transmitted via fecooral and carried particularly by rodents, being a main source of infection in aviary psittacines, raptors, and wildlife.[130–132] Acute death is the main clinical sign. Passerines have been reported to have an acute disease, while in pigeons and psittacines, disease can be acute or chronic.[130] Pseudotuberculosis is rare in poultry with some

cases reported in turkeys presenting with diarrhea, weight loss, and lameness or with peracute death due to septicemia.[133] Lesions include enteritis, hepatitis and splenitis, pneumonia, and nephritis.[131] Diagnosis is often post mortem by visualization of multifocal white foci in the liver and other coelomic organs correspondent to hepatic necrosis in histology, followed by culture of the affected tissue.[134] Due to its peracute nature, treatment is often not possible, and efforts should be focused prevention by rodent control. In flock cases, treatment can be attempted following culture and sensitivity of deceased animals.[134] The use of Y pseudotuberculosis phages obtained from mammals and birds of a zoo in Berlin was investigated for the possible treatment of pseudotuberculosis, with positive results.[135]

Viral Diseases

Poxviridae

Poxviruses are species-specific and have been reported in raptors, poultry, passerines, seabirds, and others.[136–139] Avipoxviruses can cause 2 main types of infection, cutaneous or dry form which causes dermatologic signs with papules and scab formation and is transmitted via mechanical and vector routes.[137,138,140] The wet or diphtheroid form causes caseous plaques in the oropharynx, tongue, and esophagus and is transmitted via oral route.[137,139,141] Diagnosis is based on physical examination, PCR, histology with visualization of pathognomonic Bollinger's intracytoplasmic bodies, and transmission electron microscopy.[137–139,142] There is no specific treatment for avipoxviruses, and lesions should resolve in a couple of weeks.[143] Mortality is higher in juvenile birds, due to secondary bacterial infections, because of inability to eat, and due to laryngeal obstruction.[138] Being a species-specific virus, it requires species-specific vaccines. However, a fowlpox vaccine has shown efficacy in passerines.[143]

Herpesviridae

Herpesvirus-associated disease occurs in many avian species. Mucosal papillomas have been attributed to Psittacid herpesvirus 1 (PsHV-1) in neotropical parrots, with a prevalence of 100% in a study involving a population of Amazon parrots and macaw species.[144] Psittacid herpesvirus 2 (PsHV-2) is the responsible of mucosal papillomas in gray parrots.[145,146] Mucosal papillomas develop particularly in the cloaca, but other parts of the alimentary tract may be affected such as oropharynx, esophagus, crop, or proventriculus.[144] Bile duct carcinomas and pancreatic adenocarcinomas have been also associated with PsHV-1 alongside mucosal papillomas.[147] Diagnosis should not be based on physical examination alone, as all papillomas in psittacines may not be attributed to herpesvirus infections.[148] Instead, diagnosis is based on immunohistochemistry of a tissue biopsy, and PCR of affected tissues or cloacal swabs.[144,147] Treatment is symptomatic and resection of papillomas may be attempted, however, recurrence is possible.[149] The use of imiquimod therapy did not show any regression of papillomas in Amazon parrots.[147]

In pigeons, Columbid alphaherpesvirus 1 (CoHV-1) causes caseous plaques that cover mucosal surfaces of the oropharynx, crop, and esophagus due to necrosis of epithelial cells, and it is accompanied by necrotic hepatitis.[150] Diagnosis can be made by oral swabs preferably or cloacal swabs for PCR, with similar sensitivity to tissue.[151] In great horned owl (Bubo virginianus), CoHV-1 has been associated with mortality secondary to hepatic, splenic, enteric, and gastrointestinal necrosis.[152] However, a distinct Strigid Herpesvirus 1 (StrHV-1) has recently been identified in an individual of the same species, presented with papillomatous conjunctivitis.[153]

Duck viral enteritis or duck plague is a seasonal disease caused by a herpesvirus.[154] Higher prevalence of cases was reported during summer following breeding season;

however, a recent study demonstrated a prevalence of 66.7% during autum.[91,154,155] Clinical signs include diarrhea, sometimes hemorrhagic, depression, dehydration, drop in egg production, and ocular and nasal discharge with a reported mortality rate of 75%.[154] Supportive treatment can be attempted and the use of vaccination as part of a prevention plan is possible; however, recent literature has reported higher prevalence in vaccinated flocks than unvaccinated ones.[154,156]

Bornaviridae

Bornavirus is the etiology for a neurologic and gastrointestinal condition of psittacines known as proventricular dilatation disease (PDD), proventricular dilatation syndrome, or "macaw wasting disease." An avian bornavirus (ABV) was first detected in 2008 in psittacines with PDD.[157,158] Clinical signs include apathy, anorexia, weight loss, presence of undigested seeds in feces, neurologic signs, and sudden death.[159,160]

Psittacines are the most common avian group to have ABV; however, different bornaviruses have been isolated in passerines with PDD- associated signs.[160,161] Fors this reason, the term ABV as a single virus agent has been substituted by specific names as follows: parrot bornavirus 1 to 8 (PaBV-1 to 8), canary bornavirus 1 to 3 (CnBV-1 to 3), munia bornavirus 1 (muBV-1), and aquatic bird bornavirus 1 to 2 (ABBC-1 to 2).[162] Parrot bornavirus 4 was confirmed as the causative agent of PDD following experimental reproduction of the disease.[159,163] A Himalayan monal (*Lophophorus impejanus*) with clinical signs of PDD was diagnosed with PaBV-4; however, passerines seem not to develop the disease following experimental infection with PaBV-4.[164,165] In a recent study, CnBV-1 has been detected in a barn owl with associated neurologic signs.[166] The possibility of horizontal transmission remains unknown.[165] Vertical transmission has been proven in cockatiels but seems to be age-dependent.[167]

Pathophysiology of ABV is based on lymphoplasmacytic infiltration of the myenteric ganglia of the upper and middle gastrointestinal tract.[159,168] Other histologic changes include hepatic lymphoid hyperplasia, nonpurulent encephalitis, myelitis, ganglioneuritis, and peripheral neuritis.[168] Age of infection has been proposed as an important factor in the developing of gross lesions and subsequently clinical signs, being absent in juvenile cockatiels experimentally infected.[168]

Macroscopic changes include a thin walled and distended proventriculus, and ventriculus to a lesser degree.[159] Diagnosis is based on clinical signs and imaging, with visualization of an enlarged proventriculus, and histology.[159,168,169] Confirmation of avian bornavirus is achieved by PCR on feces or cloacal swabs and serology.[157,168] Treatment is symptomatic, and the use of nonsteroidal anti-inflammatories has been proposed to reduce inflammation secondary to bornaviruses with no clear conclusion.[170]

Adenoviridae

Adenovirus infections are rare but have been reported to cause hemorrhagic gastroenteritis and high mortality in raptors, psittacine, and turkeys.[171,172] Treatment is symptomatic including antibiotics if secondary bacterial infections are present.[91]

Orthomyxoviridae

Avian influenza affects waterfowl, poultry, raptors, and other wildlife, and it is caused by a highly contagious orthomyxovirus.[173–176] Transmission occurs via feco-oral but also via aerosol.[177] Highly pathogenic avian influenza causes high mortality rates with associated clinical signs including mainly neurologic and respiratory signs, but also diarrhea, weight loss, and reduced egg laying, while low pathogenic avian influenza causes only mild clinical signs.[173,176–179] Waterfowl are asymptomatic carriers, contributing to the spread of the disease, particularly in migratory birds.[180] Necrosis and hemorrhages of the pancreas is a common macroscopic finding seen during post-mortem, with pancreatitis and multifocal necrosis in histology.[174,179] Avian influenza is part of the list of notifiable diseases of the World Organization for Animal Health.[181] If a case is suspected, authorities must be contacted, and infected confirmed poultry are typically euthanized.

Fungal Diseases

Candidiasis

Candida albicans is a common commensal of the upper alimentary tract of birds.[182] Overgrowth of C albicans is frequent in the crop, especially of domestic fowl, causing fungal ingluvitis known as sour crop. It can also be seen in other segments of the alimentary canal such as the tongue.[183,184] Esophageal ulcers have been reported in Landes geese (Anser anser domesticus).[185] Causes of this overgrowth may include alteration in alimentary tract motility, immunosuppression or the use of antimicrobials, and an inappropriate diet.[91] Clinical signs include inappetence, regurgitation, diarrhea, crop stasis, flicking of the head and food, yellow plaques in the oropharynx, and oral foul odor.[186,187] Diagnosis is based on physical examination and identification of budding yeast on plain or Gram-stained crop, cloacal or fecal cytology, culture, PCR, and histology of affected tissues.[184–187] Recent antifungal sensitivity studies have shown resistance of C albicans to itraconazole and fluconazole, and sensitivity to nystatin and amphotericin B.[186]

Macrorhabdus

Macrorhabdus ornithogaster infection has been found in different psittacines, but budgerigars seem to be predisposed.[188] M ornithogaster targets the isthmus, between the proventriculus and ventriculus, causing glandular dysplasia and mixed inflammatory infiltration of the proventriculus.[189] Psittacines may be asymptomatic carriers or develop clinical signs including weight loss, regurgitation, lethargy, and presence of undigested seed in feces.[188,190] Melena has been associated with poor prognosis in budgerigars.[190] Diagnosis is challenging due to its intermittent shedding. Fecal cytology with and without Gram stain have been used to diagnose M ornithogaster, and preparation of a fecal macro suspension prior to cytology increases the probability of detection.[191] A rod-shaped organism measuring 20 to 70 μm in length and 1 to

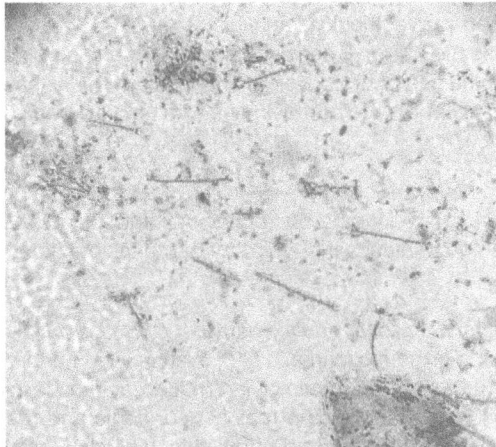

Fig. 4. Macrorhabdus ornithogaster found on fecal cytology in a budgerigar (Melopsittacus undulatus).

Table 1
Nematodes that commonly affect avian species[194–200]

Nematode Species	Birds Affected	Clinical Signs	Target Organ
Capillaria spp	Galliformes Anseriformes Psittaciformes Raptors Columbiformes	Anorexia, weight loss, death in severe burden, and poor flight performance in raptors	Oropharynx, esophagus, small and large intestines
Heterakis spp	Galliformes Anseriformes Columbiformes Psittaciformes	Asymptomatic. In pheasants (*H. Isolonche*) can cause weight loss and diarrhea. Can carry *H. meleagridis*	Caeca
Ascarids	Galliformes Anseriformes Columbiformes Psittaciformes Raptors	Asymptomatic Severe burden: weight loss, reduced egg laying, and intestinal obstruction	Small intestine

Table 2
Protozoa that commonly affect avian species[194,195,197,199–202]

Protozoa Species	Birds Affected	Clinical Signs	Target Organ
Coccidia			
Eimeria spp	Galliformes Columbiformes Anseriformes Psittaciformes Raptors	Lethargy, anorexia, weight loss, diarrhea. Melena and anemia in chickens	Intestines
Isospora spp	Passeriformes Columbiformes		
Cryptosporidium spp	Anseriformes Galliformes		
Caryospora spp	Raptors		
Trichomonas spp	Anseriformes Passeriformes Psittaciformes Raptors	White/yellow oral plaques, discomfort when eating and hyporexia, weight loss, and regurgitation	Oropharynx, esophagus, and crop
Histomonas meleagridis	Galliformes (turkeys highly susceptible) Psittaciformes	Sudden death. Sulfur yellow diarrhea	Caeca

3 μm in width is observed in cytology, stained Gram positive on Gram staining method (**Fig. 4**).[192] PCR on cloacal swabs is more likely to diagnose *M ornithogaster* than Gram-stained fecal cytology.[193]

Sparse investigations of treatment options have been performed. Amphotericin B at 10 mg/kg *per os* every 12 hours for 4 weeks showed only resolution of clinical signs in 33% of the studied budgerigar population, with later recurrence of some cases.[190] Another study using amphotericin B at a dose of 0.1 mg/mL in drinking water had a 36% of treatment failure with high levels of recurrence.[189]

Nystatin at a dose of 3,500,000 IU per liter of drinking water for 48 hours followed by 2,000,000 IU per liter of water for 28 days was used to treat a colony of budgerigars. This treatment regimen was associated with a reduction in mortality rates and post-mortem examinations revealed absence of *M ornithogaster* following treatment.[192] However, it is important to note that these birds did not undergo an antemortem diagnosis; diagnosis was inferred from postmortem findings in deceased adults within the same group.

Parasitic Diseases

Parasitic disease of the alimentary tract is common in avian species, particularly free-living birds.[194] Nematodes and protozoans are the most prevalent parasites that affect different avian groups (**Tables 1** and **2**).[106] Less species of cestodes, trematodes, and Acanthocephalans are found in birds compared to nematodes, but its prevalence may be high in some species, for example, the cestode *Raillietina echonobothrida* with a prevalence of 72% in a population of Galliformes and psittacines.[195,196]

SUMMARY

Gastrointestinal disease is common in avian patients. Practitioners must use diagnostic investigations to determine if the cause of the clinical signs is of infectious or noninfectious origin, in order to prevent further spread to other birds. Noninfectious disease often manifests with physical problems, such as thermal burns or foreign bodies. Infectious diseases can be caused by varied etiologic agents, covering viruses, bacteria, fungus, and parasites. Infectious diseases can often present with varied or vague clinical signs, so any veterinary practitioner treating birds should have a thorough understanding of possible etiologic agents in order to best direct treatment.

CLINICS CARE POINTS

- Crop burns are common in juvenile hand-raised birds, especially when the hand feeding is being carried out with someone that is not experienced. It is important to allow the tissue to 'declare itself' in order to ensure all of the damaged tissue has been removed and the edges that are to be surgically debrided are of healthy tissue.

- Foreign bodies are a common complaint of the gastrointestinal tract in parrots, who use their beaks to interact with and explore their environment. Foreign bodies may not always cause a blockage within the gastrointestinal tract, but may result in toxicity of the ingested material carries toxic materials, for example zinc, lead or other heavy metals.

- Cloacal prolapses represent intussusception of an organ and are a true emergency. The prolapsed tissue must be kept moist and lubricated until such a time that it can be replaced. The presence of a cloacal prolapse is a clinical sign of underlying pathology, and all cases of cloacal prolapse must be investigated further after emergency treatment.

- Avian chlamydiosis , caused by Chlamydia psittaci, can present with a broad range of clinical signs, and should be suspected in a lethargic bird with evidence of anorexia, biliverdinuria and diarrhoea. As this is a potentially zoonotic infection, it is important for clinicians to identify, treat and control infections.

- Bornavirus has been identified as the cause of proventricular dilatation disease, which can have very lengthy latency periods. Affected birds will often present as losing weight, regurgitating, passing undigested seed in faeces and with evidence of neurological signs such as opisthotonus. This should be considered as a differential diagnosis in any bird displaying these clinical signs that has an enlarged proventriculus on radiographs. Diagnosis can be confirmed with PCR and serology.

- Budgerigars are predisposed to Macrorhabdus ornithogaster, which targets the isthmus. Diagnosis of this fungal infection is challenging ante-mortem, and the use of a macro-suspension cytology has been shown to increase the probability of detection.

DISCLOSURE

The authors have nothing to disclose.

REFERENCES

1. Sandier P. Disorders of the digestive system. In: Samour J, editor. Avian medicine. 3rd edition. St. Louis: Elsevier; 2016. p. 373–85.
2. Mison MB, Bennett RA. Surgery- of the -avian- gastrointestinal- tract. In: Bennett RA, Pye GW, editors. Surgery of exotic animals. 1st edition. Hoboken: John Wiley & Sons, Inc.; 2021. p. 175–89.
3. Nascimento LR, Canelo EA, Rodrigues LL, et al. Ingluvolitos em periquito australiano: relato de caso. Rev Bras Ciên Vet 2015;22(1):16–8.
4. Fischer I, Curd S, Hatt JM. Chronic regurgitation in a cockatiel (Nymphicus hollandicus) with a trichobezoar. Schweiz Arch Tierheilkd 2006;148(6):309–11.
5. Rosenwax A, Cowan M. Fibrous ingluvial foreign bodies in 33 cockatiels (Nymphicus hollandicus). Aust Vet J 2015;93(10):381–4.
6. Ryan TP. Grit impaction in 2 neonatal African grey parrots (Psittacus erithacus erithacus). J Avian Med Surg 2002;16(3):230–3.
7. Laku D, Mutah A, Mohammed A, et al. Ingluviotomy in a cumulet pigeon following crop impaction: case report. Int J Vet Sci Anim Husb 2021;6(3):01–3.
8. Morishita TY, Aye PP, Harr BS. Crop impaction resulting from feather ball formation in caged layers. Avian Dis 1999;43(1):160.
9. Huang AS, Carvallo FR, Pitesky ME, et al. Gastrointestinal impactions in backyard poultry. J Vet Diagn Invest 2019;31(3):368–70.
10. Krautwald-Junghanns ME, Pees M. Gastrointestinal tract. In: Krautwald-Junghanns ME, Pees M, Reese S, et al, editors. Diagnostic imaging of exotic pets. Hannover: Schlutersche Verlagsgesellschaft mbH & Co; 2011. p. 104–13.
11. Hayati F, Ahrari Khafi MS, Salmanzadeh N, et al. Surgical removal of a tube-like foreign body from an Alexandrine parakeet (Psittacula eupatria) using a ventricular approach: a case report. Glob Vet 2012;9(6):696–9.
12. Raisi A, Amini E, Ramezani M, et al. Removing of crop foreign body in a cockatiel (Nymphicus hollandicus) by ingluviotomy technique: case report. Iran J Vet Surg 2018;13(2):71–5.
13. Roy AP, Maji AK, Mukherjee P, et al. Surgical management of oesophageal foreign body syndrome in an Indian ring-neck parakeet. Indian J Anim Health 2020;59(1):111.

14. Mesgarani H, Kazemi Mehrjerdi H, Mirshahi A, et al. Successful surgical removal of crop foreign body in a common mynah (Acridotheres tristis): a case report. Iran J Vet Sur 2014;9(1):57–60.

15. Ninu AR, Uma Rani R, Vishnugurubaran D. Esophagotomy in a domestic fowl: a rare case report. PubMed 2019;20(3):218–20.

16. Rettenmund CL, Chen S. Tracheal obstruction due to glossal entrapment by a string foreign body in a peahen (Pavo cristatus). J Exot Pet Med 2013;22(2):200–5.

17. Lin GW. Long-term prognosis and treatment of crop impaction in chickens via ingluviotomy with local infiltration anesthetic: case report. Avian Dis 2022;66(3):352–9.

18. Speer BL. Chronic partial proventricular obstruction caused by multiple gastro-intestinal foreign bodies in a juvenile umbrella cockatoo (Cacatua Alba). J Avian Med Surg 1998;12(4):271–5.

19. Salinsky J, Aguilar RF. What is your diagnosis? J Avian Med Sulakurg 2010;24(1):77–80.

20. Kinsel MJ, Briggs MB, Crang RFE, et al. Ventricular phytobezoar impaction in tree Micronesian kingfishers (Halcyon cinnamonina cinnamonina). J Zoo Wildl Med 2004;35(4):525–9.

21. Lamb SK. Obstruction by fibrous foreign object ingestion in two green-cheeked conures (Pyrrhura molinae) and a jenday conure (Aratinga jandaya). J Exot Pet Med 2019;31:127–32.

22. Cotton RJ, Divers SJ. Endoscopic removal of gastrointestinal foreign bodies in two African grey parrots (Psittacus erithacus) and a hyacinth macaw (Anodo-rhynchus hyacinthinus). J Avian Med Surg 2017;31(4):335–43.

23. Adamcak A, Hess LR, Quesenberry KE. Intestinal string foreign body in an adult umbrella cockatoo (Cacatua alba). J Avian Med Surg 2000;14(4):257–63.

24. Degernes LA, Wolf KN, Zombeck DJ, et al. Ventricular diverticula formation in captive parakeet auklets (Aethia psittacula) secondary to foreign body inges-tion. J Zoo Wildl Med 2012;43(4):889–97.

25. Hoefer H, Levitan D. Perforating foreign body in the ventriculus of an umbrella cockatoo (Cacatua alba). J Avian Med Surg 2013;27(2):128–35.

26. Applegate JR, Van Wettere A, Christiansen EF, et al. Management and case outcome of gastric impaction in four raptors: a case series. J Avian Med Surg 2017;31(1):62–9.

27. Lloyd C. Staged Endoscopic Ventricular foreign body removal in a Gyr falcon (Falco rusticolus). J Avian Med Surg 2009;23(4):314–9.

28. Miller CL, Bischoff KL, Hoff B. Polyacrylamide gel ingestion leading to fatal intes-tinal obstruction in two birds in a zoological collection. J Avian Med Surg 2009;23(4):286–9.

29. Sanchez CR, Pich A, Collinsworth S. Erosive enteritis and intestinal obstructions caused by decomposed granite in a flock of Lesser flamingos (Phoeniconaias minor). J Avian Med Surg 2019;33(1):72–81.

30. Laniesse D, Beaufrère H, Mackenzie S, et al. Perforating foreign body in the ventriculus of a pet pigeon (Columba livia domestica). J Am Vet Med Assoc 2018;253(12):1610–6.

31. Hollwarth AJ, Reese DJ, Dutton TAG. Osseous migration of a perforating gastro-intestinal foreign body in an Indian runner duck (Anas platyrhynchos domesti-cus). J Avian Med Surg 2021;35(3):361–6.

32. Hayati F, Lakzian A, Shariati E, et al. Surgical removal of a ventricular foreign body from a common myna (Acridotheres tristis): a case report. Vet Med 2011;56(2):97–100.

33. Meamar N, Asghari Beghkheirati A, Abbasi M, et al. Successful surgical removal of a perforating ventricular foreign body from a mallard duck (Anas platyrhynchos): a case report. J Poult Sci Avian Dis 2023;1(2):37–41.

34. Máinez M, Rosell J, Such R, et al. Traumatic (foreign body) pericarditis in a Toco toucan (Ramphastos toco). J Zoo Wildl Med 2016;47(4):1097–100.

35. Kim S, Kim N, Kim H, et al. Various endoscopic approaches for removal of proventricular foreign bodies in parrots—three case reports. Animals 2023;13(24):3839.

36. Mison M, Mehler S, Echols MS, et al. Approaches to the coelom and selected procedures. In: Speer B, editor. Current therapy in avian medicine and surgery. 1st edition. St. Louis: Elsevier; 2016. p. 638–45.

37. Simova-Curd S, Foldenauer U, Guerrero T, et al. Comparison of ventriculotomy closure with and without a coelomic fat patch in Japanese quail (Coturnix coturnix japonica). J Avian Med Surg 2013;27(1):7–13.

38. Lupu C, Robins S. Comparison of treatment protocols for removing metallic foreign objects from the ventriculus of budgerigars (Melopsittacus undulatus). J Avian Med Surg 2009;23(3):186–93.

39. Sabater M, Huynh M, Forbes N. Ileo-ceco-rectal intussusception requiring intestinal resection and anastomosis in a Tawny Eagle (Aquila rapax). J Avian Med Surg 2015;29(1):63–8.

40. Romagnano A. Psittacine incubation and pediatrics. Vet Clin North Am Exot Anim Pract 2012;15(2):163–82.

41. Cornelissen H. Intussusception of the intestinal tract in a white-cheeked turaco. J Assoc Avian Vet 1993;7(4):218.

42. Batista JS, de Oliveira MF, Teófilo TDS, et al. Intussusception associated with sand accumulation in a greater rhea (Rhea americana). Acta Vet 2021;71(3):344–50.

43. Reimers N, Carver D, Barnes HJ. Emaciation and sporadic mortality in older laying hens caused by intussusception of the proventriculus. Avian Dis 2018;63(1):107.

44. Ramesh S, Pazhanivel N, Meignanalakshmi S, et al. Intussusception of proventriculus in a blue & gold macaw- a case report. Res J Vet Pract 2021;9(3):21–3.

45. Cococcetta C, Binanti D, Matteucci G, et al. Antemortem diagnosis and surgical management of a rectum intussusception and cloacal wall prolapse in a hybrid falcon (F. cherrug x F. peregrinus) associated with bacterial enteritis. J Exot Pet Med 2020;33:10–3.

46. VanDerHeyden N. Jejunostomy and jejunocloacal anastomosis in macaws. Nashville, Tennessee: Proceedings of the annual conference of the association of avian veterinarians; 1993. p.72-77.

47. Greenwood A, Storm J. Intestinal intussusception in two red-tailed hawks (Buteo jamaicensis). Vet Rec 1994;134(22):578–9.

48. Dutton TAG, Forbes NA, Carrasco DC. Cloacal prolapse in raptors: review of 16 Cases. J Avian Med Surg 2016;30(2):133–40.

49. Gill KS, Helmer PJ. Cloacal diseases in companion parrots: a retrospective Study of 43 Cases (2012–2018). J Avian Med Surg 2020;34(4):364–70.

50. Beaufrère H, Nevarez J, Tully TN. Cloacolith in a blue-fronted Amazon parrot (Amazona aestiva). J Avian Med Surg 2010;24(2):142–5.

51. Christen C, Hatt JM. What is your diagnosis? J Avian Med Surg 2006;20(2): 129–31.

52. Di Nucci DL, Falzone MP. Cloacal impaction with cloacolith in a black-legged seriema (Chunga burmeisteri). Open Vet J 2018;7(4):391.

53. Wissink-Argilaga N, Pellett S. Psittacine nutrition and common deficiency diseases. Compan Anim 2015;20(9):526–31.

54. Schmidt RE, Reavill DR, Phalen DN. Gastrointestinal system and pancreas. In: Schmidt RE, Reavill DR, Phalen DN, editors. Pathology of pet and aviary birds. 2nd edition. Wiley Blackwell: Iowa; 2015. p. 55–95.

55. Koutsos E. Foundations in avian nutrition. In: Speer BL, editor. Current therapy in avian medicine and surgery. 1st edition. St. Louis: Elsevier; 2016. p. 142–50.

56. Cummings AM, Hess LR, Spielvogel CF, et al. An Evaluation of three diet conversion methods in psittacine birds converting from seed-based diets to pelleted diets. J Avian Med Surg 2022;36(2):145–52.

57. Hess L, Mauldin G, Rosenthal K. Estimated nutrient content of diets commonly fed to pet birds. Vet Rec 2002;150(13):399–404.

58. Werquin GJDL, DeCock KJS, Ghysels PGC. Comparison of the nutrient analysis and caloric density of 30 commercial seed mixtures (in toto and dehulled) with 27 commercial diets for parrots. J Anim Physiol Anim Nutr 2005;89(3–6):215–21.

59. Orosz SE. Clinical avian nutrition. Vet Clin North Am Exot Anim Pract 2014;17(3): 397–413.

60. Perpiñán D. Problems of excess nutrients in psittacine diets. Compan Anim 2015;20(9):532–7.

61. Schmidt RE, Reavill DR, Phalen DN. Liver. In: Schmidt RE, Reavill DR, Phalen DN, editors. Pathology of pet and aviary birds. 2nd edition. Wiley Blackwell: Iowa; 2015. p. 95–126.

62. Koutsos EA, Smith J, Woods LW, et al. Adult cockatiels (Nymphicus hollandicus) metabolically adapt to high protein diets. J Nutr 2001;131(7):2014–20.

63. O'Connor MR, Garner MM. Iron storage disease in african grey parrots (psittacus erithacus) exposed to a carnivorous diet. J Zoo Wildl Med 2018;49(1): 172–7.

64. Lowenstine LJ, Stasiak IM. Update on iron overload in zoologic species. In: Fowler ME, Miller ER, editors. Fowler's zoo and wild animal medicine. 8th edition. St. Louis: Elsevier Saunders; 2015. p. 674–81.

65. Olsen GP, Russell KE, Dierenfeld E, et al. A comparison of four regimens for treatment of iron storage disease using the European starling (Sturnus vulgaris) as a Model. J Avian Med Surg 2006;20(2):74–9.

66. Desmarchelier M, Langlois I. Diabetes mellitus in a Nanday conure (Nandayus nenday). J Avian Med Surg 2008;22(3):246–54.

67. Van de Weyer Y, Alan TS. Avian diabetes mellitus: a review. J Avian Med Surg 2024;38(1):21–33.

68. Dupont J, Rideau N, Simon J. Endocrine pancreas. In: Scanes CG, Dridi S, editors. Sturkie's avian physiology. 7th Edition. London: Academic Press and imprint of Elsevier; 2022. p. 915–37.

69. Rideau N. Insulin secretion in birds. In: Leclercq B, Whitehead CC, editors. Leanness in domestic birds: genetic, metabolic and hormonal aspects. London, Boston: Elsevier; 1988. p. 269–94.

70. Bonda M. Plasma glucagon, serum insulin, and serum amylase levels in normal and a hyperglycemic macaw. Tampa, Florida: Proceedings of the annual conference of the association of avian veterinarians; 1996: p. 77-88.

71. Gancz AY, Wellehan JFX, Boutette J, et al. Diabetes mellitus concurrent with hepatic haemosiderosis in two macaws (Ara severa, Ara militaris). Avian Pathol 2007;36(4):331–6.

72. McCleery B, McCready J. Management of diabetes mellitus in an eclectus parrot (Eclectus roratus) using insulin glargine. London, United Kingdom: ICARE 2019 conference proceedings; 2019: p. 107.

73. Murphy J. Diabetes in toucans. New Orleans, Louisianna: proceedings of the annual conference of the association of avian veterinarians; 1992: p. 165-170.

74. Pollock CG, Pledger T, Renner M. Diabetes mellitus in avian species. Tampa, Florida: Proceedings of the annual conference of the association of avian veterinarians; 2001: p. 151-155.

75. Doneley B. Disorders of the pancreas. In: Avian medicine and surgery in practice: companion and aviary birds. 2nd edition. Boca Raton: CRC Press Taylor & Francis Group; 2016. p. 65–269.

76. Zehnder A, Graham J, Reavill DR, et al. Neoplastic diseases in avian species. In: Speer BL, editor. Current therapy in avian medicine and surgery. 1st edition. St. Louis: Elsevier; 2016. p. 107–41.

77. Caldas Menezes R, Tortelly R, Corrêa Gomes D, et al. Nodular typhlitis associated with the nematodes Heterakis gallinarum and Heterakis isolonche in pheasants: frequency and pathology with evidence of neoplasia. Memo Inst Oswaldo Cruz 2003;98(8):1011–6.

78. Kasimov V, White RT, Foxwell J, et al. Whole-genome sequencing of Chlamydia psittaci from Australian avian hosts: a genomics approach to a pathogen that still ruffles feathers. Microb Genom 2023;9(7):001072.

79. Stalder S, Marti H, Borel N, et al. Occurrence of Chlamydiaceae in raptors and crows in Switzerland. Pathogens 2020;9(9):724.

80. Tolba HMN, Abou Elez RMM, Elsohaby I. Risks factors associated with Chlamydia psittaci infections in psittacine birds and bird handlers. J Appl Microbiol 2019;126(2):402–10.

81. Thierry S, Vorimore F, Rossignol C, et al. Oral uptake of Chlamydia psittaci by ducklings results in systemic dissemination. PLoS One 2016;11(5):e0154860.

82. Ornelas-Eusebio E, Sanchez-Godoy FD, Chavez-Maya F, et al. First identification of Chlamydia psittaci in the acute illness and death of endemic and endangered psittacine birds in Mexico. Avian Dis 2016;60(2):540–4.

83. Wang C, Li L, Xie Y, et al. Isolation and characterization of avian Chlamydia psittaci from symptomatic pet birds in southern Hunan, China. Avian Dis 2018;63(1):31–7.

84. Sanchez-Migallon Guzman D, Diaz-Figueroa O, Tully T, et al. Evaluation of 21-day doxycycline and azithromycin treatments for experimental Chlamydophila psittaci infection in cockatiels (Nymphicus hollandicus). J Avian Med Surg 2010;24(1):35–45.

85. Razmyar J, Rajabioun M, Zaeemi M, et al. Molecular identification and successful treatment of Chlamydophila psittaci (genotype B) in a clinically affected Congo African grey parrot (Psittacus erithacus erithacus). Iran J Vet Res 2016;17(4):281–5.

86. Grimes JE. Evaluation and interpretation of serologic responses in psittacine bird chlamydiosis and suggested complementary diagnostic procedures. J Avian Med Surg 1996;10(2):75–83.

87. Fowler ME, Ardans A, Reynolds B, et al. Chlamydiosis in captive raptors. Avian Dis 1990;34(3):657–62.

88. Balsamo G, Maxted AM, Midla JW, et al. Compendium of measures to control Chlamydia psittaci infection among humans (psittacosis) and pet birds (avian chlamydiosis), 2017. J Avian Med Surg 2017;31(3):262–82.

89. Kriz P, Kaevska M, Bartejsova I, et al. Mycobacterium avium subsp. Avium found in raptors exposed to infected domestic fowl. Avian Dis 2013;57(3): 688–92.

90. Nesic V, Marinkovic D, Matovic K, et al. Avian tuberculosis in a free-living Eurasian griffon vulture. J Vet Diagn Invest 2022;34(34):723–6.

91. Jackson R. Gastrointestinal disorders. In: Poland G, Raftery A, editors. BSAVA Manual of backyard poultry medicine and surgery. 1st edition. Quedgeley: British Small Animal Veterinary Association; 2019. p. 178–205.

92. Shitaye JE, Matlova L, Horvathova, et al. Mycobacterium avium subsp. Avium distribution studied in a naturally infected hen flock and in the environment by culture, serotyping and IS901 RFLP methods. Vet Microbiol 2008;127(1–2): 155–64.

93. Tsiouris V, Kiskinis K, Mantzios T, et al. Avian mycobacteriosis and molecular identification of mycobacterium avium subsp. Avium in racing pigeons (Columba livia domestica) in Greece. Animals 2011;11:291.

94. Ledwon A, Miqsko M, Napiorkowska A, et al. Case study and attempt on treatment of mycobacteriosis caused by Mycobacterium avium in a parental flock of meat-breed pigeons. Avian Dis 2020;64(3):335–42.

95. Krause KJ, Reavill D, Weldy SH, et al. Mycobacterium genavense in an African penguin (Spheniscus demersus). J Zoo Wildl Med 2015;46(4):971–5.

96. Schmitz A, Rinder M, Thiel S, et al. Retrospective evaluation of clinical signs and gross pathologic findings in birds infected with Mycobacterium genavense. J Avian Med Surg 2018;32(3):194–204.

97. Haridy M, Fukuta M, Mori Y. An outbreak of Mycobacterium genavense infection in a flock of captive diamond doves (Geopelia cuneata). Avian Dis 2014;58(3): 383–90.

98. Sattar A, Zakaria Z, Abu J, et al. Evaluation of six decontamination procedures for isolation of Mycobacterium avium complex from avian feces. PLoS One 2018;13(8):e0202034.

99. Shitaye JE, Matlova L, Horvathova A, et al. Diagnostic testing of different stages of avian tuberculosis in naturally infected hens (Gallus domesticus) by the tuberculin skin and rapid agglutination tests, faecal and egg examinations. Vet Med 2008;53(2):101–10.

100. Ledwon A, Dolka I, Dolka B, et al. Multidrug therapy of Mycobacterium avium subsp. Avium infection in experimentally inoculated budgerigars (Melopsittacus undulatus). Avian Pathol 2015;44(6):470–4.

101. Biet F, Boschiroli ML, Thorel MF, et al. Zoonotic aspects of Mycobacterium bovis and Mycobacterium avium-intracellulare complex (MAC). Vet Res 2005;36(3): 411–36.

102. Rana EA, Nizami TA, Islam MS, et al. Phenotypical identification and toxinotyping of Clostridium perfringens isolates from healthy and enteric disease-affected chickens. Vet Med Int 2023;1:2584171.

103. Lloyd C. Gastrointestinal tract disease. In: Chitty J, Lierz M, editors. BSAVA Manual of raptors, pigeons and passerine birds. 1st edition. Quedgeley: British Small Animal Veterinary Association; 2008. p. 260–9.

104. De Santi M, Schocken-Iturrino RB, Froner CM, et al. Necrotic enteritis caused by Clostridium perfringens in blue and gold macaws (Ara ararauna). J Avian Med Surg 2020;34(1):65–9.

105. Wu S, Stanley D, Rodgers N, et al. Two necrotic enteritis predisposing factors, dietary fishmeal and Eimeria infection, induce large changes in the cecal microbiota of broiler chickens. Vet Microbiol 2014;169:188–97.

106. Rossi G, Terracciano G, Cherardi R, et al. Parasites, bacteria, and associated pathological changes in the digestive system of diurnal and nocturnal raptors in central Italy. Pathogens 2021;10(12):1567.

107. Smyth JA. Pathology and diagnosis of necrotic enteritis: is it clear-cut? Avian Pathol 2016;45(3):282–7.

108. Zanu HK, Keerqin C, Kheravii SK, et al. Influence of meat and bone meal phytase and antibiotics on broiler chickens challenged with subclinical necrotic enteritis: 1.growth performance, intestinal pH, apparent ileal digestibility, cecal microbiota, and tibial mineralization. Poult Sci J 2020;99(3):1540–50.

109. Geier MS, Mikkelsen LL, Torok VA, et al. Comparison of alternatives to in-feed antimicrobials for the prevention of clinical necrotic enteritis. J Appl Microbiol 2010;109(4):1329–38.

110. Harrold D, Saunders R, Bailey J. Dietary putrescine supplementation reduces faecal abundance of Clostridium perfringens and markers of inflammation in captive azure-winged magpies. J Zoo Aquar Res 2020;8(2):114–23.

111. Shamshirgaran MA, Golchin M, Mohammadi E. Lactobacillus casei displaying Clostridium perfringens NeTB antigen protects chickens against necrotic enteritis. Appl Microbiol Biotechnol 2022;106:6441–53.

112. Iqbal S, Qureshi S, Banday MS, et al. Short variable regions flaA Gene (SVR-flaA) diversity and virulence profile of multidrug-resistant Campylobacter from poultry and poultry meat in India. J Food Prot 2024;87(7):100308.

113. Stern NJ, Svetoch EA, Eruslanov BV, et al. Paenibacillus polymyxa purified bacteriocin to control campylobacter jejuni in chickens. J Food Prot 2005; 68(7):1450–3.

114. Chiba M, Miri S, Yousuf B, et al. Dual bacteriocin and extracellular vesicle-mediated inhibition of Campylobacter jejuni by the potential probiotic candidate Ligilactobacillus salivarius UO.C249. Appl Environ Microbiol 2024;90(8): e0084524.

115. Zhuge X, Jiang M, Tang F, et al. Avian-source mcr-1-positive Escherichia coli is phylogenetically diverse and shares virulence characteristics with E. coli causing human extra-intestinal infections. Vet Microbiol 2019;239:108483.

116. Jones DM, Nisbet DJ. The gram negative bacterial flora of the avian gut. Avian Pathol 1980;9(1):33–8.

117. Sola-Gines M, Cameron-Veas K, Badiola I, et al. Diversity of multi-drug resistant avian pathogenic Escherichia coli (APEC) causing outbreaks of colibacillosis in broilers during 2012 in Spain. PLoS One 2015;10(11):E0143191.

118. Patel K, Stapleton GS, Trevejo RT, et al. Human salmonellosis outbreak linked to salmonella tiphymurium epidemic in wild songbirds, United States, 2020-2021. Emerg Infect Dis 2023;29(11):2298–306.

119. Molina-Lopez RA, Vidal A, Obon E, et al. Multidrug-resistant Salmonella enterica serovar Typhimurium monophasic variant 4,12:i:- isolated from asymptomatic wildlife in a Catalonian wildlife rehabilitation center, Spain. J Wildl Dis 2015; 51(3):759–63.

120. Millan J, Aduriz G, Moreno B, et al. Salmonella isolates from wild birds and mammals in the Basque country (Spain). Rev Sci Tech 2004;23(3):905–11.

121. Ward MP, Ramer JC, Proudfoot J, et al. Outbreak of salmonellosis in a zoologic collection of lorikeets and lories (Trichoglosus, Lorius and Eos spp). Avian Dis 2003;47(2):493–8.

122. Hall AJ, Saito EK. Avian wildlife mortality events due to salmonellosis in the United States, 1985-2004. J Wildl Dis 2008;44(3):585–93.
123. Saleem G, Farooq U, Javed MT, et al. Pathobiological and immunohistochemical findings in broilers chickens naturally infected with Salmonella enterica serotype gallinarum biotype gallinarum. Pak Vet J 2022;42(1):88.
124. Molenaar RJ, Dijkman R, teer Ven C, et al. A Salmonella pullorum outbreak with neurological signs in adult layers and outbreak investigation using whole genome sequencing. Avian Pathol 2024;53(1):44–55.
125. Pinto PN, Torres ACD, Rodriguez MP, et al. An outbreak of fatal Pullorum disease (Salmonella pullorum) in Guinea fowl keets (Numida meleagridis). Pesqui Vet Bras 2023;43:e07088.
126. Nisbet DJ, Tellez GI, Lowry VK, et al. Effect of a commercial competitive exclusion culture (Preempt™) on mortality and horizontal transmission of Salmonella gallinarum in broiler chickens. Avian Dis 1998;42(4):651–6.
127. Berchieri Jr A, Murphy CK, Marston K, et al. Observations on the persistence and vertical transmission of Salmonella enterica serovars Pullorum and Gallinarum in chickens: effect of bacterial and host genetic background. Avian Pathol 2001;30:221–31.
128. Crouch CF, Nell T, Reijnders M, et al. Safety and efficacy of a novel inactivated trivalent Salmonella enterica vaccine in chickens. Vaccine 2020;38(43): 6741–50.
129. MSD. Nobilis calenvac T suspension for injection for chickens. In: MSD animal health hub. 2024. Available at: https://www.msd-animal-health-hub.co.uk/Products/Nobilis-SalenvacT#:~:text=Nobilis%20Salenvac%20T%20is%20a,and%20Salmonella%20typhimurium%20DT%20104. Accessed August 26, 2024.
130. Cork SC, Collins-Emerson JM, Alley MR, et al. Visceral lesions caused by Yersinia pseudotuberculosis, serotype II, in different species of bird. Avian Pathol 2010;28(4):393–9.
131. Stoute ST, Cooper GL, Bickford AA, et al. Yersinia pseudotuberculosis in Eurasian collared doves (Streptopelia decaocto) and retrospective study of avian yersiniosis at the California animal health and food safety laboratory system (1990-2015). Avian Dis 2015;60(1):82–6.
132. Platt-Samoraj A, Zmudzki J, Pajdak-Czaus J, et al. The prevalence of Yersinia enterocolitica and Yersinia pseudotuberculosis in small wild rodents in Poland. Vector Borne Zoonotic Di 2020;20(8):586–92.
133. Wallner-Pendleton E, Cooper G. Several outbreaks of yersinia pseudotuberculosis in California turkey flocks. Avian Dis 1983;27(2):524–6.
134. Ceccolini ME, Macgregor SK, Spiro S, et al. Yersinia pseudotuberculosis infections in primates, artiodactyls, and birds within a zoological facility in the United Kingdom. J Zoo Wildl Med 2020;51(3):527–38.
135. Hammerl JA, Barac A, Bienert A, et al. Birds kept in the German zoo 'Tierpark Berlin' are a common source for polyvalent Yersinia pseudotuberculosis phages. Front Microbiol 2022;12:634289.
136. Wrobel ER. Seroprevalence of avian pox and Mycoplasma gallisepticum in raptors in central Illinois. J Raptor Res 2016;50(3):289–94.
137. Hydock K, Brown H, Nemeth N, et al. Evaluation of cytology for diagnosing avian pox in wild turkeys (Meleagridis gallopavo). Avian Dis 2017;62(1):45–9.
138. Fukui D, Nakamura M, Yamaguchi T, et al. An epizootic of emerging novel avian pox in carrion crows (Corvus corone) and large-billed crows (Corvus macrorhynchos) in Japan. J Wildl Dis 2016;52(2):230–41.

139. Tompkins EM, Anderson DJ, Pabilonia KL, et al. Avian pox discovered in the critically endangered Waved albatross (Phoebastria irrorata) from the Galapagos Islands, Ecuador. J Wildl Dis 2017;53(4):8910895.

140. Yeo G, Wang Y, Chong SM, et al. Characterization of fowlpox virus in chickens and bird-biting mosquitoes: a molecular approach to investigating avipoxvirus transmission. J Gen Virol 2019;100(5):838–50.

141. Catania S, Carnaccini S, Mainenti M, et al. Isolation of avipoxvirus from tongue of canaries (Serinus canaria) show severe localized proliferative glossitis. Avian Dis 2017;61(4):531–5.

142. Sarker S, Athukorala A, Raidal SR. Molecular characterisation of a novel pathogenic avipoxvirus from an Australian passerine bird, midlark (Gallina cyanoleuca). Virology 2021;554:66–74.

143. Ha HJ, Alley M, Howe L, et al. Evaluation of the pathogenicity of avipoxvirus strains isolated from wild birds in New Zealand and the efficacy of a fowlpox vaccine in passerines. Vet Microbiol 2013;165(3–4):268–74.

144. Styles DK, Tomaszewski EK, Jaeger LA, et al. Psittacid herpesviruses associated with mucosal papillomas in neotropical parrots. Virology 2004;325(1): 24–35.

145. Styles DK, Tomaszewski EK, Phalen D. A novel herpesvirus found in African grey parrots (Psittacus erithacus erithacus). Avian Pathol 2005;34(2):150–4.

146. Legler M, Kothe R, Wohlsein P, et al. First detection of psittacid herpesvirus 2 in Congo African grey parrots (Psittacus erithacus erithacus) associated with pharyngeal papillomas and cloacal inflammation in Germany. Berl Munch Tierarztl Wschr 2014;127(5–6):222–6.

147. Legler M, Kothe R, Rautenschlein S, et al. Detection of psittacid herpesvirus 1 in Amazon parrots with cloacal papilloma (internal papillomatosis of parrots, IPP) in an aviary of different psittacine species. Dtsch Tierarztl Wochenschr 2008; 115(12):461–70.

148. Jones AL, Suarez-Bonnet A, Mitchell JA, et al. Avian papilloma and squamous cell carcinoma: a histopathological, immunohistochemical and virological study. J Comp Pathol 2020;175:13–23.

149. Lierz M. Systemic infectious diseases. In: Harcourt-Brown N, Chitty J, editors. BSAVA Manual of psittacine birds. 2nd edition. Quedgeley: British Small Animal Veterinary Association; 2005. p. 155–69.

150. Gornatti-Churria CD, Loukopoulos P, Stoute ST, et al. A retrospective study of pigeon herpesviral infection in domestic pigeons in California (1991-2014) and literature review. J Vet Diagn Invest 2023;35(3):252–7.

151. Phalen DN, Alvarado C, Grillo V, et al. Prevalence of columbid herpesvirus infection in feral pigeons from new South Wales and Victoria, Australia, with spillover into a wild powerful owl (Ninox struena). J Wildl Dis 2017;53(3):543–51.

152. Rose N, Warren AL, Whiteside D, et al. Columbid herpesvirus-1 mortality in great horned owls (Bubo virginianus) from Calgary, Alberta. Can Vet J 2012;53(3): 265–8.

153. Gleeson MD, Moore BA, Edwards SG, et al. A novel herpesvirus associated with chronic superficial keratitis and proliferative conjunctivitis in a great horned owl (Bubo virginianus). Vet Ophthalmol 2018;22(1):67–75.

154. Abdullatif TM, Ghanem IA, El Bakrey RMM. Duck viral enteritis in Egypt: isolation and detection of the circulating virus during outbreaks from 2016-2018. Slov Vet Zb 2021;58(24-Suppl):21.

155. Converse KA, Gregory AK. Duck plague epizootics in the United States, 1967-1995. J Wildl Dis 2001;37(2):347–57.

156. Ahamed T, Sultana P, Rahman MZ, et al. Protection of Khaki Campbell ducks against duck plague using an inactivated duck plague vaccine. World Vet J 2023;13(2):332–40.
157. Kistler AL, Gancz A, Clubb S, et al. Recovery of divergent avian bornaviruses from cases of proventricular dilatation disease: identification of a candidate etiologic agent. Virol J 2008;5:1–15.
158. Honkavuori KS, Gancz A, Clubb S, et al. Novel borna virus in psittacine birds with proventricular dilatation disease. Emerg Infect Dis 2008;14(12):88.
159. Gancz AY, Kistler AL, Greninger AL, et al. Experimental induction of proventricular dilatation disease in cockatiels (Nymphicus hollandicus) inoculated with brain homogenates containing avian bornavirus 4. Virol J 2009;6(1):100.
160. Philadelpho NA, Davies YM, Guimaraes MB, et al. Detection of avian bornavirus in wild and captive passeriformes in Brazil. Avian Dis 2019;63(2):294–7.
161. Rinder M, Baas N, Hagen E, et al. Canary bornavirus (Orthobornavirus serini) infections are associated with clinical symptoms in common canaries (serinus canaria dom.). Viruses 2022;14(10):2187.
162. Kuhn JH, Durrwald R, Bao Y, et al. Taxonomic reorganization of the family Bornaviridae. Virol Div News 2015;160:621–32.
163. Gray P, Hoppes S, Suchodolski P, et al. Use of avian bornavirus isolates to induce proventricular dilatation disease in conures. Emerg Infect Dis 2010;16(3):473–9.
164. Bourque L, Laniesse D, Beaufrere H, et al. Identification of avian bornavirus in a Himalayan monal (Lophophorus impejanus) with neurological disease. Avian Pathol 2015;44(4):323–7.
165. Rubbenstroth D, Brosinski K, Rinder M, et al. No contact transmission of avian bornavirus in experimentally infected cockatiels (Nymphicus hollandicus) and domestic canaries (Serinus canaria forma domestica). Vet Microbiol 2014;172:146–56.
166. Aguilera-Sepulveda P, Llorente F, Rosenstierne MW, et al. Detection of a new avian bornavirus in a barn owl (Tyto alba) by pan-viral microarray. Vet Microbiol 2024;289:109959.
167. Link J, Herzog S, Gartner AM, et al. Factors influencing verticakisl transmission of psittacine bornavirus in cockatiels (Nymphicus hollandicus). Viruses 2022;14(12):2721.
168. Petzold J, Gartner AM, MAlberg S, et al. Tissue distribution of parrot bornavirus 4 (PaBV-4) in experimentally infected young and adult cockatiels (Nymphicus hollandicus). Viruses 2020;14(10):2181.
169. Dennison SE, Adams WM, Johnson PJ, et al. Prognostic accuracy of the proventriculus:keel ratio for short-term survival in psittacines with proventricular disease. Vet Radiol Ultrasound 2009;50(2):483–6.
170. Hoppes S, Heatley JJ, Guo J, et al. Meloxicam treatment in cockatiels (Nymphicus hollandicus) infected with avian bornavirus. J Exot Pet Med 2013;22(3):275–9.
171. Forbes NA, Simpson GN, Higgins RJ, et al. Adenovirus infection in Mauritius kestrels (Falco punctatus). J Avian Med Surg 1997;11(1):31–3.
172. Ramsubeik S, Carmen J, Uzal FA, et al. Necrotic enteritis in a commercial Turkey flock coinfected with hemorrhagic enteritis virus. J Vet Diagn Invest 2023;35(3):317–21.
173. Stoute S, Crossley B, Shivaprasad HL. Study of an outbreak of highly pathogenic avian influenza H5N8 in commercial pekin ducks (Anas platyrhynchos domesticus) in California. Avian Dis 2018;62(1):101–8.

174. Bozic B, Polacek V, Vucicevic I, et al. Morphological differences of pancreatic lesions in mute swans and hens naturally infected with highly pathogenic avian influenza virus H5N8. Acta Vet Beogr 2018;68(2):217–23.

175. Gunther A, Pohlman A, Globig A, et al. Continuous surveillance of potentially zoonotic avian pathogens detects contemporaneous occurrence of highly pathogenic avian influenza viruses (HPAIV H5) and flaviviruses (USUV, WNV) in several wild and captive birds. Emerg Microbes Infect 2023;12(2):2231561.

176. Mansour SMG, ElBakrey RM, Ali H, et al. Natural infection with highly pathogenic avian influenza virus H5N1 in domestic pigeons (Columba livia) in Egypt. Avian Pathol 2014;43(4):319–24.

177. Bertran K, Busquets N, Abad FX, et al. Highly (H5N1) and low (H7N2) pathogenic avian influenza virus infection in falcons via nasochoanal route and ingestion of experimentally infected prey. PLoS One 2012;7(3):E32197.

178. Nemeth N, Ruder MG, Poulson RL, et al. Bald eagle and nest failure due to clade 2.3.4.4 highly pathogenic H5N1 influenza a virus. Sci Rep 2023;13(1):191.

179. Bertran K, Lee D, Criado MF, et al. Pathobiology of Tennessee 2017 H7N9 low and high pathogenicity avian influenza viruses in commercial broiler breeders and specific pathogen free layer chickens. Vet Res 2018;49:82.

180. Prosser DJ, Densmore CL, Hindman LJ, et al. Low pathogenic avian influenza viruses in wild migratory waterfowl in a region of high poultry production, Delmarva, Maryland. Avian Dis 2016;61(1):128–34.

181. Avian influenza. In: World organization for animal health. Available at: https://www.woah.org/en/disease/avian-influenza/. Accessed October 2, 2024.

182. Abd El-Tawab AA, El-Hofy FI, El-Diasty EM, et al. Phenotypic and genotypic characterization of Candida albicans isolated from chicken. Benha Vet Med J 2020;38(2):120–4.

183. Vidal A, Baldoma L, Molina-Lopez RA, et al. Microbiological diagnosis and antimicrobial sensitivity profiles in diseased free-living raptors. Avian Pathol 2017;46(4):442–50.

184. Quist EM, Belcher C, Levine G. Disseminated histoplasmosis with concurrent oral candidiasis in an Eclectus parrot (Eclectus roratus). Avian Pathol 2011;40(2):207–11.

185. Wang H, Li X, Wang W, et al. Isolation, identification and fenotyping of Candida albicans from Landes geese. Transbound Emerg Dis 2021;69(2):349–59.

186. Talazadeh F, Ghorbanpoor M, Shahriyari A. Candidiasis in Birds (Galliformes, Anseriformes, Psittaciformes, Passeriformes, and Columbiformes); a focus on antifungal susceptibility pattern of Candida albicans and non-albicans isolates in avian clinical specimens. Top Companion Anim Med 2022;46:100598.

187. Samour JH, Naldo JL. Diagnosis and therapeutic management of candidiasis in falcons in Saudi Arabia. J Avian Med Surg 2002;16(2):129–32.

188. Blagojevic B, Davidov I, Vukomanovic G, et al. Occurrence of Macrorhabdus ornithogaster in exotic birds. Pol J Vet Sci 2024;27(1):139–42.

189. Baron HR, Stevenson BC, Phalen DN. Inconsistent efficacy of waer-soluble amphotericin B for the treatment of Macrorhabdus ornithogaster in a budgerigar (Melopsittacus undulatus) aviary. Aus Vet J 2020;98(7):333–7.

190. Pustow R, Krautwald-Junghanns ME. The incidence and treatment outcomes of Macrorhabdus ornithogaster infection in Budgerigars (Melopsittacus undulatus) in a veterinary clinic. J Avian Med Surg 2017;31(4):344–50.

191. Baron HR, Stevenson BC, Phalen DN. Comparison of in-clinic diagnostic testing methods for Macrorhabdus ornithogaster. J Avian Med Surg 2021;35(1):37–44.

192. Kheirandish R, Mahmoud S. Megabacteriosis in budgerigars: diagnosis and treatment. Comp Clin Path 2011;20:501–5.
193. Sullivan PJ, Ramsay EC, Greenacre CB, et al. Comparison of two methods for determining prevalence of Macrorhabdus ornithogaster in a flock of captive budgerigars (Melopsittacus undulatus). J Avian Med Surg 2017;21(2):128–31.
194. Salavati A, Khalilzade-Houjagan M, Haddadmarandi M, et al. A cross-sectional survey of gastrointestinal parasites in an ornithological garden. J Avian Med Surg 2023;36(4):380–7.
195. Noor R, Javid A, Hussain A, et al. Prevalence of parasites in selected captive bird species. Braz J Biol 2024;84:E254251.
196. Dezfuli BS, Manera M, Rubini S. Intestinal histopathology due to an Acantho-cephalan in two corvid species from Northern Italy. J Wildl Dis 2021;57(1): 215–9.
197. Ola-Fandunsin SD, Ganiyu IA, Musa R, et al. Gastrointestinal parasites of different avian species in Ilorin, North Central Nigeria. J Ad Vet Anim Res 2019;6(1):108–16.
198. Oyarzun-Ruiz P, Cifuentes-Castro C, Varas F, et al. Helminth and ectoparasitic faunas of the Harris's hawk, Parabuteo unicinctus (Accipitriformes: accipitridae), in Chile: new data on host-parasite associations for neotropical raptors. Rev Bras Parasitol Vet 2022;31(3):e007522.
199. Santana-Sanchez G, Flores-Valle IT, Gonzalez-Gomez M, et al. Caryospora neo-falconis and other enteroparasites in raptors from Mexico. Int J Parasitol Para-sites Wildl 2015;4(3):351–5.
200. Adhikari RB, Badahur AP, Adhikari Dhakal M, et al. Prevalence and diversity of intestnial parasites in household and temple pigeons (Columba livia) in central Nepal. Vet Med Sci 2022;8(4):1528–38.
201. Garner MM, Sturtwvant FC. Trichomoniasis in a blue-fronted Amazon parrot (Amazona aestiva). J Assoc Avian Vet 1992;6(1):17–20.
202. Echenique JVZ, Soares MP, Bruni M, et al. Oral trichomoniasis in raptors in Southern Brazil. Braz J Vet Res Anim Sci 2019;39(12):983–8.

Therapies in Exotic Animal Gastroenterology

Julianne E. McCready, DVM, DVSc, DACZM

KEYWORDS

- Birds • Gastroenterology • Gastroprotectants • Rabbits • Reptiles • Rodents
- Therapeutics

KEY POINTS

- Gastrointestinal (GI) stasis in hindgut fermenters is a syndrome that occurs secondary to pain, stress, inappropriate diet, or underlying disease.
- Treatment of GI stasis involves fluid therapy, analgesics, nutritional support, and correcting the underlying condition. The use of prokinetic agents is controversial.
- In rabbits, lidocaine continuous rate infusions improve GI motility, food intake, and fecal output; result in more normal behaviors; and improve survival in obstruction cases.
- Maropitant may have a role in visceral analgesia as part of a multimodal analgesic protocol.

INTRODUCTION

Gastrointestinal (GI) disorders are a common presentation in exotic animal medicine.[1-10] In particular, GI stasis (also known as GI tract dysfunction, rabbit GI syndrome, or GI hypomotility syndrome) is one of the most common conditions treated by exotic animal veterinarians. However, as this syndrome is a secondary condition, it is important that the underlying disorder is diagnosed in order to direct treatment appropriately. For instance, non-GI conditions, such as liver lobe torsions in domestic rabbits (*Oryctolagus cuniculus*), are a common cause of GI stasis. Treatment of GI stasis involves fluid therapy, analgesia (often multimodal), nutritional support, and other more targeted treatments as indicated. Inflammatory and neoplastic GI disorders are common in certain species, such as ferrets.[10] This review focuses mainly on management of non-infectious GI disorders of exotic animals. Treatment of infectious GI disorders is more specifically addressed in another article in this issue.

Zoological Medicine Service, Department of Veterinary Clinical Sciences, College of Veterinary Medicine, Oklahoma State University, 2065 W. Farm Road, Stillwater, OK 74078, USA
E-mail address: julianne.mccready@okstate.edu

Vet Clin Exot Anim 28 (2025) 453–483
https://doi.org/10.1016/j.cvex.2024.11.011   vetexotic.theclinics.com

Abbreviations	
CRI	continuous rate infusion
ECM	exotic companion mammal
FB	foreign body
GDV	gastric dilatation-volvulus
GI	gastrointestinal
HT	hydroxytryptamine
ICe	intracoelomic
IM	intramuscularly
IO	intraosseous
IV	intravenous
NSAID	non-steroidal anti-inflammatory drug
PO	*per os*
PPI	proton pump inhibitor
SC	subcutaneous fluid therapy

FLUID THERAPY

Fluid therapy is often indicated for animals with GI signs. Animals may become dehydrated due to decreased intake or from fluid losses resulting from vomiting or diarrhea. Even if hindgut fermenters do not appear clinically dehydrated on physical examination, their gut contents may become dehydrated following periods of decreased intake, which can exacerbate decreased GI motility.

Intravenous Fluid Therapy

Intravenous (IV) fluid therapy is indicated for exotic animals with moderate to severe dehydration. There are some important considerations associated with IV catheterization that are not typically considered in canine and feline medicine.

In some species, there is a risk that IV catheter self-removal may lead to fatal exsanguination.[11] This is particularly a concern in parrots, due to their strong beaks, curious nature, and relatively small size. Parrots with indwelling IV catheters require Elizabethan collars and constant supervision. Larger birds with weaker beaks, such as poultry and waterfowl, generally tolerate IV catheters well with less concern regarding self-removal.

In rabbits, IV catheters are commonly placed in the marginal ear vein (**Fig. 1**), cephalic vein, or lateral saphenous vein (**Table 1**). Marginal ear vein catheters are often

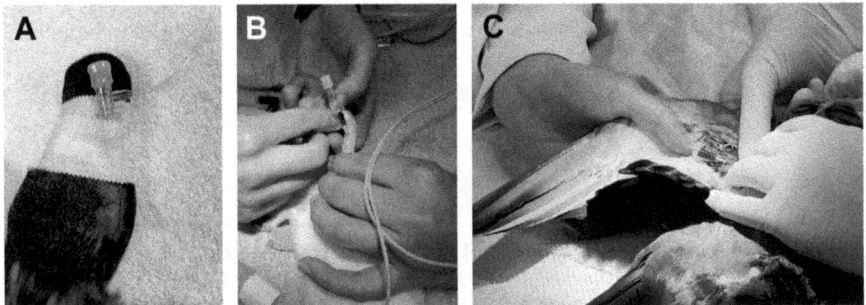

Fig. 1. Intravenous catheters in the process of being placed in some exotic companion animal species. (*A*) Marginal ear vein of a rabbit. (*B*) Lateral tail vein of a rat. (*C*) Basilic vein of a pigeon.

Table 1
Intravenous catheterization sites in various species[12-14,124]

Species	Intravenous Catheterization Sites
Mammals	
Rabbit	Marginal ear vein, cephalic vein, lateral saphenous vein, jugular vein
Rat	Cephalic vein, lateral saphenous vein, lateral coccygeal vein
Guinea pig, chinchilla	Cephalic vein, lateral saphenous vein
Ferret	Cephalic vein, lateral saphenous vein, omobranchial vein
Birds	Basilic vein, medial metatarsal vein, jugular vein
Reptiles	
Lizards	Ventral coccygeal vein
Snakes	Palatine vein, jugular vein
Chelonians	Jugular vein

well-tolerated by hospitalized rabbits, but do carry a risk of pinnal necrosis. However, in a recent randomized prospective study of complications associated with IV catheterization in rabbits, no major complications such as pinnal necrosis and phlebitis were encountered.[12] The failure rate for IV catheter placement was significantly higher for the cephalic (59%) compared to the marginal ear vein (27.8%).[12] Minor complications, such as twisted tubing, chewed tubing, and self-removal, were occasionally noted.[12]

The ventral coccygeal vein is a common catheterization site in lizards, and in one study, no complications were reported associated with placement.[13]

IV catheterization is difficult in snakes due to their lack of limbs. Jugular vein catheterization can be considered but typically requires a cut-down. The palatine vein can be catheterized, but due to its location in the oral cavity, cannot be maintained in an unsedated patient.

There are certain species in which it is very difficult to maintain an IV catheter due to their anatomy and behavior; this includes hedgehogs, which tend to curl up into a ball, and chelonians, which tend to retreat into their shells. Jugular central venous catheter placement for long-term venous access has been described in chelonians.[14]

IV catheter sites in other species are listed in **Table 1** and some examples are shown in **Fig. 1**.

Intraosseous Fluid Therapy

Intraosseous (IO) fluid therapy can be considered in animals with severe dehydration or shock and in which IV access is unable to be obtained. A benefit of this route is that IO catheters can be placed in very small animals, such as small birds and rodents, in which IV catheterization would be extremely challenging. An important consideration of IO catheter placement in birds is that certain bones are pneumatized, which precludes their use as IO catheter sites. These bones include the humerus and femur in most birds, but there are variations and the ulna is pneumatized in certain species, such as pelicans, turkey vultures, and California condors.[15,16]

IO catheterization can be painful, and sedation, anesthesia, or a local block should be considered prior to placement. There is also a concern that infusion of fluids via an IO catheter may be even more painful than insertion of the catheter itself, as is reported in humans.[17] Therefore, analgesics should be considered not just for IO catheter placement, but for the duration for which the IO catheter is maintained for fluid therapy.

Subcutaneous Fluid Therapy

Subcutaneous (SC) fluid therapy is indicated for mild dehydration in mammals. It is a useful route for patients whose owners decline hospitalization and elect outpatient care. It is also useful in patients that are too alert and active to tolerate IV fluid therapy, which is commonly the case in ferrets.

SC fluid therapy is commonly used in birds, particularly in those species in which IV catheter self-removal could lead to fatal hemorrhage. In contrast to mammals, in which severe dehydration should be treated via IV or IO fluids, birds are able to absorb SC fluids very well and some argue that SC fluids are appropriate even for birds in shock, due to birds' ability to recruit interstitial fluid extremely well.[18]

As with birds, it is proposed that reptiles given SC fluids can restore their vascular and interstitial fluid volumes well and SC fluids may be a viable option for hypovolemic reptiles.[18] In a study in central bearded dragons (*Pogona vitticeps*), increased blood glucose following 2.5% dextrose administration either SC or intracoelomic (ICe) was used to demonstrate the efficacy of absorption of SC fluids in this study.[19] While the blood glucose increased significantly more following ICe administration at 15 and 30 minutes, by 1 hour, there was no significant difference in blood glucose between the 2 administration routes.[19] Therefore, SC fluids are generally recommended over ICe in reptiles, due to similar absorption rates but a lower risk of complications. In this species, lactated Ringer's solution or Plasma-Lyte A are acceptable fluid options; however, reptile Ringer's solution (ie, mixture of 5% dextrose solution and isotonic crystalloid solution) is not recommended as it induces severe hyperglycemia and significantly reduced plasma osmolarity.[20]

Amphibians have little SC space, and administering injectable fluid therapy can be challenging. SC injections in anurans are essentially lymphatic injections.[18,21] Similarly, fish have very little SC space and SC fluids are not practical in these animals.[18]

Soaking and Immersion Fluid Therapy

Soaking is often indicated for dehydrated reptiles, although it is unclear how much fluids reptiles can actually absorb through their cloacae. Reptiles experiencing dehydration or being kept in an enclosure with inappropriately low humidity can also have secondary dysecdysis, which soaking can help alleviate.

Fluid baths can aid in osmotic balance in amphibians and fish. For amphibians with fluid loss (often seen in terrestrial amphibians), mildly hypotonic baths may help the animal to retain fluid.[21] In contrast, in amphibians with fluid overload, hydrocoelom, or edema (often seen in aquatic amphibians or in animals with renal disease), hypertonic baths may be indicated to remove excess fluid.[21,22]

Freshwater fish are hypertonic to their environment and excrete large volumes of dilute urine.[23] In ill freshwater fish, low-level salt immersion can be helpful to relieve osmotic stress.[24] In contrast, saltwater fish are hypotonic to their environment and are easily dehydrated.[23] In these fish, hyposalinity can be a useful treatment to aid in osmoregulation.

NUTRITIONAL SUPPORT

Animals with GI disorders are commonly anorexic; therefore, nutritional support is often indicated.

Mammals

In dogs and cats, syringe-feeding is generally not recommended due to the risk of creating food aversions. However, due to their different nutritional physiology, many exotic companion mammal (ECM) patients cannot tolerate periods of anorexia longer than 8 to 12 hours. Syringe-feeding is often well-tolerated in many ECMs and is used more frequently than nasogastric or esophagostomy tubes.

Several common ECMs are hindgut fermenters, including rabbits, guinea pigs (*Cavia porcellus*), degus (*Octodon degus*), and chinchillas (*Chinchilla lanigera*). These species can suffer from GI stasis, which is a secondary condition that can be caused by pain, stress, improper diet, dental malocclusion, or underlying disease. Although the underlying cause should be corrected and treated, it is important to ensure that the animal continues to intake adequate fiber to prevent dysbiosis and worsening of its condition. Guinea pigs are prone to hepatic lipidosis following periods of anorexia, and adequate nutritional intake is critical in this species.[25] **Table 2** summarizes treatment options for GI stasis.

Domestic ferrets (*Mustela putorius furo*) have a short GI transit time and are prone to insulinomas. Therefore, anorexia can rapidly lead to hypoglycemia. Most ferrets presenting with GI signs will require some degree of nutritional support, often in the form of hand-feeding or syringe-feeding a high-protein diet. Feeding tubes can be considered for ferrets experiencing prolonged anorexia. The use of a gastrostomy and jejunostomy tube has been reported in a ferret.[26]

Birds

Many bird species have high metabolic rates and cannot tolerate long periods of anorexia. This is particularly true in small psittacine species, passerine species, and hummingbirds. Birds can often easily be tube or gavage fed into the crop (in taxa with a crop, such as parrots, pigeons, chickens, passerines, falcons, and hawks) or proventriculus (in taxa lacking a crop, such as owls and ducks). Metal gavage tubes are indicated in species with strong beaks, such as parrots, while soft tubes (such as red rubber tubes) can be used in species with weaker beaks, such as poultry, waterfowl, and pigeons.

Reptiles

Reptiles, due to their lower metabolic rates, often eat far less frequently than mammals and birds. Consequently, when they are ill from GI disorders, they often present with far more prolonged anorexia than mammals and birds do. Snakes, depending on the species, often eat only every few weeks, so they are easy to tube feed every few weeks as needed until the patient's appetite improves (and the underlying condition is treated). Lizards generally eat more frequently, but often can be syringe-fed by owners. It is important that clinicians and owners are careful when opening the animal's jaws and take care to prevent the animal from biting the syringe. Metabolic bone disease is common in lizards with poor husbandry, and iatrogenic jaw fractures can occur from poor syringe-feeding technique. It may be wise to use a red rubber tube or other soft tube at the end of the syringe to lessen the risk of inadvertent jaw trauma.

Chelonians are often very difficult to tube feed. Most chelonians can retreat in their shells, and some species have a hinge that results in them being able to fully enclose their head within their shell. Extracting the head of a chelonian from its shell can be extremely challenging even in small, young, or sick animals. Opening the beak can also be very difficult in an uncooperative chelonian. Chelonians tend to not eat when hospitalized and aquatic species often will not eat when dry-docked. Therefore, esophagostomy tubes are often indicated in anorexic chelonians (**Fig. 2**). Complications associated with esophagostomy tube placement in chelonians are common (40/98, or 40.82% of patients), but most complications are minor, such as tube obstruction and dislodgement.[27]

Table 2
Treatment options for gastrointestinal stasis in hindgut fermenters

Treatment	Dose	Indication
Recommended		
Fluid therapy[21]	Weight (kg) x % dehydration x 1000 mL = fluid deficit	Dehydration, anorexia
Norepinephrine[125]	0.5–1.0 mcg/kg/min	Hypotension
Nutritional support Oxbow Animal Health Critical Care Herbivore[126] Lafeber EmerAid Herbivore Sustain or Intensive Care Herbivore[127]	1 Tbsp/kg dry + 2 Tbsp/kg water PO q 8h or divided into smaller, more frequent feedings if desired	Anorexia >8–12 h
	30 mL/kg PO q 6-8h	
Opioid analgesia		Moderate to severe pain
Buprenorphine[89,128,129]	0.03–0.06 mg/kg (R), 0.2 mg/kg IV q 7h (GP), 0.2 mg/kg SC q 6h (C)	
Hydromorphone[130,131]	0.1–0.4 mg/kg (R), 0.3 mg/kg IV q 2-3h or IM q 4-5h (GP), 0.5–2 mg/kg SC q 4h (C)	
Fentanyl	3–5 mcg/kg/h (R)	
NSAIDs Meloxicam[132,133]	1 mg/kg q 24h (R), 1.5 mg/kg PO or IV q 12–24h (GP; *long-term safety of this dose not evaluated*)	Mild pain in well-hydrated, non-azotemic patient
Lidocaine[88,89]	75–100 mcg/kg/min IV ± 2 mg/kg IV loading dose (R)	Improved food intake and fecal output, visceral analgesia
Maropitant[29,31,32]	1–4 mg/kg PO or SC q 24 h (R)	Improved fecal output, visceral analgesia
As indicated		
Antibiotics[36]	Various; note that penicillins, lincosamides, amoxicillin, cephalosporins, and erythromycin cannot be given PO to hindgut fermenters	Bacterial enteritis, other confirmed bacterial infections, severe GI stasis leading to enterotoxemia or sepsis
Cholestyramine[21,36,50]	0.5 g/kg PO q 12–24h, 2 g/animal in 20 mL water PO q 24h (R), 1 g/animal in water PO q 24h (GP)	Enterotoxemia

Gastroprotectants		Prolonged anorexia, evidence of GI bleeding or ulceration
Famotidine[21]	0.5–1 mg/kg PO, SC, or IV (R)	
Ranitidine[36,61,105]	2–5 mg/kg PO q 12h, 2 mg/kg IV q 24h (R); withdrawn from market in United States	
Omeprazole[134]	0.5–1 mg/kg PO q 12h (dog dosing), 20 mg/kg SC q 12h (R)	
Pantoprazole	1 mg/kg IV q 12h (dog dosing)	
Sucralfate[43]	25–100 mg/kg PO q 8–12h (R, GP, C)	
Questionable or not recommended		
Metoclopramide[21,36,38,105]	0.2–2 mg/kg PO, SC, IM q 6–12h, 0.01–0.09 mg/kg/h IV CRI (R)	Increasing GI motility; limited evidence of efficacy
Cisapride[36,44]	0.5 mg/kg PO q 8–12h (R; *did not affect GI transit or fecal output in rabbits at this dose*), 10 mg/kg PO q 12h (C)	Increasing GI motility; limited evidence of efficacy, especially at commonly recommended doses
Simethicone[21,50]	65–130 mg/animal PO q 1h x 2–3 treatments (R)	Reducing abdominal discomfort associated with excessive gas; limited evidence of efficacy but unlikely to be harmful
Proteolytic enzymes (bromelain, pineapple juice, papain)[50]	Not recommended	Previously advocated for treatment of trichobezoars but not currently recommended as efficacy is questionable and may be irritating to oral and gastric mucosa

Abbreviations: C, chinchillas; CRI, continuous rate infusion; GI, gastrointestinal; GP, guinea pigs; IM, intramuscularly; IV, intravenously; PO, orally; R, rabbits; SC, subcutaneously.

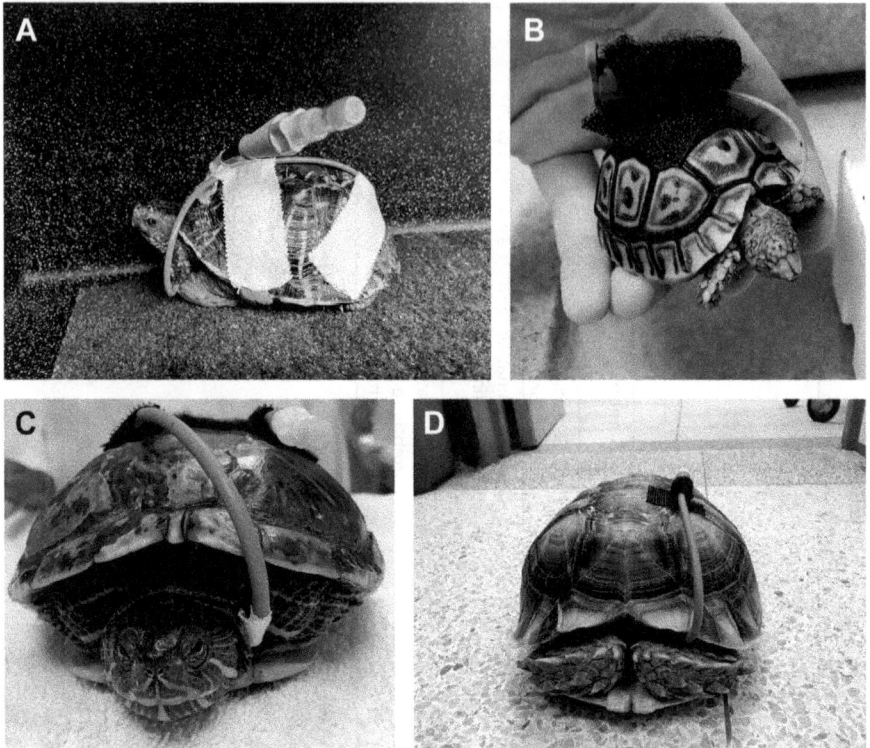

Fig. 2. Esophagostomy tubes in place in various chelonian species, including (*A*) an ornate box turtle (*Terrapene ornata ornata*), (*B*) a debilitated juvenile leopard tortoise (*Stigmochelys pardalis*), (*C*) a red-eared slider (*Trachemys scripta elegans*), and (*D*) a sulcata tortoise (*Centrochelys sulcata*). Note that the esophagostomy tube is accessible even with the sulcata tortoise enclosed in his shell.

ANTI-EMETICS
Maropitant

Maropitant is a neurokinin-1 receptor antagonist that may be used to treat nausea and vomiting.[28] A common ECM species that may present for vomiting is the ferret, and maropitant may be indicated as part of supportive therapy for gastroenteritis. However, before deciding to administer any medication that may mask continued clinical signs, it is important to rule out surgical conditions such as a foreign body (FB) obstruction. Abdominal imaging should always be recommended in any ferret presenting with vomiting. Non-GI illness can lead to signs of nausea in ferrets, particularly hypoglycemia due to an insulinoma. Therefore, any ferret presenting signs of nausea (eg, salivation, pawing at the mouth) should have a blood glucose measurement performed.

Rabbits and rodents are incapable of vomiting; however, maropitant may still have some potential benefits in these species. In rabbits, maropitant 1 mg/kg IV or SC was associated with increased fecal production on the day of treatment and 1 day after treatment, indicating that it may be a useful adjunct in the management of GI stasis.[29] A pharmacokinetic study showed that a higher dose (10 mg/kg SC) may be required to reach plasma concentrations similar to those found in dogs at 1 and 2 mg/kg SC.[30] However, a non-significant trend toward decreasing food intake and fecal output was noted with high dose (10 mg/kg SC) maropitant in rabbits.[31] Maropitant at 2 and 10 mg/kg SC also failed to significantly reduce pain post-operation ovariohysterectomy and orchiectomy in rabbits in that study.[31] Another study found that rabbits that received maropitant 4 mg/kg SC post-ovariohysterectomy or orchiectomy had lower pain scores at 5 to 8 hours and behavior scores at 12 to 24 hours compared to saline controls, and no adverse effects associated with maropitant were noted.[32] Therefore, doses of 1 to 4 mg/kg maropitant can be considered as part of supportive care for GI stasis and other painful conditions in rabbits. In rats, maropitant appeared to have an additive effect for analgesia when combined with morphine.[33]

In a pharmacokinetic study of maropitant in chickens, a dose of 1 to 2 mg/kg SC every 12 to 24 hours was suggested; pharmacodynamic studies in birds are required to determine efficacy in preventing emesis.[34] Empiric maropitant use based on mammal dosing has been suggested in reptiles, but further research is needed.[35]

Ondansetron

An anecdotal dose of 0.5 mg/kg intramuscularly (IM), IV, or orally/*per os* (PO) q 8 hours is suggested for ondansetron in ferrets.[10]

PROKINETICS
Metoclopramide

Metoclopramide is a dopamine receptor antagonist and serotonin 5-hydroxytryptamine $(HT)_4$ (HT) receptor agonist/5-HT_3 antagonist.[36] It functions mainly on the upper GI tract with little to no effect on the lower GI tract. It is often anecdotally recommended as part of management of GI stasis in rabbits, guinea pigs, and chinchillas.[36,37] In a pharmacokinetic study of metoclopramide in rabbits, bioavailability was high after IM and SC administration, but plasma concentrations were variable and bioavailability was low following rectal administration.[38] PO administration, likely the most common route to be utilized in outpatient management of GI stasis, was not evaluated in the study.[38] The efficacy of the drug was also not evaluated in this study.[38] There is concern that metoclopramide may be less effective in young rabbits compared to adults based on *in vitro* research.[36]

Overall, there is little evidence of efficacy to support metoclopramide use for GI stasis. In one study, metoclopramide administration was not significantly associated with short-term outcome and rabbits with GI tract dysfunction.[37] In addition, there is a concern that the use of prokinetic agents when a GI obstruction is present could lead to an intestinal perforation and/or pain. It is recommended that treatment of GI stasis should focus on rehydration, nutritional support, analgesia, and treating the underlying cause of the condition. Therefore, metoclopramide is rarely, if ever, indicated for GI stasis in hindgut fermenters.

The efficacy of metoclopramide is also questionable in birds and reptiles. In Hispaniolan Amazon parrots (*Amazona ventralis*), metoclopramide 0.5, 0.75, and 1 mg/kg IM did not significantly affect GI motility as measured by fluoroscopy.[39] In Mojave Desert tortoises (*Gopherus agassizii*), metoclopramide 1 mg/kg PO did not significantly affect GI transit time.[40]

Metoclopramide may have efficacy in elasmobranchs. Gastric emptying time was significantly shorter in whitespotted bamboo sharks (*Chiloscyllium plagiosum*) treated with metoclopramide 0.4 mg/kg PO q 24h x 10 days compared to controls.[41] Metoclopramide is used for stimulating ovulation in teleosts, but further research is needed regarding its GI effects in teleost fish.

Cisapride

Cisapride functions by binding serotonin 5-HT receptors and exerting antagonist effects on enteric cholinergic neurons.[36,42] Unlike metoclopramide, cisapride may also affect colonic motility.[42]

Cisapride is another prokinetic that has been anecdotally recommended for management of GI stasis with little evidence to support its use.[42] The common recommended dose range is 0.5 mg/kg PO q 8-12h.[36,42,43] However, cisapride 0.5 mg/kg PO q 8h x 2 d did not significantly affect GI transit, fecal output, or food and water intake in rabbits.[44] Cisapride at doses up to 10 mg/kg did not affect colonic transit significantly in rats (*Rattus norvegicus*) and guinea pigs.[45] Chinchillas given 10 mg/kg PO q 12h for 4 doses had a slight, but not clinically relevant, attenuation of fecal output reduction compared to syringe feeding alone.[46] However, without concurrent administration of syringe feeding, which is one of the mainstays of treatment of GI stasis, cisapride had no effect on fecal output.[46]

Cisapride is currently not recommended for management of GI stasis for similar reasons to metoclopramide, although some authors still advocate for its use.[36,42] Cisapride can be associated with stomach cramps and diarrhea in some species, and with fatal adverse drug reactions in humans.[36,42] Overall, there is insufficient evidence of efficacy, and it is recommended to direct management of GI stasis to identifying and treating the underlying cause rather than targeting the secondary effect of decreased GI motility. GI motility can instead be stimulated by syringe-feeding a high-fiber diet until the animal is eating on its own.

Cisapride has been anecdotally recommended in birds to reduce vomiting or regurgitation associated with conditions such as avian ganglioneuritis and severe aspergillosis.[42]

Cisapride 1 mg/kg PO did not significantly affect the GI transit time in Mojave Desert tortoises.[40] In fact, cisapride was associated with a slower transit time, although this result was not statistically significant.[40] Cisapride 1 to 4 mg/kg PO q 24h has been suggested in other reptile species,[47] but this is anecdotal.

Trimebutine

Trimebutine is a motility-stimulating drug that is used in humans for the treatment of irritable bowel syndrome and other disorders. Trimebutine 1.5 mg/kg PO or IV has been anecdotally suggested for use in enhancing GI motility in rabbits with GI stasis.[48] The drug is not available in the United States but an oral form is available in Canada.[48] It has been studied *in vitro* in rabbits but research is needed regarding its clinical efficacy.[49]

Erythromycin

The macrolide antibiotic erythromycin is sometimes used for motility enhancement in mammals such as dogs at subantimicrobial doses. Erythromycin is contraindicated in hindgut fermenters due to the risk of dysbiosis.[36,50] It can be used in ferrets, but it is unknown if it stimulates GI motility in this species. Erythromycin 2 mg/kg PO did not significantly affect the GI transit time of Mojave Desert tortoises.[40]

APPETITE STIMULANTS

Appetite stimulants (**Table 3**) can be considered to improve the appetite of anorexic animals, potentially reducing the need for time-consuming and potentially stressful assisted feedings. However, it is important to investigate and address the underlying cause of the anorexia rather than relying on these drugs. These drugs can be considered as an adjunct treatment for anorexic animals in certain cases but should not be

Table 3
Appetite stimulating drugs that have been found to be effective or ineffective in various exotic companion mammal and bird species

Appetite Stimulating Drug	Effective	Ineffective
Mirtazapine[51–54]	Rabbits	Chinchillas, budgerigars
Capromorelin[52–54,56,57]	Rabbits (less than mirtazapine), chinchillas, budgerigars, pigeons	four-toed hedgehogs
Cyprohepatidine[54]		Budgerigars
Midazolam[59,60]	Budgerigars	
Lorazepam[60]	Budgerigars	

the sole treatment or take the place of nutritional support if voluntary intake is inadequate.

Mirtazapine

Mirtazapine is commonly used in anorexic cats to stimulate their appetite. There are several recent studies evaluating its efficacy in ECMs. In one study, 1 and 3 mg/kg PO mirtazapine were compared with control treatment in rabbits.[51] There was an increase in fecal output with the 3 mg/kg dose on treatment days but there was no significant difference between baseline and post-treatment fecal output.[51] Food intake was unaffected by treatment. Body weight decreased in the week following treatment in the 3 mg/kg group.[51] In another study assessing the efficacy of transdermal mirtazapine, mirtazapine 0.5 and 1 mg/kg transdermal once a day increased feed intake and fecal output compared with saline controls and with capromorelin.[52] However, following surgery, feed intake and fecal output were not significantly different following mirtazapine 1 mg/kg transdermal once a day compared with capromorelin or saline control.[52] A noted side effect of transdermal mirtazapine was erythema/petechiae of the pinna. Mirtazapine may increase fecal output and has inconsistent effects on feed intake, depending on the route of administration, but these effects may not be seen in rabbits suffering from painful conditions such as surgery.

In chinchillas, mirtazapine at 5 and 20 mg/kg PO q 24h was ineffective at stimulating the appetite.[53]

In budgerigars (*Melopsittacus undulatus*), mirtazapine 1 and 5 mg/kg PO via gavage did not result in a significant effect on food intake.[54] Mirtazapine 1 mg/kg transdermal was anecdotally reported to improve the appetite of an anorexic eastern indigo snake (*Drymarchon couperi*) receiving chemotherapy.[55]

Capromorelin

In rabbits, capromorelin 4 or 8 mg/kg PO twice a day increased food intake and fecal output compared to saline controls, while once daily dosing did not.[52] The increase in feed intake and fecal output was less with capromorelin compared to mirtazapine. Following surgery, there was no significant difference in feed intake and fecal output between capromorelin 8 mg/kg PO twice a day and saline control.[52] The authors recommended mirtazapine over capromorelin for appetite stimulation in rabbits as mirtazapine appeared more efficacious.

In chinchillas, capromorelin at 3 and 10 mg/kg PO q 24h significantly increased food intake.[53] In contrast, capromorelin at 10 mg/kg PO q 24h did not lead to a statistically significant increase in food intake in four-toed hedgehogs (*Atelerix albiventris*).[56]

In budgerigars, capromorelin at 10 and 40 mg/kg PO via gavage resulted in a significant increase in food intake compared to control.[54] Because there were no dose-dependent effects on food intake, and because the higher dose resulted in more frequent regurgitation (25% with control, 42% with 10 mg/kg, and 92% with 40 mg/kg), the 10 mg/kg dose was recommended.[54] In pigeons (*Columba livia*), capromorelin 12 mg/kg PO once daily resulted in increased food intake and weight gain compared to controls, without adverse effects.[57]

Cyproheptadine

Cyproheptadine is an antihistamine with antiserotonin properties that has been used in cats as an appetite stimulant.[58] Cyproheptadine 0.5 and 2.5 mg/kg PO via gavage was unsuccessful at increasing food intake in budgerigars.[54] A dose of 1 to 4 mg/animal PO q 12 to 24h has been suggested as a possible appetite stimulant in rabbits based on a personal communication.[21] Further research is needed regarding this drug's efficacy.

Benzodiazepines

Benzodiazapines, which are commonly used as sedatives in exotic animal medicine, may also be useful in stimulating the appetite. Midazolam 1 mg/kg IM and lorazepam 1 mg/kg IM significantly increased food intake in budgerigars but resulted in mild sedation.[59,60]

GASTROPROTECTANTS

Gastroprotectants may be indicated for patients with evidence of GI bleeding or confirmed GI ulceration or erosion. GI ulceration or bleeding is a common condition in ferrets with GI infections such as *Helicobacter*, in anorexic rabbits,[61] and in small psittacine birds with prolonged anorexia.[62] Rabbits secrete higher amounts of gastric acid compared to dogs, cats, rats, and guinea pigs, and prophylactic anti-ulcer therapy should be considered in anorexic rabbits.[61]

Small psittacine birds (such as budgerigars and lovebirds) with low fat stores that are anorexic for greater than 24 hours may experience hemorrhagic diathesis.[62] On necropsy, reflux of blood from the intestines into the stomach may be noted.[62] Another condition that may lead to GI bleeding in budgerigars is disease caused by the fungus *Macrorhabdus ornithogaster*. Melena may be commonly seen with this infection and is associated with a poorer prognosis.[63] This author commonly sees positive fecal occult blood tests in small psittacine birds, especially budgerigars, presenting with anorexia, and recommends performing this test in these birds when they present with anorexia, vomiting, or diarrhea.

There are many challenges to the appropriate use of gastroprotectants in exotic companion animal medicine. Many of the studies involving gastroprotectants in rodents, rabbits, and birds were conducted in a laboratory setting as human models and can be difficult to translate to clinical practice. Consensus statements regarding the evidence-based use of gastroprotectants are not available in exotic animal medicine, as there are in canine and feline medicine.[64] Commercially available tablets of omeprazole may not contain appropriate milligram strength for small patients. Unfortunately, crushing enteric-coated delayed-release tablets or compounding omeprazole may decrease its efficacy.[64] There is a concern that delayed-release formulations may be less effective in dogs and cats due to their faster intestinal transit times compared to humans[64]; some exotic companion animal species, such as ferrets and birds, have even faster intestinal transit times than dogs and cats, so this is likely even more of a concern in these species.

Histamine H₂-Receptor Antagonists

Histamine H_2-receptor antagonists block H_2 receptors on parietal cells to inhibit gastric acid secretion and decrease pepsin output.[61,64] Histamine H_2-receptor antagonists commonly used in veterinary medicine include famotidine, ranitidine, and cimetidine.

In canine and feline internal medicine, famotidine is considered to have limited efficacy unless given as a continuous rate infusion (CRI). Famotidine given as an IV CRI was more successful in raising the intragastric pH compared to famotidine 1 mg/kg IV q 12 hours in dogs.[65] In dogs, proton pump inhibitors (PPIs) are considered to have superior efficacy to H_2 receptor antagonists for increasing intragastric pH.[64,66] In dogs and cats, once daily dosing of H_2 receptor antagonists is not considered beneficial and twice daily dosing is inferior to twice daily dosing with a PPI.[64] In a study in rabbits' gastric glands, omeprazole inhibited hydrogen-potassium adenosine triphosphatase (H^+/K^+ ATPase) activity and dibutyryl cyclic AMP-stimulated gastric acid secretion, while famotidine did not.[67] This may also indicate that PPIs may also be more useful clinically than H_2 receptor antagonists in rabbits, but further research is needed in other ECMs to determine if these findings hold true in other species.

In a formulary, famotidine doses of 0.25 to 0.5 mg/kg or 2.5 mg PO, SC, or IV q 24 hour have been anecdotally suggested in ferrets and 0.5 to 1 mg/kg PO, SC, or IV has been anecdotally recommended in rabbits.[21] The efficacy of H_2 antagonists in birds is questionable; famotidine was ineffective in chickens, even at high doses.[68]

Ranitidine is an anti-ulcer medication that may also act as a prokinetic and is sometimes used as part of management of GI stasis in rabbits and other hindgut fermenters.[61] However, a few years ago, the drug was withdrawn from the market in the United States due to concerns about an association with neoplasia risk in humans.[36] A potential replacement for ranitidine is nizatidine, another H_2 antagonist; use of this drug is currently anecdotal.[36]

Proton Pump Inhibitors

PPIs are substituted benzimidazole drugs targeting the final stage in acid production.[64] PPIs commonly used in veterinary medicine include omeprazole and pantoprazole. Indications for PPIs in human medicine include duodenal ulcers, *Helicobacter pylori*, gastroesophageal reflux, and gastric ulcers.[64] They are considered superior to H_2-receptor antagonists, sucralfate, and misoprostol for treating gastroduodenal ulceration and erosion in humans.[64] These drugs are most effective when given 30 to 45 minutes before or with a meal.[64] In dogs and cats, it is recommended that PPIs be gradually tapered if given for greater than 3 to 4 weeks to avoid rebound gastric acid secretion.[64] Various side effects associated with PPIs have been reported in humans, but there is a lack of evidence showing that they cause serious side effects in dogs and cats.[64] Dysbiosis is possible, so animals administered PPIs should be monitored closely for diarrhea.

Omeprazole reduces gastric acid production by inhibiting the H^+/K^+ ATPase system of parietal cells in the stomach.[36] Recommended dose of omeprazole in ferrets range from 0.7 mg/kg PO q 24h to 4 mg/kg PO q 24h.[21] An omeprazole dose of 20 mg/kg SC q 12 hour has been suggested in rabbits due to this dose's ability to reduce gastric ulcer formation induced by indomethacin; it is unknown if lower doses may also be useful.[21,36] Higher doses of omeprazole may be required in birds compared to mammals; a dose range of 10 to 100 mg/kg PO q 24h in birds has been suggested and the authors recommended 20 mg/kg PO q 24h.[68]

Sucralfate

Sucralfate is a complex salt of sucrose octasulfate and aluminum hydroxide that binds to ulcers by forming complexes with proteins associated with the damaged mucosa.[64] Sucralfate is indicated for animals with esophagitis and potentially for GI ulceration. A sucralfate dose of 25 to 125 mg/kg PO q 6-12h is anecdotally suggested in ECMs.[21,69] In a study in 3 to 5 kg rabbits, esophageal administration of 1 g sucralfate prevented acid-induced and pepsin-induced esophagitis.[70] In a flock of lorikeets (*Trichoglossus* spp.) with a *Synhimantus* (*Dispharynx*) *nasuta* proventricular nematodiasis outbreak, fecal occult blood tests were positive in all confirmed cases and lorikeets were treated with sucralfate 100 mg/kg PO q 12h.[71] A green iguana was given 200 mg/kg PO q 24h sucralfate following duodenoileal anastomosis.[72]

ANTI-INFLAMMATORIES AND IMMUNOSUPPRESSIVES

Anti-inflammatory drugs such as non-steroidal anti-inflammatory drugs (NSAIDs) and immunosuppressives such as corticosteroids may be indicated for certain GI disorders in exotic animal medicine. It is important to be aware of the potential risk factors of these drugs and only use them when indicated. Importantly, GI ulceration is a known side effect of NSAIDs, so they should be avoided when the patient has known or suspected GI ulceration. Some exotic animal patients tolerate NSAIDs relatively well; for instance, at a very high dose of 20 mg/kg meloxicam PO, only 2 out of 9 kestrels developed gastric ulcers, and the result was not significantly different from saline treatment.[73] Note that this study was not advocating for the use of such high doses, but instead demonstrating the resistance of this bird species to meloxicam-related adverse effects. In contrast, small mammalian carnivores like ferrets are expected to be more sensitive to the GI adverse effects of NSAIDs, similar to dogs and cats.

Corticosteroids should be judiciously in exotic pets, as with all animals. Some taxa, including birds, are sensitive to the immunosuppressive effects of steroids,[74] raising concern for patients developing opportunistic infections, such as aspergillosis, during treatment. Corticosteroids should never be used concurrently with NSAIDs due to the increased risk of GI ulceration. The appropriate wash-out period between the 2 drug types is unknown for exotic animal species, but guidelines from canine and feline medicine can be followed. Hemolymphatic neoplasia such as lymphoma is common in many exotic pet species. It is recommended to perform a thorough evaluation for this and other neoplasms before starting corticosteroids, as the use of these drugs could hamper diagnosis of neoplasia in the future.

Treatment of Gastrointestinal Neoplasia

For diffuse GI neoplasia, such as lymphoma, surgery is usually not indicated (unless there is an obstruction or perforation) and treatment generally involves corticosteroids and chemotherapy. Lymphoma is a very common neoplasm in ferrets, and GI lymphoma has been reported.[75,76]

Diffuse large B-cell lymphoma was the most common type of lymphoma noted in rabbits in a retrospective study.[77] Various treatments have been reported for rabbits with diffuse large B-cell lymphoma with GI involvement, including L-asparaginase, vincristine or vinblastine, prednisone, cyclophosphamide, doxorubicin, and lomustine.[77] Two reported cases of enteropathy-associated T-cell lymphoma in rabbits were euthanized without specific treatment for the lymphoma.[77] A rat with lymphoma (suspected large cell and thought to have arisen from the thymus) with peripheral invasion of heart and spread to the colon was treated with L-asparaginase, corticosteroids (initially dexamethasone, then prednisolone), and lomustine.[78]

In bearded dragons, the most common intestinal neoplasm was disseminated lymphoma, and it was associated with a poor to grave prognosis.[79] Gastric neuroendocrine carcinoma is the most common gastric neoplasm in bearded dragons; it is highly metastatic and associated with a grave prognosis.[79]

Treatment of Inflammatory Bowel Disease

In ECM medicine, inflammatory bowel disease is most likely to be encountered in a ferret. Treatment may involve immunosuppressives such as prednisone or azathioprine and a hypoallergenic diet.[10]

A pet rabbit with diarrhea, transudative effusion, weight loss, and small intestinal muscularis thickening was treated with enrofloxacin, metronidazole, and prednisolone.[80] Mild to moderate chronic diffuse lymphoplasmacytic enteritis consistent with inflammatory bowel disease was noted on necropsy.[80]

Inflammatory bowel disease is rare in birds. In a case report, a harpy eagle was treated with prednisone 1 mg/kg PO q 24h, which resulted in improvement of the clinical signs.[81] Concurrent terbinafine was administered due to the risk of mycoses in birds undergoing corticosteroid therapy.

Treatment of Eosinophilic Gastroenteritis

Eosinophilic gastroenteritis has been reported in ferrets, although it is uncommon. Reported treatments include prednisone and ivermectin.[10] Eosinophilic gastroenteritis in a four-toed hedgehog was managed with prednisolone, omeprazole, psyllium supplementation, a feline hypoallergenic diet, antibiotics as needed for dysbiosis, and a course of fenbendazole.[82]

TREATMENT OF DYSBIOSIS
Toxin Binders

Cholestyramine is an ion-exchange resin that can bind bacterial toxins and is indicated for treatment of enterotoxemia in hindgut fermenters.[36,50] It has been shown to be effective in preventing mortality from clindamycin-associated enterotoxemia in rabbits.[36]

Probiotics

Probiotics could theoretically be helpful for treatment of dysbiosis or for replenishing GI flora following antimicrobial treatment. However, consider the normal flora in each species and whether the selected probiotic contains similar microorganisms. For instance, rabbits possess little to no *Lactobacillus*, a common constituent of many commercial probiotics.[83,84] Common GI bacterial phyla in rabbits include Firmicutes and Bacteroidota.[83,84] *Streptococcus* and *Escherichia coli* are common in neonatal rabbits prior to weaning but uncommon in adults.[83] *Enterococcus* spp. is reported to make up a large portion of the rabbit gut microflora by some authors and is found in several commercial probiotics (**Table 4**).[36] However, *Enterococcus* was not reported as 1 of the 15 most abundant bacterial genera in the rabbit foregut and hindgut microbiota in a recent study that utilized 16S rRNA gene amplicon sequencing.[84] Ideally, species-specific probiotics would be developed, but it is recommended to at least choose a probiotic that does not exclusively contain *Lactobacillus* spp. when selecting a probiotic for rabbits.

The predominant phyla found in ferret fecal samples were Firmicutes, Proteobacteria, and Actinobacteriota.[85] Probiotics designed for dogs and cats could be assumed to be more appropriate for other carnivorans, such as ferrets, than they are for herbivores such as rabbits. However, the ferret fecal microbiota composition and diversity

Table 4
The species of microorganisms reported in several common commercially available veterinary probiotics

Probiotic	Species Included
PetAg Bene-Bac Plus[135]	Lactobacillus casei, fermentum, acidophilus, and plantarum Enterococcus faecium Bifidobacterium bifidum Pediococcus acidilactici
Purina FortiFlora[136]	E. faecium
Nutramax Proviable[137]	E. faecium B. bifidum Streptococcus thermophilus Lactobacillus helveticus, delbrueckii, casei, and plantarum
VetriScience Vetri Mega Probiotic[138]	Lactobacillus acidophilus, plantarum, casei, and brevis B. bifidum and longum S. thermophilus

has been found to differ from that of cats.[85] The ferret microbiota does contain bacterial genera such as *Lactobacillus* and *Enterococcus* that are commonly found in probiotics, which could suggest some utility to these products.[85] Overall, ferret gut flora is fairly simple and dysbiosis is much less likely in this species compared to herbivores.[10]

Transfaunation

Transfaunation with cecotrophs or feces from a healthy conspecific has anecdotally been reported in rabbits and rodents for treatment of dysbiosis and enterotoxemia.[50] However, the efficacy of this treatment has not been critically evaluated. There are some logistical considerations regarding transfaunation. The cecotrophs must be collected from a healthy donor, which may require placing an e-collar on the donor to prevent immediate cecotroph ingestion.[36] Cecotrophs could be blenderized and syringe-fed to the recipient, but there is concern that this may disrupt the cecotrophs' mucus coating and reduce their efficacy.[36]

ANALGESICS

GI disease can often be very painful. Although most clinicians would not hesitate to give analgesics to an animal with a fractured limb, sometimes clinicians fail to recognize just how debilitating visceral pain can be to an animal. Analgesia is part of the mainstay of treatment of GI stasis. Almost any rabbit or rodent experiencing GI stasis is experiencing some degree of pain and could benefit from analgesia. In addition, GI stasis is secondary to other underlying disease, the underlying disease itself is often painful.

Opioids

Opioids are indicated for moderate to severe pain, including pain related to GI disease. Although a common concern is that opioids can negatively affect GI motility, potentially worsening GI stasis, it is crucial to understand that GI stasis is often secondary to a painful condition and GI stasis can lead to pain itself through gas distension of GI tract. Therefore, the patient is unlikely to improve and start eating without appropriate analgesia. Options for opioid analgesia include buprenorphine, hydromorphone, and fentanyl.

In one study, rabbits were given methadone 0.3 mg/kg IV, 0.6 mg/kg IM, and 1 mg/kg SC. Food intake decreased on day 2 after administration, but fecal production was unaffected.[86] However, control rabbits that did not receive methadone were also not handled, so the decreased in food intake may have been due to handling stress or the drug itself.[86] Human analgesic concentrations were reached with IV dosing but not with SC and inconsistently with IM.[86] Another study found that food intake and fecal output was decreased after buprenorphine 0.1 mg/kg SC and also affected to a lesser extent by hydromorphone 0.2 mg/kg SC.[87] Methadone did not affect food intake and fecal production in this study, but the dose used (0.2 mg/kg SC)[87] may have been sub-therapeutic based on the results of the more recent aforementioned pharmacokinetic study.[86]

Non-steroidal Anti-inflammatory Drugs

NSAIDs can be considered for treatment of mild pain in well-hydrated, non-azotemic patients with no evidence of GI bleeding or ulceration. Benefits of NSAIDs include the fact that they are non-controlled drugs and do not cause sedation and are therefore an attractive option for outpatient management of GI stasis. Although rabbits and rodents generally tolerate NSAIDs such as meloxicam well, side effects are possible, especially in dehydrated patients. Rabbits can develop severe pre-renal azotemia secondary to dehydration from GI stasis. Therefore, ideally any rabbit presenting with GI stasis should have renal values evaluated prior to prescribing an NSAID. Rabbits and rodents require much higher doses of meloxicam compared to dogs and cats (see **Table 2**).

Lidocaine

Lidocaine is a sodium channel blocker that has anti-inflammatory and anti-endotoxin properties and that functions as a prokinetic.[88] It is also believed to provide analgesia by reducing ectopic activity of afferent neurons through its action at sodium, calcium, potassium, and N-methyl-D-aspartic acid receptors.[88] In rabbits undergoing ovario-hysterectomies, those receiving a lidocaine CRI (100 mcg/kg/min) had significantly higher GI motility, food intake, and fecal output, and significantly lower blood glucose, compared to those receiving buprenorphine (0.06 mg/kg IV q 8h).[89] Although pain scores did not differ between groups, rabbits receiving lidocaine had higher numbers of normal behaviors (sprawling and frolicking) postoperatively, compared to the buprenorphine group.[89] In a study of rabbits with GI obstruction, survival was significantly greater in rabbits treated with a lidocaine CRI (75–100 mcg/kg/min ± loading dose of 2 mg/kg IV) than those that were not.[88] Due to its beneficial effects and analgesic properties, lidocaine administration should be considered for rabbits presenting with moderate to severe GI stasis.

One potential side effect of lidocaine administration is hypotension, so obtain a blood pressure measurement on rabbits prior to starting a lidocaine CRI, especially for rabbits showing signs of shock. Be sure to calculate the lidocaine CRI dose accurately, as accidental overdose can lead to cardiovascular and neurologic side effects, including arrhythmias, tachycardia, opisthotonus, and seizures.[90] Treatment of lidocaine toxicity may include oxygen supplementation, IV lipid emulsion, and midazolam for seizure activity; potential cardiovascular complications were seen after lipid emulsion in 2 rabbits.[90,91]

Limited information is available regarding the use of lidocaine as an analgesic in other exotic companion animals. Lidocaine at 3 mg/kg/h and 6 mg/kg/h IV as CRIs did not significantly change the minimum anesthetic concentration of isoflurane in chickens.[92]

Other Analgesics

Gabapentin is sometimes used for managing neuropathic pain related to avian ganglioneuritis.[93]

Metamizole (also known as dipyrone) is a nonsteroidal antipyretic analgesic that is sometimes used in the management of GI stasis and other painful conditions in rabbits and rodents.[21,94–96] It inhibits cyclooxygenase but also has other mechanisms of action.[96,97] It may be useful for treating pain associated with spastic conditions of the GI tract.[97] This drug has been withdrawn from the market in several countries, including the United States, due to concerns about myelotoxicity in humans.[97]

As noted previously, maropitant may have visceral analgesic properties[33] and can be considered an adjunct treatment in the management of GI disorders. Additional adjunct analgesics that can be considered for GI pain that does not respond to other drugs include low doses of ketamine and low doses of an alpha-2 adrenergic agonist such as dexmedetomidine.[98,99]

MEDICAL MANAGEMENT OF CONSTIPATION AND IMPACTIONS

Constipation is fairly common in reptiles, and often due to underlying husbandry problems, such as inappropriate or inadequate temperature, humidity, water sources, substrate, vitamin and mineral supplementation, or diet. Correcting the husbandry is a key in managing this condition. Other treatments that may be helpful include parenteral fluid therapy, soaking, vibrational therapy, enemas, and laxatives.[100]

Compaction and dehydration of the cecal contents leading to cecolith formation can occur in rabbits.[50] This can be related to altered GI motility, an inappropriate diet (short fiber length or indigestible fiber), or a congenital disorder.[50] A disorder of sodium transport into the cecum has been reported in English Spot and Checkered Giant rabbits and is often called "megacolon syndrome" despite involving the cecum rather than the colon.[50] Treatment of cecal impaction/cecoliths involves rehydration, feeding an appropriate high-fiber diet, analgesia, and potentially promotility agents and careful enemas.[50]

ENDOSCOPY AND SURGERY
Gastrointestinal Endoscopy

GI endoscopy (**Fig. 3**) may be indicated as a non-invasive method of removing FBs from the upper GI tract.[69,101–103] Refer to the Norin Chai's article, "Gastrointestinal Endoscopy," in this issue for further information.

Gastrointestinal Surgery

Gastrointestinal obstruction
Surgery may be indicated to remove FBs in locations that are not amenable to endoscopic removal. This is most commonly performed in ferrets, which tend to tolerate GI surgery well.

GI surgery is less commonly performed in hindgut fermenters due to the risk of complications. The most common FB in rabbits is actually usually the patient's own hair, which is referred to by some as a trichobezoar[94] and by others as a compressed hair pellet.[104] Risks associated with GI surgery in hindgut fermenters include intestinal dehiscence leading to septic peritonitis, adhesion formation, intestinal stricture, and post-operative GI stasis.

Several studies have demonstrated that rabbits with confirmed GI obstructions can be managed medically (**Table 5**).[88,105] In one study, rabbits were managed medically with orogastric decompression.[105] Of the 35 rabbits, 3 died shortly after presentation,

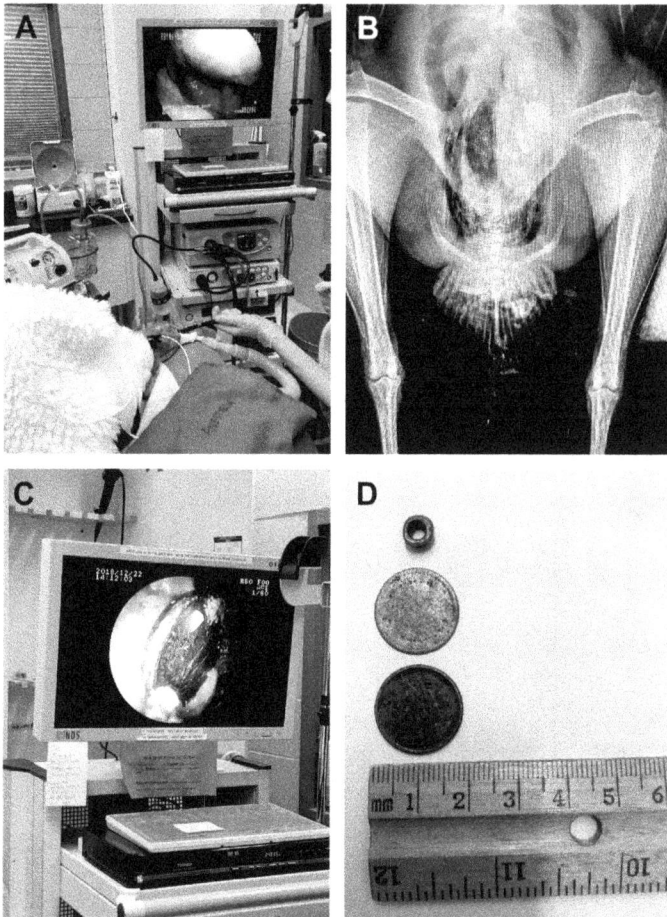

Fig. 3. Use of flexible endoscopy to remove metallic foreign bodies from the ventriculus of a domestic turkey (*Meleagris gallopavo domesticus*). Note that it was challenging to enter the highly muscular ventriculus with the flexible endoscope in this gallinaceous bird. (*A*) The turkey anesthetized and positioned for endoscopy. (*B*) Ventrodorsal radiograph showing the metallic foreign bodies (FB). (*C*) One of the metallic FBs visible on the endoscopy monitor. (*D*) The removed FBs.

while the rest survived (32/35, 91% overall, or 32/32, 100% of treated patients) with medical management alone. In another study, rabbits treated with a lidocaine CRI had increased odds of survival (89.7%) compared to those not treated with lidocaine (56%).[88] In 155 rabbits with gastric dilation on radiographs, 105 survived to discharge, 4 were euthanized at admission, 31 died, 7 were euthanized without further treatment due to surgery being declined, and 8 underwent surgery. All of the surgically treated rabbits died intra-operatively or post-operatively or were euthanized due to inoperable disease.[94]

In contrast, another study showed fairly good survival with surgically-treated small intestinal obstructions in rabbits.[104] Overall survival was 75.2%, but age was a significant factor in survival.[104] Note that the majority of rabbits in this study had their obstructions extraluminally manipulated into the cecum without GI tract incision. This was successful in 87.9% of cases, and only a few rabbits required enterotomy,

Table 5
Summary of recent studies evaluating survival rates in domestic rabbits with gastrointestinal dilation or obstruction

Study	Survival with Medical Management Alone	Summary of Medical Management	Survival with Surgical Treatment	Summary of Surgical Treatment
Steinagel & Ogslebee,[105] 2023	91% (32/35) overall or 100% (35/35) that received orogastric decompression; 3 died shortly after presentation without orogastric decompression	Orogastric decompression, IVF, analgesia, metoclopramide, ranitidine, maropitant, lidocaine CRI	n/a	n/a
Huckins et al,[88] 2024	89.7% (35/39) with lidocaine CRI 56% (14/25) without lidocaine CRI	Lidocaine CRI, IVF, buprenorphine IVF, opioids	n/a n/a	n/a n/a
Böttcher & Müller,[94] 2024	71.4% (105/147) non-surgically-treated cases	IV or SC fluids, metamizole, metoclopramide	0% (0/8)	All surgically-treated rabbits died or euthanized
Sheen et al,[104] 2023	n/a	IVF, opioids, orogastric decompression	75.2% (106/141) overall; 95.7% (22/23) for rabbits <25 m, 80.2% (65/81) for rabbits 25–72 m, 51.4% (19/37) for rabbits >72 m	Obstruction manipulated into cecum whenever possible (87.9%); enterectomy, gastronomy, and R&A in select cases

Abbreviations: CRI, continuous rate infusion; IV, intravenous; IVF, intravenous fluids; n/a, not applicable; R&A, resection and anastomosis; SC, subcutaneous.

gastrotomy, or resection and anastomosis.[104] This technique likely avoids some serious complications associated with GI surgery in rabbits. However, iatrogenic perforation during attempted manipulation of the obstruction did occur in a small number of cases.[104] Surgical treatment of GI obstructions can be considered for rabbits that fail to respond to 2 or 3 attempts at orogastric decompression.[105] Please refer to the Isabelle Desprez and Lucile Chassang's article, "Rabbit Gastroenterology," in this issue for further information on GI surgery in rabbits.

Surgical removal of FBs may also be indicated in certain cases in birds,[106,107] reptiles, and amphibians,[108] especially if medical management or endoscopic removal is not feasible or successful, or if there is a GI perforation. There is a high risk of dehiscence and leakage of gastric contents following ventriculotomy due to the thickness of the muscular walls of the ventriculus.[107] Therefore, a proventricular incision is preferred in order to gain access to the ventriculus.

Risks associated with GI surgery in all species include hemorrhage, infection, skin dehiscence (**Fig. 4**), delayed wound healing, surgical site dehiscence and septic peritonitis/coelomitis, and anesthetic risks.

Gastric dilatation-volvulus

Guinea pigs are the ECM most likely to be presented with a gastric dilatation-volvulus (GDV).[109–111] The prognosis for GDV in guinea pigs is poor to grave. In one report, 2/8 (25%) guinea pigs survived, with one euthanized and the others dying intra-operatively or post-operatively.[110] In another report, 5/18 (28%) guinea pigs survived, with 33% surviving with surgery and 25% with medical management.[111] GDV has also been reported in rabbits[112,113] and a rat.[114]

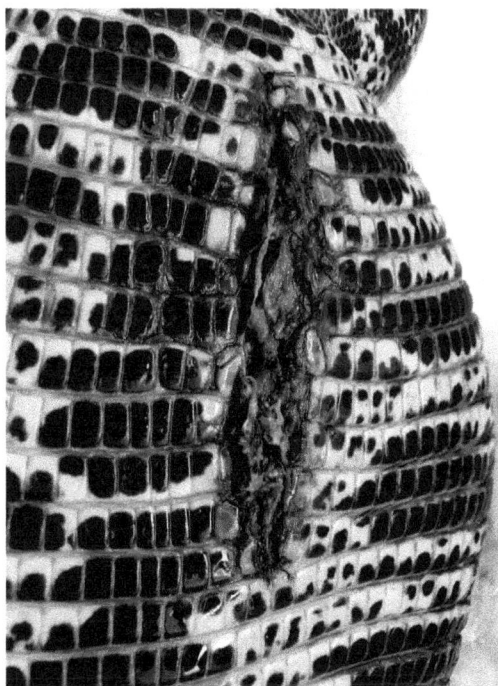

Fig. 4. Severe incisional dehiscence and infection following a ventral coeliotomy and colotomy in an Argentine black and white tegu (*Salvator merianae*).

Rectal and cloacal prolapse

Prior to surgical treatment of a prolapse, protect the prolapse with lubricant, apply dextrose to reduce swelling, assess the stability of the patient, and investigate the cause of the prolapse. In mild cases, often the prolapse can be easily manually reduced with the patient sedated or anesthetized. Retaining sutures can then be placed (purse-string suture in mammals, 2 transverse vent sutures in birds and reptiles).

In cases of intestinal prolapse, abdominal/coelomic surgery is typically required to identify and correct the underlying cause. Prolapse of the intestine has a poorer prognosis than simple rectal or cloacal prolapse.[115]

Rectal or cloacal prolapse is not always related to primary GI disease.[115] This is particularly true in birds and reptiles, in which the cloaca is the common opening for the urinary, reproductive, and GI systems. However, this is also true in mammals, as excessive straining due to urinary disease can result in rectal prolapse.[116] Therefore, perform a thorough evaluation of the patient to identify any predisposing causes.

Mesenteric torsion and volvulus

Mesenteric torsion or volvulus has been reported in a rabbit[117] and in macropods.[118,119]

Gastrointestinal infections

Although most GI infections are managed medically, there are certain cases in which surgery may be indicated, such as for chronic, encapsulated GI abscesses. The author observed an almost 2-year-old castrated male Sprague Dawley rat that underwent

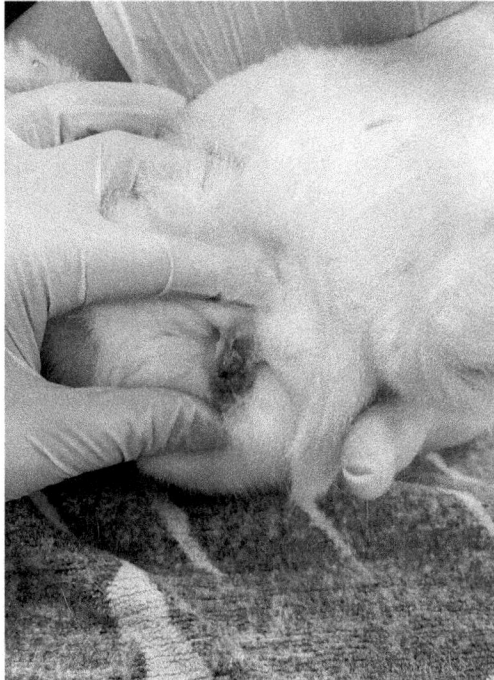

Fig. 5. Anorectal mass in a domestic rabbit. The mass was resected and histopathology revealed an inflammatory anorectal polyp.

resection and anastomosis for a large jejunal abscess (*Enterobacter* and *Pseudomonas* spp. on culture). The rat recovered well and lived for over a year following surgery, with no recurrence noted on necropsy.

Several cases of appendicitis have been reported in rabbits, and both medical and surgical management have been described.[120] Medical management involved antimicrobials, fluids, analgesics, and medications such as ranitidine, clebopride, and trimebutine.[120] Surgical treatment involved appendectomy with cauterization or suturing o the ileocecofold.[120]

Gastrointestinal neoplasia

Surgical resection may be indicated for focal neoplasms or those causing an obstruction or perforation. Resection and anastomosis may be indicated for intestinal adenocarcinomas in ferrets, with prognosis dependent on whether the tumor has metastasized.[76] In a rat with a colonic adenocarcinoma, resection and anastomosis was curative.[121]

Anorectal papillomas or polyps (**Fig. 5**) are common benign tumors arising from the mucocutaneous junction of the rectum and anus in rabbits.[122] They are treated surgically via sharp dissection or via laser or electro/radiosurgery.[122] Malignant rectal neoplasms have also been described in rabbits, so histopathology is warranted for any resected masses.[123]

SUMMARY

GI problems are common in exotic companion animal medicine. Treatment often involves fluid therapy, nutritional support, and analgesia. Maropitant may be useful as an anti-emetic in species that can vomit and may also function as an adjunct analgesic in many species. Certain appetite stimulants appear effective in various species, but it is important to treat the underlying cause of the anorexia and not rely solely on these drugs as the mainstay of treatment. Endoscopic removal of FBs is less invasive than surgery and should be considered when appropriate. Surgery may be indicated in certain situations, such as for FBs that are not amenable to endoscopic removal and for focal neoplasms.

CLINICS CARE POINTS

- There is limited evidence to support the use of prokinetic agents in management of GI stasis in hindgut fermenters. Treatment should instead focus on rehydration, syringe-feeding, analgesia, and correcting the underlying cause. Alternative analgesics such as lidocaine and maropitant may be helpful as part of a multimodal analgesic plan.

- Perform fecal occult blood testing and initiate gastroprotectants as indicated in small anorexic parrots, as GI bleeding can be fatal in these small birds.

- Rabbits with GI obstructions can often be successfully managed medically without surgery. When surgery is performed, it may be preferable to manually manipulate the foreign body into the cecum, or into the stomach in the case of proximal duodenal foreign bodies, rather than performing an enterotomy.

DISCLOSURE

The author declares that they have no known competing financial or commercial interests that could have appeared to influence the work reported in this article. No funding was provided for this article.

REFERENCES

1. Shiga T, Nakata M, Miwa Y, et al. Age at death and cause of death of pet rabbits (*Oryctolagus cuniculus*) seen at an exotic animal clinic in Tokyo, Japan: a retrospective study of 898 cases (2006–2020). J Exot Pet Med 2022;43:35–9.
2. Tokashiki EY, Rahal SC, Melchert A, et al. Retrospective study of conditions grouped by body systems in pet rabbits. J Exot Pet Med 2019;29:207–11.
3. O'Neill DG, Craven HC, Brodbelt DC, et al. Morbidity and mortality of domestic rabbits (*Oryctolagus cuniculus*) under primary veterinary care in England. Vet Rec 2020;186(14):451.
4. Thas I, Wagner RA, Thas O. Clinical diseases in pet black-tailed prairie dogs (*Cynomys ludovicianus*): a retrospective study in 206 animals. J Small Anim Pract 2019;60(3):153–60.
5. O'Neill DG, Kim K, Brodbelt DC, et al. Demography, disorders and mortality of pet hamsters under primary veterinary care in the United Kingdom in 2016. J Small Anim Pract 2022;63(10):747–55.
6. Godwin L, Rao S, Sadar MJ. Causes of morbidity and mortality in sugar gliders (*Petaurus breviceps*) presented to a veterinary teaching hospital in Colorado. In: *AEMV and ARAV proceedings*. AEMV and ARAV. 2024. p. 46.
7. Viere A, Wright L, Schwartz H, et al. A retrospective review of mortality in lorikeets and lories under human care in North America, 1995-2022. In: Proceedings of the 2024 joint AAZV EAZWV conference. American Association of Zoo Veterinarians and European Association of Zoo and Wildlife Veterinarians. 2024. p. 144.
8. Reed K, Anderson K, Wolf K. Mortality trends for budgerigars (*Melopsittacus undulatus*) housed in a walk-through aviary in a zoo in North America, 2009–2019. J Zoo Wildl Med 2021;52(4). https://doi.org/10.1638/2021-0036.
9. Magnotti JM, Garner MM, Stahl SJ, et al. Retrospective review of histologic findings in captive Gila monsters (*Heloderma suspectum*) and beaded lizards (*Heloderma horridum*). J Zoo Wildl Med 2021;52(1). https://doi.org/10.1638/2020-0058.
10. Hoefer H. Gastrointestinal diseases of ferrets. In: Quesenberry K, Orcutt C, Mans C, et al, editors. Ferrets, rabbits, and rodents: clinical medicine and surgery. 4th edition. St. Louis, MO: Elsevier; 2021. p. 27–38.
11. Lichtenberger M, Lennox A. Critical care. In: Speer BL, editor. Current therapy in avian medicine and surgery. 1st edition. St. Louis, MO: Elsevier; 2016. p. 582–8.
12. Cojean O, Duhamelle A, Larrat S. Success rate and complication prevalence of peripheral catheterization of the cephalic, lateral saphenous and marginal ear veins in pet rabbits. J Exot Pet Med 2024;50:42–8.
13. Liles M, Brandão J, Di Girolamo N. Retrospective evaluation of intravenous catheterization in client-owned lizards at a veterinary teaching hospital: 21 cases (2018–2021). J Vet Emerg Crit Care 2023;33(2):236–41.
14. Pardo MA, Divers S. Jugular central venous catheter placement through a modified Seldinger technique for long-term venous access in chelonians. J Zoo Wildl Med 2016;47(1):286–90.
15. Duerr RS. Medical and surgical management of seabirds and allies. In: Hernandez SM, Barron HW, Miller EA, et al, editors. Medical management of wildlife species: a guide for practitioners. Hoboken, NJ: John Wiley & Sons, Inc.; 2020. p. 247–57.
16. Stringfield C. The California condor (*Gymnogyps californianus*) veterinary program: 1997-2010. In: Miller ER, Fowler M, editors. Fowler's zoo and wild animal

medicine: current therapy, vol. 7. St. Louis, MO: Elsevier Saunders; 2012. p. 286–96.

17. Cummings CO. Are we providing adequate analgesia for intraosseous infusion in exotic animal practice? J Exot Pet Med 2023;44:27.

18. Parkinson L. Fluid therapy in exotic animal emergency and critical care. Vet Clin Exot Anim Pract 2023;26(3):623–45.

19. Minor RL, Doss GA, Mans C. Evaluation of glucose absorption rates following intracoelomic or subcutaneous administration in experimentally dehydrated inland bearded dragons (*Pogona vitticeps*). Am J Vet Res 2021;82(11):920–3.

20. Parkinson LA, Mans C. Evaluation of subcutaneously administered electrolyte solutions in experimentally dehydrated inland bearded dragons (*Pogona vitticeps*). Am J Vet Res 2020;81(5):437–41.

21. Carpenter JW, Harms CA, editors. Carpenter's exotic animal formulary. 6th edition. Elsevier; 2023.

22. Parker-Graham C, Clayton LA, Mangus LM. Amphibian renal disease. Vet Clin Exot Anim Pract 2020;23(1):215–30.

23. Mylniczenko ND. Anatomy and taxonomy. In: Hadfield CA, Clayton LA, editors. Clinical guide to fish medicine. Hoboken, NJ: John Wiley & Sons, Inc.; 2021. p. 3–34.

24. Stevens BN, Michel A, Liepnieks ML, et al. Outbreak and treatment of carp edema virus in koi (*Cyprinus carpio*) from northern California. J Zoo Wildl Med 2018;49(3):755–64.

25. Pignon C, Mayer J. Guinea pigs. In: Quesenberry K, Orcutt CJ, Mans C, et al, editors. Ferrets, rabbits, and rodents: clinical medicine and surgery. St. Louis, MO: Elsevier; 2021. p. 270–97.

26. Adamovicz L, Applegate J, Harris J, et al. Use of a gastrostomy and jejunostomy tube for management of gastric distention following pyloric outflow obstruction in a ferret (*Mustela putorius furo*). J Exot Pet Med 2019;28:105–10.

27. Hedley J, Fayers B, Abou-Zahr T. Complications associated with esophagostomy tube placement in chelonian patients. J Exot Pet Med 2021;37:24–6.

28. Le K. Maropitant. J Exot Pet Med 2017;26(4):305–9.

29. Ozawa SM, Hawkins MG, Drazenovich TL, et al. Pharmacokinetics of maropitant citrate in New Zealand White rabbits (*Oryctolagus cuniculus*). Am J Vet Res 2019;80(10):963–8.

30. Sadar MJ, McGee WK, Au GG, et al. Pilot pharmacokinetics of a higher dose of subcutaneous maropitant administration in healthy domestic rabbits (*Oryctolagus cuniculus*). J Exot Pet Med 2022;41:1–2.

31. Roeder M, Boscan P, Rao S, et al. Use of maropitant for pain management in domestic rabbits (*Oryctolagus cuniculus*) undergoing elective orchiectomy or ovariohysterectomy. J Exot Pet Med 2023;47:14–20.

32. Grayck M, Sullivan MN, Boscan P, et al. Use of subcutaneous maropitant at two dosages for pain management in domestic rabbits (*Oryctolagus cuniculus*) undergoing elective ovariohysterectomy or orchiectomy. Top Companion Anim Med 2024;61:100888.

33. Karna SR, Kongara K, Singh PM, et al. Evaluation of analgesic interaction between morphine, dexmedetomidine and maropitant using hot-plate and tail-flick tests in rats. Vet Anaesth Analg 2019;46(4):476–82.

34. Mones AB, Petritz OA, Knych HK, et al. Pharmacokinetics of maropitant citrate in Rhode Island Red chickens (*Gallus gallus domesticus*) following subcutaneous administration. J Vet Pharmacol Therapeut 2022;45(5):495–500.

35. Carpenter JW, Klaphake E, Gibbons PM, et al. Reptile formulary. In: Divers SJ, Stahl SJ, editors. Mader's reptile and Amphibian medicine and surgery. 3rd edition. St. Louis, MO: Elsevier; 2019. p. 1191–211.

36. Smith MV. Therapeutics. In: Smith MV, editor. Textbook of rabbit medicine. 3rd edition. St. Louis, MO: Elsevier; 2023. p. 100–37.

37. Oparil KM, Gladden JN, Babyak JM, et al. Clinical characteristics and short-term outcomes for rabbits with signs of gastrointestinal tract dysfunction: 117 cases (2014–2016). J Am Vet Med Assoc 2019;255(7):837–45.

38. Vito VD, Kim TW, Rota S, et al. Pharmacokinetics of metoclopramide after intra-ARTERIAL, intramuscular, subcutaneous, and perrectal administration in rabbits. J Exot Pet Med 2015;24(3):361–6.

39. Bowman MR, Paré JA, Ziegler LE, et al. Effects of metoclopramide on the gastrointestinal tract motility of Hispaniolan parrots (*Amazona ventralis*). In: American Association of Zoo Veterinarians Conference 2002. Milwaukee, WI: American Association of Zoo Veterinarians; 2002.

40. Tothill A, Johnson J, Branvold H, et al. Effect of cisapride, erythromycin, and metoclopramide on gastrointestinal transit time in the desert tortoise, *Gopherus agassizii*. J Herpetol Med Surg 2000;10(1):16–20.

41. Joblon MJ, Flower JE, Thompson LA, et al. Radiographic determination of gastric emptying and gastrointestinal transit time in cownose rays (*Rhinoptera bonasus*) and whitespotted bamboo sharks (*Chiloscyllium plagiosum*) and the effect of metoclopramide on gastrointestinal motility. J Zoo Wildl Med 2020; 51(2):326.

42. Wangen K. Therapeutic review: cisapride. J Exot Pet Med 2013;22(3):301–4.

43. Morrisey JK, Carpenter JW. Appendix: formulary. In: Quesenberry K, Orcutt CJ, Mans C, et al, editors. Ferrets, rabbits, and rodents: clinical medicine and surgery. 4th edition. St. Louis, MO: Elsevier; 2021. p. 620–30.

44. Feldman ER, Singh B, Mishkin NG, et al. Effects of cisapride, buprenorphine, and their combination on gastrointestinal transit in New Zealand white rabbits. J Am Assoc Lab Anim Sci 2021;60(2):221–8.

45. Jekl V, Hauptman K, Knotek Z. Evidence-based advances in rodent medicine. Vet Clin Exot Anim Pract 2017;20(3):805–16.

46. Mans C, Fink DM, Ciarrocchi C. Effects of oral cisapride administration in chinchillas (*Chinchilla lanigera*) with experimentally induced fecal output reduction. J Exot Pet Med 2021;38:21–5.

47. Sladakovic I, Schnellbacher RW. Miscellaneous drug therapy. In: Divers SJ, Stahl SJ, editors. Mader's reptile and Amphibian medicine and surgery. 3rd edition. St. Louis, MO: Elsevier; 2019. p. 1185.

48. Fisher P, Graham J. Rabbits. In: Carpenter JW, Marion CJ, editors. Exotic animal formulary. 5th edition. St. Louis, MO: Elsevier; 2018. p. 494–531.

49. Li C, Qian W, Hou X. Effect of four medications associated with gastrointestinal motility on Oddi sphincter in the rabbit. Pancreatology 2009;9(5):615–20.

50. Oglesbee BL, Lord B. Gastrointestinal diseases of rabbits. In: Quesenberry K, Orcutt CJ, Mans C, et al, editors. Ferrets, rabbits, and rodents: clinical medicine and surgery. 4th edition. St. Louis, MO: Elsevier; 2021. p. 174–87.

51. Ozawa S, Thomson A, Petritz O. Safety and efficacy of oral mirtazapine in New Zealand White rabbits (*Oryctolagus cuniculus*). J Exot Pet Med 2022;40:16–20.

52. Draper JM, Savson DJ, Lavin ES, et al. Comparison of effects of capromorelin and mirtazapine on appetite in New Zealand white rabbits (*Oryctolagus cuniculus*). J Am Assoc Lab Anim Sci 2022;61(5):495–505.

53. Mans C, Hamilton E. Effects of capromorelin and mirtazapine on food intake in chinchillas. In: ExoticsCon 2023 proceedings. Boston, MA: ExoticsCon; 2023. p. 128.
54. Mans C, Titel CE, Doss GA. Effects of capromorelin, mirtazapine, and cyproheptadine on food intake in budgerigars (*Melopsittacus undulatus*). In: ExoticsCon 2023 proceedings. Boston, MA: ExoticsCon; 2023. p. 26.
55. Bogan JE, Sones E, Mason AK. Chemotherapy in two snakes as an adjunctive therapy to surgical treatment of neoplasia. In: ExoticsCon 2023 proceedings. Boston, MA: ExoticsCon; 2023. p. 300.
56. Huckins GL, Mans C, Doss GA. Effects of oral capromorelin on food intake and body weight in healthy, four-toed hedgehogs (*Atelerix albiventris*). J Exot Pet Med 2024;52:1–3.
57. Trumpp K, Burns L, Jacobson C, et al. Effect of capromorelin (Entyce®) on appetite and weight gain of domestic pigeons (*Columba livia domestica*). In: ExoticsCon 2023 Proceedings. Boston, MA: ExoticsCon; 2023. p. 96.
58. Plumb DC. Plumb's veterinary drug handbook. 6th edition. Ames, IA: Blackwell Publishing; 2008.
59. Martel A, Berg C, Doss G, et al. Effects of midazolam on food intake in budgerigars (*Melopsittacus undulatus*). J Avian Med Surg 2022;36(1). https://doi.org/10.1647/20-00096.
60. Scagnelli A, Titel C, Doss G, et al. Effects of midazolam and lorazepam on food intake in budgerigars (*Melopsittacus undulatus*). J Exot Pet Med 2022;41:42–5.
61. Smith MV. Digestive disorders. In: Smith MV, editor. Textbook of rabbit medicine. 3rd edition. St. Louis, MO: Elsevier; 2023. p. 156–91.
62. Reavill DR, Dorrestein G. Psittacines, Coliiformes, Musophagiformes, Cuculiformes. In: Terio KA, McAloose D, St. Leger J, editors. Pathology of wildlife and zoo animals. London, UK: Academic Press; 2018. p. 775–98.
63. Püstow R, Krautwald-Junghanns ME. The incidence and treatment outcomes of *Macrorhabdus ornithogaster* infection in budgerigars (*Melopsittacus undulatus*) in a veterinary clinic. J Avian Med Surg 2017;31(4):344–50.
64. Marks SL, Kook PH, Papich MG, et al. ACVIM consensus statement: support for rational administration of gastrointestinal protectants to dogs and cats. J Vet Intern Med 2018;32(6):1823–40.
65. Hedges K, Odunayo A, Price JM, et al. Evaluation of the effect of a famotidine continuous rate infusion on intragastric pH in healthy dogs. J Vet Intern Med 2019;33(5):1988–94.
66. Tolbert K, Bissett S, King A, et al. Efficacy of oral famotidine and 2 omeprazole formulations for the control of intragastric pH in dogs. J Vet Intern Med 2011;25(1):47–54.
67. Tomoi M, Itoh H, Ueda S, et al. Effects of omeprazole and famotidine on (H+-K+) ATPase and acid secretion in rabbit gastric glands [Article in Japanese]. Nihon Yakurigaku Zasshi 1988;92(2):105–11.
68. Barron HW. Appendix II: formulary for common wildlife species. In: Hernandez SM, Barron HW, Miller EA, et al, editors. Medical management of wildlife species: a guide for practitioners. Hoboken, NJ: John Wiley & Sons, Inc.; 2020. p. 449–65.
69. Webb J, Graham J, Fordham M, et al. Diagnosis and treatment of esophageal foreign body or stricture in three ferrets (*Mustela putorius furo*). J Am Vet Med Assoc 2017;251(4):451–7.
70. Schweitzer EJ, Bass BL, Johnson LF, et al. Sucralfate prevents experimental peptic esophagitis in rabbits. Gastroenterology 1985;88(3):611–9.

71. Pouillevet H, Langlois I, Lamglait B, et al. Evaluation of clinical diagnostics for proventricular nematodiasis due to *Synhimantus nasuta* in lorikeets (*Trichoglossus* spp.). J Zoo Wildl Med 2022;53(2).

72. Wills S, Beaufrère H, Watrous G, et al. Proximal duodenoileal anastomosis for treatment of small intestinal obstruction and volvulus in a green iguana (*Iguana iguana*). J Am Vet Med Assoc 2016;249(9):1061–6.

73. Summa NM, Guzman DSM, Larrat S, et al. Evaluation of high dosages of oral meloxicam in American kestrels (*Falco sparverius*). J Avian Med Surg 2017; 31(2):108–16.

74. Crouch EEV, Reinoso-Perez MT, Vanderstichel RV, et al. The effect of dexamethasone on hematologic profiles, hemosporidian infection, and splenic histology in house finches (*Haemorhous mexicanus*). J Wildl Dis 2022;58(3).

75. Suran JN, Wyre NR. Imaging findings in 14 domestic ferrets (*Mustela putorius furo*) with lymphoma. Vet Radiol Ultrasound 2013;54(5):522–31.

76. Williams BH, Wyre NR. Neoplasia in ferrets. In: Quesenberry K, Orcutt CJ, Mans C, et al, editors. Ferrets, rabbits, and rodents: clinical medicine and surgery. 4th edition. St. Louis, MO: Elsevier; 2021. p. 92–108.

77. Robertson JA, Guzman DSM, Willcox JL, et al. Clinical and pathological findings of rabbits with lymphoma: 16 cases (1996–2019). J Am Vet Med Assoc 2022; 260(9):1–10.

78. Faye-Fierman S, Gardhouse S, McCready JE, et al. Clinical presentation and treatment of lymphoma in companion rats (*Rattus norvegicus*; 2008–2020). J Am Vet Med Assoc 2022;260(12):1533–40.

79. LaDouceur EE, Argue A, Garner MM. Alimentary tract neoplasia in captive bearded dragons (*Pogona* spp). J Comp Pathol 2022;194:28–33.

80. Farris KH, Mans C. A case of inflammatory bowel disease in a rabbit (*Oryctolagus cuniculus*). In: *AEMV and ARAV proceedings*. AEMV and ARAV. 2024. p. 33.

81. Doss GA, Mans C, Johnson L, et al. Diagnosis and management of inflammatory bowel disease in a harpy eagle (*Harpia harpyja*) with suspected fenbendazole toxicosis. J Am Vet Med Assoc 2018;252(3):336–42.

82. Hrysyzen TMS, Malmberg JL, Johnston MS. Diagnosis and clinical management of eosinophilic gastroenteritis in an African pygmy hedgehog (*Atelerix albiventris*). J Exot Pet Med 2019;30:88–91.

83. Smith SM. Gastrointestinal physiology and nutrition of rabbits. In: Quesenberry K, Orcutt CJ, Mans C, Carpenter JW, editors. Ferrets, rabbits, and rodents: clinical medicine and surgery. 4th edition. St. Louis, MO: Elsevier; 2021. p. 162–73.

84. Rahic-Seggerman FM, Rosenthal K, Miller C, et al. Effects of diet on the bacterial and eukaryotic microbiota across the gastrointestinal tract of healthy rabbits (*Oryctolagus cuniculus*). Am J Vet Res 2024;85(4):1–11.

85. Scarsella E, Fay JS, Jospin G, et al. Characterization and description of the fecal microbiomes of pet domestic ferrets (*Mustela putorius furo*) living in homes. Animals 2023;13(21):3354.

86. Pujol J, Vergneau-Grosset C, Beaudry F, et al. Pharmacokinetics and innocuity of a single dose of intravenous, intramuscular, and subcutaneous methadone in the domestic rabbit (*Oryctolagus cuniculus*). J Exot Pet Med 2023;47:41–6.

87. Pathak D, Di Girolamo N, Maranville R, et al. Effects of injectable analgesics on selected gastrointestinal physiological parameters in rabbits. In: ExoticsCon 2021 proceedings. Nashville, TN: ExoticsCon; 2021. p. 342–3.

88. Huckins GL, Tournade C, Patson C, et al. Lidocaine constant rate infusion improves the probability of survival in rabbits with gastrointestinal obstructions: 64 cases (2012–2021). J Am Vet Med Assoc 2024;262(1):61–7.

89. Schnellbacher RW, Divers SJ, Comolli JR, et al. Effects of intravenous administration of lidocaine and buprenorphine on gastrointestinal tract motility and signs of pain in New Zealand White rabbits after ovariohysterectomy. Am J Vet Res 2017;78(12):1359–71.

90. Di Girolamo N. Accidental acute lidocaine toxicity in two pet rabbits treated using intravenous lipid emulsion. In: International conference on avian, herpetological, exotic mammal, zoo and wildlife medicine. Ghent, Belgium: ICARE; 2024. p. 272.

91. Moreno AA, Thielen L, Liles M, et al. Accidental acute lidocaine toxicity in four pet rabbits and treatment with intravenous lipid emulsion. In: AEMV and ARAV proceedings. AEMV and ARAV. 2024. p. 131.

92. Escobar A, Dzikiti BT, Thorogood JC, et al. Effects of two continuous infusion doses of lidocaine on isoflurane minimum anesthetic concentration in chickens. Vet Anaesth Analg 2023;50(1):91–7.

93. Hoppes SM, Shivaprasad HL. Update on avian bornavirus and proventricular dilatation disease. Vet Clin Exot Anim Pract 2020;23(2):337–51.

94. Böttcher A, Müller K. Radiological and laboratory prognostic parameters for gastric dilation in rabbits (Oryctolagus cuniculus). Vet Rec 2024;194(5):e3827.

95. Brezina T, Fehr M, Neumüller M, et al. Acid-base-balance status and blood gas analysis in rabbits with gastric stasis and gastric dilation. J Exot Pet Med 2020; 32:18–26.

96. Bauer C, Schillinger U, Brandl J, et al. Comparison of pre-emptive butorphanol or metamizole with ketamine +medetomidine and s-ketamine + medetomidine anaesthesia in improving intraoperative analgesia in mice. Lab Anim 2019; 53(5):459–69.

97. Jasiecka A, Maślanka T, Jaroszewski JJ. Pharmacological characteristics of metamizole. Pol J Vet Sci 2014;17(1):207–14.

98. Strigo IA, Duncan GH, Bushnell CM, et al. The effects of racemic ketamine on painful stimulation of skin and viscera in human subjects. Pain 2005;113(3): 255–64.

99. Rankin DC. Sedatives and tranquilizers. In: Grimm KA, Lamont LA, Tranquilli WJ, et al, editors. Veterinary anesthesia and analgesia: the fifth edition of Lumb and Jones. 5th edition. Ames, IA: John Wiley & Sons, Inc.; 2015. p. 196–205.

100. Nicholas E, Warwick C. Alleviation of a gastrointestinal tract impaction in a tortoise using an improvised vibrating massager. J Herpetol Med Surg 2011; 21(4):93.

101. Pignon C, Crescence L. Upper gastrointestinal flexible endoscopy in rabbits: a pilot study. In: ExoticsCon 2023 proceedings. ExoticsCon. 2023.

102. Cotton RJ, Divers SJ. Endoscopic removal of gastrointestinal foreign bodies in two African grey parrots (Psittacus erithacus) and a hyacinth macaw (Anodorhynchus hyacinthinus). J Avian Med Surg 2017;(31):4.

103. Burns PM, Langlois I, Dunn M. Endoscopic removal of a foreign body in a Mexican axolotl (Ambystoma mexicanum) with the use of MS222-induced immobilization. J Zoo Wildl Med 2019;50(1):282.

104. Sheen JC, Sladakovic I, Finch S. Prognostic indicators for survival in surgically managed small intestinal obstruction in pet rabbits: 141 presentations (2011–2021). J Am Vet Med Assoc 2023;1–10.

105. Steinagel AC, Oglesbee BL. Clinicopathological and radiographic indicators for orogastric decompression in rabbits presenting with intestinal obstruction at a referral hospital (2015–2018). Vet Rec 2023;192(5):e2481.

106. Lamb SK. Obstruction by fibrous foreign object ingestion in two green-cheeked conures (*Pyrrhura molinae*) and a jenday conure (*Aratinga jandaya*). J Exot Pet Med 2019;31:127–32.

107. Laniesse D, Beaufrère H, Mackenzie S, et al. Perforating foreign body in the ventriculus of a pet pigeon (*Columba livia domestica*). J Am Vet Med Assoc 2018;253(12).

108. Nascimento GM, Vieu S, Phouratsamay A. Chronic intestinal impaction by coconut fiber and sphagnum moss in a Cranwell's horned frog (*Ceratophrys cranwelli*). J Exot Pet Med 2023;45:26–7.

109. Mitchell EB, Hawkins MG, Gaffney PM, et al. Gastric dilatation-volvulus in a Guinea pig (*Cavia porcellus*). J Am Anim Hosp Assoc 2010;46(3):174–80.

110. Nógrádi AL, Cope I, Balogh M, et al. Review of gastric torsion in eight Guinea pigs (*Cavia porcellus*). Acta Vet Hung 2017;65(4):487–99.

111. Pignon C, Kuypers M, Robert C, et al. Gastric dilatation and volvulus in Guinea pigs: a retrospective study. In: AEMV and ARAV proceedings. Dallas, TX: AEMV and ARAV; 2017. p. 77.

112. Vasyliev A, Jew N. Surgical treatment and resolution of gastric dilatation and volvulus (GDV) in a rabbit (*Oryctolagus cuniculus*). In: International conference on avian, herpetological, exotic mammal, zoo and wildlife medicine. Ghent, Belgium: ICARE; 2024. p. 259–64.

113. Chan SC. Surgical and medical management of gastric dilation and volvulus in pet rabbits: two cases. AEMV and ARAV Proceedings. AEMV and ARAV 2023; 2024:37.

114. Woodhall H, Barrow K, Brown S, et al. Successful surgical treatment of gastric dilatation and volvulus in a pet domestic rat (*Rattus norvegicus*). J Exot Pet Med 2024;51:9–12.

115. Gill KS, Helmer PJ. Cloacal diseases in companion parrots: a retrospective study of 43 cases (2012–2018). J Avian Med Surg 2020;34(4). https://doi.org/10.1647/1082-6742-34.4.364.

116. Di Girolamo N, Huynh M. Disorders of the urinary and reproductive systems in ferrets. In: Quesenberry K, Orcutt CJ, Mans C, et al, editors. Ferrets, rabbits, and rodents: clinical medicine and surgery. 4th edition. St. Louis, MO: Elsevier; 2021. p. 39–54.

117. Gleeson M, Chen S, Fabiani M, et al. Mesenteric root and cecal torsion in a domestic rabbit (*Oryctolagus cuniculus*). J Exot Pet Med 2019;28:76–81.

118. Knafo SE, Rosenblatt AJ, Morrisey JK, et al. Diagnosis and treatment of mesenteric volvulus in a red kangaroo (*Macropus rufus*). J Am Vet Med Assoc 2014; 244(7):844–50.

119. Glassman A, Hallman C, Clary E, et al. Mesenteric volvulus in a Bennett's wallaby (*Notamacropus rufogriseus*). J Exot Pet Med 2020;32:56–7.

120. Di Girolamo N, Petrini D, Szabo Z, et al. Clinical, surgical, and pathological findings in client-owned rabbits with histologically confirmed appendicitis: 19 cases (2015–2019). J Am Vet Med Assoc 2022;260(1):82–93.

121. Applegate JR, Troan BV, Chen LR, et al. Surgical management of colonic adenocarcinoma in a rat (*Rattus norvegicus*). J Exot Pet Med 2017;26(1):47–52.

122. Guzman DSM, Szabo Z, Steffey MA. Soft tissue surgery: rabbits. In: Quesenberry K, Orcutt CJ, Mans C, et al, editors. Ferrets, rabbits, and rodents: clinical medicine and surgery. 4th edition. St. Louis, MO: Elsevier; 2021. p. 446–66.

123. Flenghi L, Bernhard C, Levrier C, et al. Rectal prolapse in two rabbits (*Oryctolagus cuniculi* [sic]) with rectal neoplasia. J Exot Pet Med 2021;39:64–7.

124. Tai C, Knafo SE. Novel placement of an omobrachial vein catheter in a ferret (*Mustela putorius furo*). J Exot Pet Med 2020;34:24–5.

125. Uccello O, Sanchez A, Valverde A, et al. Cardiovascular effects of increasing dosages of norepinephrine in healthy isoflurane-anesthetized New Zealand White rabbits. Vet Anaesth Analg 2020;47(6):781–8.

126. Critical care herbivore anise. Oxbow Animal Health. Available at: https://oxbowanimalhealth.com/product/critical-care-herbivore-anise/.

127. EmerAid intensive care Herbivore®. EmerAid. Available at: https://emeraid.com/vet/emeraid-herbivore/.

128. Sadar MJ, Knych HK, Drazenovich TL, et al. Pharmacokinetics of buprenorphine after intravenous and oral transmucosal administration in Guinea pigs (*Cavia porcellus*). Am J Vet Res 2018;79(3):260–6.

129. Fox L, Mans C. Analgesic efficacy and safety of buprenorphine in chinchillas (*Chinchilla lanigera*). J Am Assoc Lab Anim Sci 2018;57(3):286–90.

130. Ambros B, Knych HK, Sadar MJ. Pharmacokinetics of hydromorphone hydrochloride after intravenous and intramuscular administration in Guinea pigs (*Cavia porcellus*). Am J Vet Res 2020;81(4):361–6.

131. Evenson EA, Mans C. Analgesic efficacy and safety of hydromorphone in chinchillas (*Chinchilla lanigera*). J Am Assoc Lab Anim Sci 2018;57(3):282–5.

132. Moeremans I, Devreese M, De Baere S, et al. Pharmacokinetics and absolute oral bioavailability of meloxicam in Guinea pigs (*Cavia porcellus*). Vet Anaesth Analg 2019;46(4):548–55.

133. Delk KW, Carpenter JW, KuKanich B, et al. Pharmacokinetics of meloxicam administered orally to rabbits (*Oryctolagus cuniculus*) for 29 days. Am J Vet Res 2014;75(2):195–9.

134. Chandranath S, Bastaki S, Singh J. A comparative study on the activity of lansoprazole, omeprazole and PD-136450 on acidified ethanol- and indomethacin-induced gastric lesions in the rat. Clin Exp Pharmacol Physiol 2002;29(3):173–80.

135. Bene-Bac® plus small animal gel. PetAg. Available at: https://www.petag.com/products/bene-bac-plus-small-animal-gel?gad_source=1&gclid=Cj0KCQjwiOy1BhDCARIsADGvQnC-6BQVChFwIDMleeFlxn8BQjx35tPeEfZLwxi3fAKMpm9ozi3znmUaAu1AEALw_wcB.

136. Purina pro plan veterinary supplements FortiFlora canine nutritional supplement. Purina. Available at: https://www.purina.com/dogs/shop/pro-plan-veterinary-supplements-fortiflora.

137. Proviable-DC capsules multi-strain probiotic for cats and dogs. Proviable. Available at: https://www.proviable.com/proviable-dc-capsules-for-dogs.

138. Vetri mega Probiotic™ digestive supplement for dogs & cats. VetriScience. Available at: https://www.vetriscience.com/vetri-mega-probiotic-153-digestive-supplement-for-dogs-cats.html.

Treatment of Gastrointestinal Infectious Diseases in Exotic Animals

Julianne E. McCready, DVM, DVSc, DACZM

KEYWORDS

- Antimicrobials • Birds • Gastroenterology • Infectious diseases • Rabbits • Reptiles
- Rodents

KEY POINTS

- Certain antibiotics, including penicillins, lincosamides, ampicillin, amoxicillin, cephalosporins, and erythromycin, are contraindicated in hindgut fermenters when administered orally.
- Treatment options for *Macrorhabdus ornithogaster* include amphotericin B, sodium benzoate, and nystatin, but recurrence following treatment is very common.
- Currently, there is no cure for avian ganglioneuritis, but various treatments have been attempted, including nonsteroidal anti-inflammatory drugs such as celecoxib and robenacoxib, cyclosporine, and antivirals.
- There are several different reported treatment protocols for gastric and intestinal cryptosporidiosis in reptiles, but recurrence following immunosuppression is common.

INTRODUCTION

Appropriate antimicrobial use is crucial when managing exotic animal patients with gastrointestinal (GI) disorders to prevent adverse effects and antimicrobial resistance. A thorough diagnostic work-up should be performed in a patient presenting with GI signs to ensure that antimicrobials are indicated. Not all GI signs in exotic animals are caused by infectious diseases and antimicrobials are not required in every case. Primary infectious GI disorders are common in certain species, such as ferrets, hamsters, and some bird species. GI helminth parasites are fairly uncommon in captive-bred pet mammals and birds housed exclusively indoors but are more common in reptiles and in any animals with outdoor access.[1] Some GI parasites in reptiles are commensal or even beneficial and may not require treatment.[1]

Zoological Medicine Service, Department of Veterinary Clinical Sciences, College of Veterinary Medicine, Oklahoma State University, 2065 W. Farm Road, Stillwater, OK 74078, USA
E-mail address: julianne.mccready@okstate.edu

Vet Clin Exot Anim 28 (2025) 485–501
https://doi.org/10.1016/j.cvex.2024.11.012
1094-9194/25/© 2024 Elsevier Inc. All rights are reserved, including those for text and data mining, AI training, and similar technologies.
vetexotic.theclinics.com

Abbreviations	
IM	intramuscular
IV	intravenous
PCR	polymerase chain reaction
PO	per os
qPCR	quantitative polymerase chain reaction
SC	subcutaneous

ANTIMICROBIALS
Antibiotics

Antibiotics may be indicated for patients with bacterial infections of the GI tract. However, it is important to use antibiotics judiciously and avoid administering antibiotics empirically to any animal presenting with nonspecific GI signs. Routine use of antimicrobials is not indicated for stable, normothermic rabbits and rodents presenting with GI stasis. However, antibiotics can be considered for animals with evidence of severe disease or sepsis, such as hypothermia, bradycardia, hypoglycemia or severe hyperglycemia, hypercholesterolemia, hypertriglyceridemia, and band heterophils, or with confirmed GI infections.[2–6]

Certain antibiotics are contraindicated when administered orally to hindgut fermenters due to the risk of dysbiosis. These are antibiotics that target mainly Gram-positive and anaerobic bacteria and can destroy the animal's normal GI flora, allowing for *Clostridium* spp. overgrowth.[7] A useful mnemonic to remember the antibiotics that should not be used orally in hindgut fermenters is "PLACE" (**Box 1**).

Antibiotics that are generally well tolerated orally by hindgut fermenters include sulfonamides, fluoroquinolones, azithromycin, metronidazole, chloramphenicol, and doxycycline.[7,8] However, chinchillas seem more prone to anorexia with antibiotic treatment compared to other small mammals; anorexia has been reported following treatment with the fluoroquinolone pradofloxacin[9] and with metronidazole[10–12] in chinchillas.

There are numerous bacteria capable of causing a GI infection in exotic companion animals; however, this review only focuses on a few common ones.

Treatment of Helicobacter mustelae in ferrets
Helicobacter mustelae-associated gastritis is very common in pet ferrets. A variety of protocols have been reported for treatment of this condition, including amoxicillin, metronidazole, and bismuth subsalicylate; clarithromycin and ranitidine bismuth citrate; clarithromycin and omeprazole; and enrofloxacin and colloidal bismuth subcitrate.[13]

Treatment of proliferative ileitis in hamsters
Although it is important to be judicious with antibiotics, as stated earlier, for young hamsters presenting with diarrhea, it is often best to start empiric antibiotics

---

Box 1
Mnemonic (PLACE) for antibiotics contraindicated orally in hindgut fermenters such as rabbits, guinea pigs, and chinchillas

- P: Penicillins
- L: Lincosamides (including lincomycin and clindamycin)
- A: Ampicillin and amoxicillin
- C: Cephalosporins
- E: Erythromycin

immediately due to the severity of the disease process. Proliferative ileitis, also known as "wet tail," is caused by *Lawsonia intracellularis*. This disease tends to have a poor prognosis.[14] Therefore, aggressive supportive care, including fluid therapy, nutritional support, and antibiotics (such as tetracyclines, enrofloxacin, or chloramphenicol), is indicated.

Treatment of clostridial infections
Clostridium spp. can cause several important enteric and non-enteric infections of gallinaceous birds. Necrotic enteritis is caused by *Clostridium perfringens* types A and C and causes fibrinonecrotic enteritis with diphtheritic pseudomembrane formation, leading to depression, dehydration, and death in chickens and turkeys.[15,16] Predisposing factors may include concurrent coccidiosis and dietary issues (such as feeds containing wheat).[15] Treatment involves antibiotics that target Gram-positive bacteria, such as penicillin or bacitracin. Prevention includes controlling coccidial infections, environmental sanitation, and appropriate diet. Clostridial enteritis has also been reported in psittacine birds, especially lorikeets.[17]

Ulcerative enteritis is caused by *Clostridium colinum* and involves ulcers, hemorrhage, and potentially perforation of the intestinal tract in quail, grouse, turkeys, chickens, and partridges.[16] Clinical signs include diarrhea, depression, and death.[15] Treatment may involve bacitracin, penicillin, or tetracyclines.[15]

Treatment of salmonellosis
GI carriage of *Salmonella* spp. without clinical signs is common in many exotic companion animal species, especially reptiles and poultry. Treatment of clinical *Salmonella* spp. infections is controversial and often not recommended due to the risk of animals becoming carriers and the zoonotic potential of *Salmonella* spp. If treatment is elected, it should be based on culture and sensitivity and given for 3 to 8 weeks.[18]

Antifungals

There are 2 fungal infections of the GI tract that are commonly encountered in parrots, namely candidiasis and macrorhabdosis.

Antifungals for treatment of candidiasis
Candida infections, especially infections due to *Candida albicans*, are common GI infections in birds. Prior broad-spectrum antibiotic use may be a risk factor for candidiasis in many species, including in birds.[18] Commonly used antifungals for treatment of candidiasis include fluconazole, itraconazole, ketoconazole, and nystatin.[18,19] Toxicity has been reported with fluconazole in budgerigars (*Melopsittacus undulatus*) and with itraconazole in gray parrots (*Psittacus erithacus*); these drugs should be avoided in these species if possible.[19] Some authors recommended the use of apple cider vinegar in drinking water (10 mL/L of water) to reduce the crop pH, as the yeast grows best in an alkaline environment.[18]

Recently, non-*albicans* candidiasis has been increasingly identified in birds.[20,21] In a case series of non-*albicans Candida* in 6 birds (5 psittacine birds and 1 ring-necked dove), 2 cases died, 1 was lost to follow-up, and 3 resolved with treatment.[20] Five of the cases involved *Candida glabrata* and one involved *Candida krusei*. A variety of antifungals were used, including fluconazole, voriconazole, terbinafine, and nystatin.[20] In an eclectus parrot (*Eclectus roratus*) with *C glabrata* proventriculitis, multimodal treatment with nystatin, fluconazole, antibiotics, gastroprotectants, maropitant, analgesics, and supportive care was ultimately successful, but long-term antifungal treatment was needed.[21] *C glabrata* is often resistant to antifungals.[21]

Antifungals for treatment of macrorhabdosis

Macrorhabdus ornithogaster is a yeast that colonies the GI tract, particularly the isthmus (ie, junction between proventriculus and ventriculus), of several bird species.[18,22] It is also known as avian gastric yeast and was previously known as megabacteria, before it was determined to be a fungal organism.[22] Commonly affected psittacine bird species include budgerigars,[23–28] cockatiels,[24] lovebirds,[25] and parrotlets.[29] It has also been reported in non-psittacine birds, including zebra finches, canaries, ostriches, and chickens.[18,22,30] Diagnosis and treatment of this organism can be very challenging. The organism can be harbored without causing clinical signs. In addition, due to its location in the GI tract, it is intermittently shed in the feces and may require repeated fecal examinations to identify its presence. It can cause clinical signs ranging from chronic weight loss to vomiting, diarrhea, and even death (**Fig. 1**). This organism is rarely eradicated with treatment and recurrence is common. Repeat treatment or prolonged treatment may be required. Reported treatments (**Table 1**) for macrorhabdosis include amphotericin B,[23–26,30] nystatin,[22] and sodium benzoate.[31,32] Ketoconazole, terbinafine, and itraconazole are reported to be ineffective.[18] Gentian violet and fluconazole have been evaluated for treatment of *M ornithogaster* but toxicity occurred in budgerigars.[29]

Amphotericin B: One study reported the use of amphotericin B 100 mg/kg per os (PO) q 12 hour x 4 weeks in affected budgerigars.[23] Results indicated that 36% of birds recovered, 17% improved but had a recurrence, 20% died without improvement, and 9% were euthanized.[23] Overall, the authors considered 53% of birds treated successfully but noted that treatment was stressful due to the handling required for treatment.[23]

In another study, affected budgerigars and cockatiels (*Nymphicus hollandicus*) were treated with amphotericin B 0.1 mg/mL in drinking water alone or combined with oral administration at 100 mg/kg PO q 12 hour.[24] Following treatment, 56.4% of flocks tested negative for *M ornithogaster* DNA, while 43.6% were still positive. When comparing drinking water treatment versus oral and drinking water treatment, 52.2% were negative after drinking water treatment, while 62.5% were negative after drinking water and oral treatment. However, the difference was not statistically significant.

Another study used amphotericin B at 0.9 mg/mL and found that shedding decreased during treatment.[26] Drinking water treatment may be a reasonable option

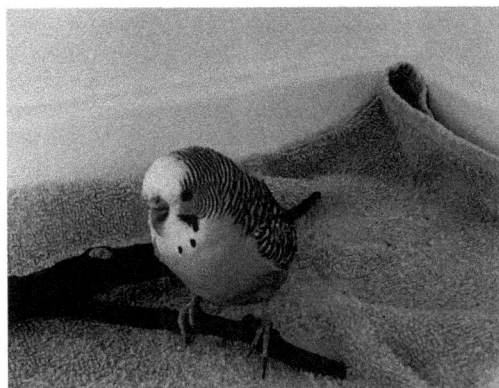

Fig. 1. *Macrorhabdus ornithogaster* is a common gastrointestinal infection in budgerigars (*Melopsittacus undulatus*). This 4-year-old budgerigar presented for hematochezia, and a fecal PCR was positive for *Macrorhabdus ornithogaster*. The patient arrested before treatment could be initiated, and necropsy was declined.

Table 1
Some reported dosing regimes for *Macrorhabdus ornithogaster*

Drug	Dose and Route	Species
Amphotericin B	100 mg/kg PO q 12 h x 30 d[23,25]	Budgerigars, peach-faced lovebirds, various other psittacine birds, chickens
	25 mg/kg PO q 12–24 h[25,30]	Various psittacine birds, chickens, American white ibis
	0.1 mg/mL in drinking water ± 100 mg/kg PO q 12 h[24]	Budgerigars, cockatiels
	0.9–1 mg/mL in drinking water[25,26]	Budgerigars, various psittacine birds
Nystatin	3,500,000 IU/L in drinking water x 48 h, then 2,000,000 IU/L drinking water x 28 d[22]	Budgerigars
Sodium benzoate	0.5–1 tsp/L (~2.5–5 mL/L) in drinking water x 5 wk[31]	Budgerigars
	500–1000 mg/L in drinking water x 4–8 wk[32]	Budgerigars

in large flocks or for birds that are very stressed with handling. However, for individual pet birds that are accustomed to handling, direct oral administration is likely preferred to ensure they are receiving the appropriate dose of the medication.

In a retrospective case series, poor treatment success (16.67%) was noted, with 63.8% of birds dying or being euthanized within 3 months of diagnosis.[25] Doses used in this study included 5 mg/kg PO q 12 hours (1 bird, 0% success rate), 25 mg/kg PO q 12 hours (25 birds, 16% success rate), 50 mg/kg PO q 12 hours (2 birds, 0% success rate), 100 mg/kg PO q 12 hours (5 birds, 20% success rate), and 1 mg/mL in water (3 birds, 33.33% success rate).[25] In a pilot study, 2 birds were treated with amphotericin B 100 mg/kg PO q 12 hours x 30 days. Treatment significantly decreased *M ornithogaster* shedding in the feces, but after discontinuation of treatment, birds had a rebound in fecal shedding and began shedding in even higher numbers.[25] The authors also compared the efficacy of 25 and 100 mg/kg amphotericin B in chickens and found that there was significantly more *M ornithogaster* per slide in the control and 25 mg/kg groups compared to the 100 mg/kg group.[25] The 25 mg/kg dose was ineffective and did not cure any of the birds or reduce the concentration of *M ornithogaster* in the isthmus. The 100 mg/kg dose reduced the concentration of the organism but only cured 3 out of 10 birds.[25] Therefore, if amphotericin B is used to treat *M ornithogaster* in birds, 100 mg/kg is generally recommended, but some authors report success with lower doses.[29] Be aware that birds may relapse after treatment and repeated treatment may be needed.

Amphotericin B, especially when administered intravenous (IV), has been associated with renal adverse effects in mammals, but this has yet to be reported in birds.[33]

Nystatin: In one study, an *M ornithogaster* outbreak occurred in a flock of around 500 budgerigars. Following treatment with nystatin 3,500,000 IU/L drinking water for 48 h and then 2,000,000 IU/L drinking water for 28 d, no further mortality occurred.[22] Other authors reported the use of nystatin at 500 mg/kg feed without major success.[32] Resistance is common with nystatin.[18,29]

Sodium benzoate: Sodium benzoate at 1 tsp/L (~5 mL/L) in drinking water x 5 weeks cleared a *Macrorhabdus* infection in nonbreeding budgerigars. However, in breeding budgerigars, neurologic signs and death occurred due to increased water consumption, even at a lower dose (½ tsp/L or ~2.5 mL/L).[31] Therefore, this treatment should be used cautiously in breeding flocks, as breeding birds ingest more water, or if birds may be polydipsic for other reasons, such as high environmental temperatures. Other authors used sodium benzoate at 500 to 1000 mg/L in drinking water; treatment reduced mortality but the authors noted depression and decreased water consumption with the higher dose.[32] Some authors have reported toxicity in finches and canaries as well.[18] An alternative option that could potentially be less toxic than sodium benzoate is potassium benzoate, but this has not yet been evaluated.[29]

Antiparasitics

GI parasite infections are fairly common in some exotic companion animal species. Some GI parasites may be commensal or even beneficial in some reptile species, so treatment is not always indicated based on the identification of the parasite on a fecal flotation.[1,34] It is important to take into account the type of parasite identified, magnitude of the infection, the clinical status of the patient, and any potential environmental factors that need to be addressed.

Antiparasitics for helminth infections

Benzimidazoles: Benzimidazoles function by binding to beta-tubulin and are effective against nematodes, cestodes (tapeworms), and trematodes (flukes). In green iguanas (*Iguana iguana*), oxfendazole 25 mg/kg PO once was 100% effective at eliminating oxyurid nematodes by 4 weeks, without any obvious adverse effects.[35] Oxfendazole is an active metabolite and may be more effective and safer than other benzimidazoles, such as fenbendazole.[35] Oxyurid nematodes may function as commensals in some reptile species, such as bearded dragons, so treatment is not always necessary.[36] Treatment should generally be reserved for animals experiencing clinical signs or with very high burdens.[36]

Histomoniasis is a disease caused by the protozoal parasite *Histomonas meleagridis*, which is carried by the cecal nematode *Heterakis gallinarum*. Chickens may act as a reservoir for histomoniasis, while turkeys may suffer high mortality rates. There is currently no approved treatment of histomoniasis in the United States. It is recommended to avoid housing chickens with turkeys; if chickens are housed with turkeys, frequent fecal flotations or deworming of the chickens with benzimidazoles are recommended.

Although they are commonly used antiparasitic drugs, benzimidazole toxicity has been reported in several exotic animal species. This includes pigeons, doves, vultures, a harpy eagle, storks, pelicans, porcupines, and rabbits.[37–39] Potential toxic effects of benzimidazoles in rabbits include bone marrow hypoplasia leading to hematologic abnormalities (leukopenia, anemia, thrombocytopenia, or pancytopenia), bacteremia, hemorrhage, and death.[40] Benzimidazoles are commonly used for treatment of non-GI *Encephalitozoon cuniculi*-related disease in rabbits and can be used with caution if hematology is frequently monitored during treatment. Weekly complete blood counts are recommended.[40] Benzimidazole use is not recommended in certain taxa, such as Columbiformes, due to the high mortality rates associated with their use.[39] Hematologic and biochemical changes have been noted in Hermann's tortoises treated with fenbendazole, including heteropenia, hypoglycemia, hyperuricemia, and hyperphosphatemia.[34] Although these tortoises did not show any clinical signs associated with these blood work changes, caution may be warranted regarding the use of fenbendazole in tortoises.[34] The listed doses of fenbendazole in formularies are often fairly high, and dose reduction should be considered when treating clinically ill animals.

Pyrantel: Pyrantel is a pyrimidine anthelmintic that causes paralysis of the worms through depolarizing muscular blockade.[7,41] Pyrantel can be safely used to treat nematode infections in taxa that cannot safely receive benzimidazoles, such as Columbiformes (**Fig. 2**). Because it does not directly kill the worms, reinfection is common. This author has used a combination of pyrantel and selamectin to successfully treat ascarid infections in pigeons, after treatment with pyrantel alone resulted in recurrence.

Macrocyclic lactones: Macrocyclic lactones are effective against nematodes and arthropod parasites. These drugs enhance the release of gamma amino butyric acid at presynaptic neurons, causing paralysis and death of the parasite.[41] Lorikeets (*Trichoglossus* spp.) with proventricular nematodiasis due to *Synhimantus nasuta* were treated with 1.15 to 1.2 mg/kg ivermectin subcutaneous (SC) followed by 0.6 to 0.8 mg/kg q 2 to 4 d x 5 doses and selamectin 14.5 to 20 mg/kg topically monthly x 6 doses.[42] Mild transient ataxia and lethargy were noted after the higher dose of ivermectin.[42] Toxicity associated with ivermectin has been reported in other avian species, including budgerigars, finches, king pigeons, and a nanday conure (*Aratinga nenday*).[19,41] Therefore, caution is warranted regarding the use of higher doses of ivermectin in birds. Selamectin has been less well studied in birds, but some suggest that it is relatively safe.[19] Ivermectin is contraindicated in chelonians due to the high risk of toxicity.[34] There are also some concerns regarding ivermectin toxicity in other reptile species, including skinks and indigo snakes.[34]

Levamisole: Levamisole functions by stimulating the parasite's parasympathetic and sympathetic ganglia and interfering with carbohydrate metabolism; it also has

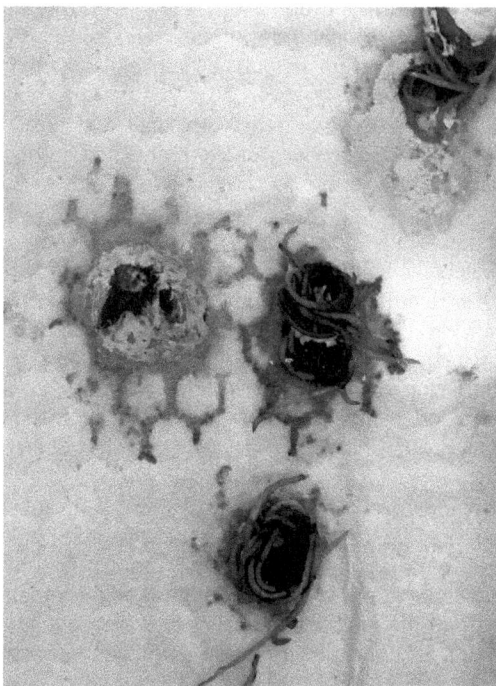

Fig. 2. Ascarid nematodes in the feces of domestic pigeons following treatment with pyrantel. Pyrantel paralyzes worms, but does not kill them, and may result in whole worms being passed in the feces.

immunostimulating effects.[41] The empiric use of levamisole in iguanas has been reported.[34] This drug has a narrow margin of safety and should not be used in debilitated animals. Adverse effects in reptiles and amphibians may include neurologic signs. Toxicity after SC or intramuscular (IM) injection has been reported in pet birds, such as cockatoos, budgerigars, and mynah birds.[41] Signs of toxicity in birds may include depression, ataxia, paralysis, mydriasis, regurgitation, and death.[41]

Praziquantel: A prazinoisoquinoline derivative anthelmintic, praziquantel occurs as a white to practically white, hygroscopic, bitter tasting, crystalline powder, either odorless or having a faint odor.[43] It has been used to clear trematode infections in green sea turtles (*Chelonia mydas*).[34] Reported side effects include elevated alanine aminotransferase and aspartate aminotransferase in green sea turtles, necrotizing skin lesions in a loggerhead sea turtle (*Caretta caretta*), and anaphylactic-like reactions in ball pythons (*Python regius*).[34]

Emodepside: Emodepside attaches presynaptically at the neuromuscular junction and results in an increase in intracellular calcium and diacylglycerol. It ultimately causes flaccid paralysis and parasite death.[41] A topical emodepside/praziquantel formulation (Profender, Bayer) had a slow onset effect and moderate efficacy (59.7% reduction in eggs per gram by day 33) against oxyurids in captive tortoises.[44] The authors were unable to make any definitive conclusions regarding the efficacy of this formulation against ascarids due to the small number of affected tortoises and one of the posttreatment fecal samples being unavailable, but there was a nonsignificant reduction in the ascarid eggs per gram by day 14.[44]

Antiparasitics for giardiasis and trichomoniasis

Metronidazole is an antiprotozoal drug that mainly has activity against trophozoites rather than cyst stages.[34] Potential side effects associated with metronidazole in exotic animal species include central nervous system signs such as ataxia, opisthotonus, tremors, seizures, and death.[34]

Metronidazole is commonly used to treat giardiasis in chinchillas but is often associated with anorexia in this species.[10–12] An alternative treatment option is tinidazole, which does not appear to cause anorexia in chinchillas at a lower dose of 20 mg/kg PO q 12 hour.[45]

Trichomoniasis is caused by protozoal parasites (typically *Trichomonas gallinae* and *Trichomonas columbae* in birds) that cause vomiting, diarrhea, and diphtheritic membranes in the upper GI tract. It is commonly reported in pigeons and birds of prey and occasionally parrots. Treatment is with nitroimidazoles, such as metronidazole, dimetridazole, ronidazole, or carnidazole.[18] It should be noted that nitroimidazoles, such as metronidazole, are prohibited in food-producing animal species in some countries. Some report that lentogenic strains of *Trichomonas* spp. may provide pigeons protection against velogenic strains.[18] Drug resistance of *Trichomonas* spp. in pigeons has been noted.

Antiparasitics for coccidiosis

Coccidiosis is a common GI infection in several exotic companion animal species, including poultry, bearded dragons, and domestic rabbits. There are several species of *Eimeria* in chickens that each affects different parts of the intestinal tract.[15] Several species of *Eimeria* affect the intestines of rabbits, while *Eimeria stiedae* affects the liver. Treatment options for coccidiosis include amprolium, ponazuril, toltrazuril, and sulfonamides.[8,19,46–48]

Amprolium is a coccidiostat that is often used prophylactically in poultry feed. It is also used to control coccidiosis in farmed rabbits.[7] Amprolium has a narrow margin of safety and side effects associated with overdoses include hemorrhagic diathesis and death.[48] Amprolium is a thiamine analog and the use of prolonged high doses of the drug can result in thiamine deficiency.[41] Some strains of coccidia in toucans and mynahs are reported to be resistant to amprolium.[41]

Ponazuril and toltrazuril are coccidiocidal triazinetriones that target nuclear division. Ponazuril is the active metabolite of toltrazuril. Ponazuril 40 mg/kg PO was effective at stopping coccidial oocyst shedding in peafowl (Pavo cristatus).[46] Use caution when administering toltrazuril 2.5% solution to birds; this solution is very alkaline and should not be administered directly into the crop.[19] Ponazuril 15 to 40 mg/kg PO q 24h x 21 d has been used to treat coccidiosis in bearded dragons. A combination of toltrazuril and clindamycin was used to treat Choleoeimeria spp. infections in a black-soil bearded dragon (also known as Lawson's or Rankin's dragon; Pogona henrylawsoni).[49] In a case report of 2 rabbits with hepatic coccidiosis, both rabbits died despite treatment with toltrazuril and trimethoprim-sulfamethoxazole.[50]

Environmental control is a crucial component of management of coccidiosis, especially in poultry, and may involve removing and replacing the top layer of litter to prevent poultry from contacting viable oocysts.[15]

Treatment of cryptosporidiosis in reptiles

Cryptosporidiosis is an important GI infection in several reptile species. In particular, Cryptosporidium serpentis is often associated with the stomach in snakes and C varanii with the intestines in lizards, especially leopard geckos.[51] Treatment often has a very poor success rate in clearing the infection, and euthanasia may be recommended for animals exhibiting clinical signs. However, various treatment options have been evaluated and can be considered if the owner wishes to attempt treatment.

Paromomycin, an aminoglycoside antibiotic, was used to treat a king cobra (Ophiophagus hannah) at a dose of 360 mg/kg PO twice weekly x 6 weeks and resulted in negative fecal PCRs for Cryptosporidium following treatment.[52] Using the same treatment protocol, paromomycin-treated eastern indigo snakes (Drymarchon couperi) were significantly more likely to test qPCR negative than control snakes (8 out of 17 vs 1 out of 17 snakes, respectively).[53] Following immunosuppression with high-dose (4 mg/kg) dexamethasone sodium phosphate, only 2 out of 17 of the treated snakes were qPCR negative, indicating the infection has the potential to recrudesce following treatment if patients are immunosuppressed.[53] Similarly, in leopard geckos, clinical signs improved with paromomycin 50 to 800 mg/kg PO q 24h, but recrudescence was noted following treatment discontinuation.[51] In bearded dragons treated with paromomycin, no organisms were noted on histopathology or in the feces of treated animals.[51]

Eastern indigo snakes infected with C serpentis were treated with 20 mg/kg nitazoxanide, 10 mg/kg azithromycin, and 5 mg/kg rifabutin PO twice weekly for 6 weeks, which resulted in a significant decrease in C serpentis DNA shedding compared to the control group.[54] However, only 2 of 12 snakes from each group were qPCR negative following treatment.[54]

Antivirals

Compared to other types of antimicrobial drugs, antivirals are used less commonly in exotic animal medicine.

Antivirals for avian bornavirus

Antivirals, including ribavirin and favipiravir, have been investigated for treatment of avian bornavirus.[55] In one study, favipiravir was more effective at reducing parrot bornavirus-4 RNA than ribavirin.[55] The use of anti-inflammatory and immunosuppressive drugs for the treatment of avian ganglioneuritis is discussed in the next section.

ANTI-INFLAMMATORIES AND IMMUNOSUPPRESSIVES

In exotic animal gastroenterology, immunosuppressive drugs are most often used for treatment of inflammatory bowel disease or GI neoplasia; however, there are certain infectious diseases in which their use may be indicated.

Treatment of Chronic Enteric Coronavirus in Ferrets

Ferret enteric coronavirus causes epizootic catarrhal enteritis, a common GI disease of ferrets. Initial treatment consists of fluid therapy, antibiotics for secondary infections, and supportive care. However, some ferrets may continue to have persistent diarrhea from malabsorption, in which case a short course of prednisone (1 mg/kg q 12 hours x 14 d) may help with recovery.[13]

Treatment of Avian Ganglioneuritis

Avian ganglioneuritis (**Fig. 3**) is a disease associated with lymphoplasmacytic inflammation in the myenteric ganglia and nerves of the proventriculus and ventriculus.[56] Research has indicated that it is associated with avian bornavirus, but not all birds with the virus go on to develop ganglioneuritis and many birds can be positive for the virus without clinical signs. Commonly affected species include macaws, gray parrots, Amazon parrots, and cockatoos, but it has also been reported in non-psittacine birds. The GI and nervous systems are the most commonly affected body systems. Currently, there is no cure for this disease, but supportive care and certain medications can be used to help improve the quality of life of affected birds. Aside from supportive care (nutritional support, analgesics, antimicrobials as needed for secondary infections), the 2 main types of drugs (**Table 2**) that have been attempted for treatment of avian ganglioneuritis are nonsteroidal anti-inflammatory drugs (NSAIDs) and an immunosuppressive (cyclosporine).

Meloxicam, a commonly used NSAID in avian medicine, does not appear beneficial in the treatment of avian ganglioneuritis. Experimentally infected cockatiels given meloxicam 0.5 mg/kg PO q 12 hour became ill and had more severe lesions than controls.[57] In another study, treatment with meloxicam 1 mg/kg PO q 24 h did not appear to alter the disease course or lesions associated with avian bornavirus; 1 bird died and 1 was euthanized in the meloxicam group, and 2 birds were euthanized in the placebo group.[58]

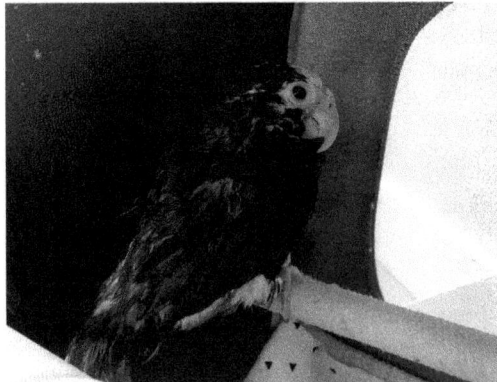

Fig. 3. Poor feather condition in a white-crowned pionus (*Pionus senilis*) with avian ganglioneuritis.

Table 2
Some reported drug protocols for management of avian ganglioneuritis

Drug	Dose and Route	Species	Outcome
Immunosuppressives			
Cyclosporine	10 mg/kg PO q 12 h[57]	Cockatiels	Birds appeared clinically normal but did not prevent infection; less severe lesions than meloxicam-treated birds
	0.2 mg/bird[63]	Cockatiels	Survived challenge; no clinical signs or gross lesions; 1 out of 8 had histologic lesions; did have high levels of viral RNA
Nonsteroidal Anti-inflammatory Drugs			
Celecoxib	10 mg/kg PO q 24 h[60]	Various bird species including blue and yellow macaw	Clinical improvement
	20 mg/kg PO q 24 h[61]	Various	Anecdotal
	40 mg/kg on seed mix[61]	Macaws (Ara spp.), cockatoos (Cacatua spp.), Amazon parrots (Amazona spp.)	Seven out of 9 birds negative on repeat crop biopsies
	10 mg/kg q 24 h[58]	Cockatiels	Did not appear to alter clinical presentation, shedding, lesions; black intestinal contents in some birds
	15–20 mg/kg PO q 12h; higher dose of 60–80 mg/kg divided q 12h if central nervous system involvement[56]	Various	Anecdotal
Robenacoxib	10 mg/kg IM weekly, then monthly, along with Mycobacterium bovis extracts[59]	Parrots	Suppressed periganglia infiltrates and reduced clinical signs
	2–10 mg/kg IM weekly, then monthly[56]	Various	Anecdotal
Tepoxalin	Unknown dose on seed mix or on hypoallergenic diet[61]	Cockatoos (palm, red-tailed black, and Cacatua spp.), macaws, Derbyan parakeet	Two out of 8 birds negative on repeat biopsies when tepoxalin given on seed mix; 14 out of 14 when given on hypoallergenic diet

(continued on next page)

Table 2
(continued)

Drug	Dose and Route	Species	Outcome
Meloxicam	0.5 mg/kg PO q 12 h[57]	Cockatiels	Became clinically ill, more severe lesions; not recommended
	1 mg/kg PO q 24 h[58]	Cockatiels	Did not appear to alter clinical presentation, shedding, lesions; black intestinal contents in some birds

Some authors have reported success with other NSAIDs, including celecoxib, robenacoxib, and tepoxalin. In a conference proceeding, parrots with avian ganglio-neuritis were treated with robenacoxib 10 mg/kg IM weekly, and then monthly, along with *Mycobacterium bovis* extract.[59] The authors observed suppressed peri-anglia infiltrates and a reduced clinical signs in most of the treated birds.[59] A dose range of 2 to 10 mg/kg IM weekly, then monthly, has been reported for robenacoxib.[56]

Celecoxib at 10 mg/kg PO q 24h was used in a conference proceeding describing greater than 14 birds diagnosed with avian ganglioneuritis via crop biopsy, with most of the birds reportedly showing clinical improvement.[60] In another conference pro-ceeding, parrots were treated with celecoxib 40 mg/kg given on food and 7 out of 9 were negative on repeat biopsy.[61] Those authors noted that they use a lower dose of 20 mg/kg PO q 24h if the bird is medicated directly orally.[61] In contrast to those pos-itive results with celecoxib, another study found that celecoxib 10 mg/kg PO q 24h did not improve the clinical course in experimentally infected cockatiels, and 1 bird died and 3 were euthanized in the celecoxib group (compared to 2 birds died or euthanized in the meloxicam group and in the control group).[58] Pharmacokinetic data for cele-coxib are available in cockatiels and a dose of 10 mg/kg PO was associated with high to complete oral absorption.[62]

In a conference proceeding, another NSAID, tepoxalin was given either on seed mix or a hypoallergenic diet; on repeat biopsy, 2 out of 8 birds were negative following treatment with tepoxalin on the seed mix, while 14 out of 14 were negative following treatment with the drug on the hypoallergenic diet.[61]

Cyclosporine is an immunosuppressive medication that has also been suggested as a potential treatment of avian ganglioneuritis. In one study, experimentally infected cockatiels were given cyclosporine 0.2 mg/bird, and all treated birds survived chal-lenge and had no clinical signs or gross lesions. One out of 8 birds did have histologic birds and treated birds still had high levels of viral RNA. In contrast, most challenged, untreated birds died or were euthanized, had proventricular dilatation, and had histo-logic lesions.[63] In a conference proceeding, experimentally infected cockatiels were treated with cyclosporine 10 mg/kg PO q 12 hour; treated cockatiels appeared clini-cally normal but cyclosporine did not prevent infection.[57]

SUMMARY

Common GI infections in exotic animal medicine include various bacterial infections (eg, *L intracellularis* in hamsters, *H mustelae* in ferrets), fungal infections (eg, *M orni-thogaster* and *Candida* sp. in birds), parasitic infections (eg, helminths, coccidiosis), and viral infections (eg, enteric coronavirus in ferrets, avian ganglioneuritis associated with avian bornavirus in birds). Antimicrobials should be used appropriately in exotic animal gastroenterology, and it is important to be aware of which infectious diseases may require prolonged or repeat treatment.

CLINICS CARE POINTS

- Penicillins, lincosamides (including lincomycin and clindamycin), ampicillin, amoxicillin, cephalosporins, and erythromycin are contraindicated orally in rabbits, guinea pigs, chinchillas, and degus.
- Some GI infections in exotic pets, such as *M ornithogaster* in birds and *Cryptosporidium* spp. in reptiles, are difficult to clear, so discuss prognosis and the risk of recurrence with clients.

- Benzimidazole toxicity has been reported in a variety of exotic animal species. These drugs should be avoided in pigeons and doves. They can be used with caution in rabbits, but complete blood counts should be monitored before, during, and after treatment.
- Ivermectin is contraindicated in chelonians.
- Recommend that clients do not house chickens and turkeys together, as chickens can act as reservoir for histomoniasis in turkeys.

DISCLOSURE

The authors declare that they have no known competing financial or commercial interests that could have appeared to influence the work reported in this study. No funding was provided for this study.

REFERENCES

1. Rossi JV. Husbandry and captive management. In: Divers SJ, Stahl SJ, editors. Mader's reptile and Amphibian medicine and surgery. 3rd edition. St. Louis, MO: Elsevier; 2019. p. 109–30.
2. Steinagel AC, Oglesbee BL. Clinicopathological and radiographic indicators for orogastric decompression in rabbits presenting with intestinal obstruction at a referral hospital (2015–2018). Vet Rec 2023;192(5):e2481.
3. Harcourt-Brown FM, Harcourt-Brown SF. Clinical value of blood glucose measurement in pet rabbits. Vet Rec 2012;170(26):674.
4. Sharma D, Hill AE, Christopher MM. Hypercholesterolemia and hypertriglyceridemia as biochemical markers of disease in companion rabbits. Vet Clin Pathol 2018;47(4):589–602.
5. Böttcher A, Müller K. Radiological and laboratory prognostic parameters for gastric dilation in rabbits (*Oryctolagus cuniculus*). Vet Rec 2024;194(5):e3827.
6. Frame J, Adamovicz L, Keller K, et al. Utilization of systemic inflammatory response syndrome (SIRS) scoring system as a prognostic indicator in *Oryctolagus cuniculus*. In: AEMV and ARAV proceedings. New Orleans, LA: AEMV and ARAV; 2024. p. 118.
7. Smith MV. Therapeutics. In: Smith MV, editor. Textbook of rabbit medicine. 3rd edition. St. Louis, MO: Elsevier; 2023. p. 100–37.
8. Oglesbee BL, Lord B. Gastrointestinal diseases of rabbits. In: Quesenberry K, Orcutt CJ, Mans C, et al, editors. Ferrets, rabbits, and rodents: clinical medicine and surgery. 4th edition. St. Louis, MO: Elsevier; 2021. p. 174–87.
9. Mans C. Effects of pradofloxacin on food intake in healthy chinchillas. J Exot Pet Med 2021;37:22–3.
10. Thomas L, Doss G, Mans C. Presumptive metronidazole benzoate induced anorexia in two healthy chinchillas (*Chinchilla lanigera*). J Exot Pet Med 2021; 36:52.
11. Mans C, Fink D. Effects of commercial metronidazole and metronidazole benzoate suspensions on food intake in chinchillas. J Small Anim Pract 2021;62(3):174–7.
12. Mans C, Fink DM, Giammarco HE, et al. Effects of compounded metronidazole and metronidazole benzoate oral suspensions on food intake in healthy chinchillas (*Chinchilla lanigera*). J Exot Pet Med 2021;36:75–9.
13. Hoefer H. Gastrointestinal diseases of ferrets. In: Quesenberry K, Orcutt C, Mans C, et al, editors. Ferrets, rabbits, and rodents: clinical medicine and surgery. 4th edition. St. Louis, MO: Elsevier; 2021. p. 27–38.

14. O'Neill DG, Kim K, Brodbelt DC, et al. Demography, disorders and mortality of pet hamsters under primary veterinary care in the United Kingdom in 2016. J Small Anim Pract 2022;63(10):747–55.

15. Morishita TY, Porter REJ. Gastrointestinal and hepatic diseases. In: Greenacre CB, Morishita TY, editors. Backyard poultry medicine and surgery: a guide for veterinary practitioners. 1st edition. Ames, IA: Wiley-Blackwell; 2015. p. 181–203.

16. Crespo R, França MS, Fenton H, et al. Galliformes and Columbiformes. In: Terio KA, McAloose D, St. Leger J, editors. Pathology of wildlife and zoo animals. London, UK: Academic Press; 2018. p. 747–73.

17. De Santi M, Schocken-Iturrino RP, Casagrande MF, et al. Necrotic enteritis caused by *Clostridium perfringens* in blue and gold macaws (*Ara ararauna*). J Avian Med Surg 2020;34(1):65.

18. Doneley B. Diseases of the gastrointestinal tract. In: Avian medicine and surgery in practice: companion and aviary birds. 2nd edition. Boca Raton, FL: CRC Press; 2016. p. 229–50.

19. Carpenter JW, Harms CA, editors. Carpenter's exotic animal formulary. 6th edition. St. Louis, MO: Elsevier; 2023.

20. Donnelly KA, Wellehan JFX, Quesenberry K. Gastrointestinal disease associated with non-*albicans Candida* species in six birds. J Avian Med Surg 2019; 33(4):413.

21. Berg KJ, Guzman DSM, Paul-Murphy J, et al. Diagnosis and treatment of *Candida glabrata* proventriculitis in an eclectus parrot (*Eclectus roratus*). J Am Vet Med Assoc 2022;260(4):442–9.

22. Kheirandish R, Salehi M. Megabacteriosis in budgerigars: diagnosis and treatment. Comp Clin Pathol 2011;20(5):501–5.

23. Püstow R, Krautwald-Junghanns ME. The incidence and treatment outcomes of *Macrorhabdus ornithogaster* infection in budgerigars (*Melopsittacus undulatus*) in a veterinary clinic. J Avian Med Surg 2017;31(4):344–50.

24. Poleschinski JM, Straub JU, Schmidt V. Comparison of two treatment modalities and PCR to assess treatment effectiveness in macrorhabdosis. J Avian Med Surg 2019;33(3):245.

25. Baron HR, Leung KCL, Stevenson BC, et al. Evidence of amphotericin B resistance in *Macrorhabdus ornithogaster* in Australian cage-birds. Med Mycol 2019;57(4):421–8.

26. Baron HR, Stevenson BC, Phalen DN. Comparison of in-clinic diagnostic testing methods for *Macrorhabdus ornithogaster*. J Avian Med Surg 2021;35(1). https://doi.org/10.1647/1082-6742-35.1.37.

27. Reed K, Anderson K, Wolf K. Mortality trends for budgerigars (*Melopsittacus undulatus*) housed in a walk-through aviary in a zoo in North America, 2009–2019. J Zoo Wildl Med 2021;52(4). https://doi.org/10.1638/2021-0036.

28. Fulton RM, Mani R. Avian gastric yeast (*Macrorhabdus ornithogaster*) and *Mycobacterium genavense* infections in a zoo budgerigar (*Melopsittacus undulatus*) flock. Avian Dis 2020;64(4). https://doi.org/10.1637/0005-2086-64.4.561.

29. Wellehan JFX, Lierz M, Phalen D, et al. Infectious disease. In: Speer BL, editor. Current therapy in avian medicine and surgery. 1st edition. St. Louis, MO: Elsevier; 2016. p. 22–106.

30. Hernandez SM, Curry SE, Murray MH, et al. An acute mortality event associated with novel *Macrorhabdus ornithogaster* infection and underlying factors in a newly-established captive group of American white ibis (*Eudocimus albus*) nestlings. J Wildl Dis 2023;59(4). https://doi.org/10.7589/JWD-D-22-00141.

31. Hoppes S. Treatment of *Macrorhabdus ornithogastor* with sodium benzoate in budgerigars (*Melopsittacus undulates* [sic]). In: Proc annu conf assoc avian vet. AAV; 2011. p. 67.
32. Madani SA, Ghorbani A, Arabkhazaeli F. Successful treatment of macrorhabdosis in budgerigars (*Melopsittacus undulatus*) using sodium benzoate. J Mycol Res 2014;1(1):21–7.
33. Antonissen G, Martel A. Antifungal therapy in birds: old drugs in a new jacket. Vet Clin Exot Anim Pract 2018;21(2):355–77.
34. Rockwell K, Mitchell MA. Antiparasitic therapy. In: Divers SJ, Stahl SJ, editors. Mader's reptile and Amphibian medicine and surgery. 3rd edition. St. Louis, MO: Elsevier; 2019. p. 1165–70.
35. Kehoe S, Divers S, Mayer J, et al. Efficacy of single-dose oxfendazole to treat oxyurid nematodiasis in the green iguana (*Iguana iguana*). J Herpetol Med Surg 2020;30(3). https://doi.org/10.5818/19-06-203.1.
36. Eatwell K, Richardson J. Gastroenterology—small intestine, exocrine pancreas, and large intestine. In: Divers SJ, Stahl SJ, editors. Mader's reptile and Amphibian medicine and surgery. 3rd edition. St. Louis, MO: Elsevier; 2019. p. 761–74.
37. Petritz OA, Chen S. Therapeutic contraindications in exotic pets. Vet Clin Exot Anim Pract 2018;21(2):327–40.
38. Doss GA, Mans C, Johnson L, et al. Diagnosis and management of inflammatory bowel disease in a harpy eagle (*Harpia harpyja*) with suspected fenbendazole toxicosis. J Am Vet Med Assoc 2018;252(3):336–42.
39. Gozalo AS, Schwiebert RS, Lawson GW. Mortality associated with fenbendazole administration in pigeons (*Columba livia*). J Am Assoc Lab Anim Sci 2006;45(6).
40. Graham JE, Garner MM, Reavill DR. Benzimidazole toxicosis in rabbits: 13 cases (2003 to 2011). J Exot Pet Med 2014;23(2):188–95.
41. Plumb DC. Plumb's veterinary drug handbook. 6th edition. Ames, IA: Blackwell Publishing; 2008.
42. Pouillevet H, Langlois I, Lamglait B, et al. Evaluation of clinical diagnostics for proventricular nematodiasis due to *Synhimantus nasuta* in lorikeets (*Trichoglossus* spp.). J Zoo Wildl Med 2022;53(2). https://doi.org/10.1638/2021-0030.
43. Plumb DC. Veterinary drug handbook. 4th edition. Hoboken, NJ: Wiley-Blackwell; 2002.
44. Tang PK, Pellett S, Blake D, et al. Efficacy of a topical formulation containing emodepside and praziquantel (Profender®, Bayer) against nematodes in captive tortoises. J Herpetol Med Surg 2017;27(3):116.
45. Tournade CM, Fink DM, Williams SR, et al. Effects of tinidazole on food intake in chinchillas (*Chinchilla lanigera*). J Am Assoc Lab Anim Sci 2021;60(5):587–91.
46. Zec SH, Papich MG, Oehler DA, et al. Pharmacokinetics of a single oral dose of ponazuril in the Indian peafowl (*Pavo cristatus*). J Zoo Wildl Med 2021;52(2). https://doi.org/10.1638/2020-0026.
47. Marroquin SC, Eshar D, Browning GR, et al. Diagnosis and successful treatment of *Eimeria* infection in a pair of pet domestic rats (*Rattus norvegicus*) with ponazuril. J Exot Pet Med 2020;33:31–3.
48. Wakenell P. Management and medicine of backyard poultry. In: Speer BL, editor. Current therapy in avian medicine and surgery. St. Louis, MO: Elsevier; 2016. p. 550–65. https://doi.org/10.1016/B978-1-4557-4671-2.00024-0.
49. Stöhr AC, Globokar-Vrhovec M, Pantchev N. Choleoeimeria spp. prevalence in captive reptiles in Germany and a new treatment option in a Lawson's dragon (*Pogona henrylawsoni*). J Herpetol Med Surg 2021;30(4). https://doi.org/10.5818/19-09-211.1.

50. Mlakar Hrženjak N, Zadravec M, Švara T, et al. Hepatic coccidiosis in two pet rabbits. J Exot Pet Med 2021;36:53–6.
51. Bogan JE. Gastric cryptosporidiosis in snakes, a review. J Herpetol Med Surg 2019;29(3–4):71.
52. Rivas AE, Boyer DM, Torregrosa K, et al. Treatment of *Cryptosporidium serpentis* infection in a king cobra (*Ophiophagus hannah*) with paromomycin. J Zoo Wildl Med 2018;49(4):1061.
53. Bogan JE, Hoffman M, Dickerson F, et al. Evaluation of paromomycin treatment for *Cryptosporidium serpentis* infection in eastern indigo snakes (*Drymarchon couperi*). J Herpetol Med Surg 2021;31(4). https://doi.org/10.5818/JHMS-D-21-00010.
54. Bogan JE, Hoffman M, Mitchell MA, et al. Evaluation of the drug combination nitazoxanide, azithromycin, and rifabutin as a treatment for *Cryptosporidium serpentis* infection in eastern indigo snakes (*Drymarchon couperi*). J Herpetol Med Surg 2022;32(4). https://doi.org/10.5818/JHMS-D-22-00014.
55. Hoppes SM, Shivaprasad HL. Update on avian bornavirus and proventricular dilatation disease. Vet Clin Exot Anim Pract 2020;23(2):337–51.
56. Rossi G, Dahlhausen RD, Galosi L, et al. Avian ganglioneuritis in clinical practice. Vet Clin Exot Anim Pract 2018;21(1):33–67.
57. Hoppes S, Tizard I, Shivaprasad HL, et al. Treatment of avian bornavirus-infected cockatiels (*Nymphicus hollandicus*) with oral meloxicam and cyclosporine. In: Proc annu conf assoc avian vet. Louisville, KY: AAV; 2012. p. 27.
58. Escandon P, Heatley JJ, Tizard I, et al. Treatment with nonsteroidal anti-inflammatory drugs fails to ameliorate pathology in cockatiels experimentally infected with parrot bornavirus-2. Vet Med Auckl 2019;10:185–95.
59. Rossi G, Crosta L, Ceccherelli R, et al. PDD: our point of view after 7 years of research. In: Proc annu conf assoc avian vet. Louisville, KY: AAV; 2012. p. 80.
60. Dahlhausen B, Aldred S, Colaizz E. Resolution of clinical proventricular dilatation disease by cyclooxygenase 2 inhibition. In: Proc annu conf assoc avian vet. Monterey, CA: AAV; 2002. p. 9–12.
61. Clubb SL. Clinical management of psittacine birds affected with proventricular dilatation disease. In: Proc annu conf assoc avian vet. AAV; 2006. p. 85–90.
62. Dhondt L, Devreese M, Croubels S, et al. Comparative population pharmacokinetics and absolute oral bioavailability of COX-2 selective inhibitors celecoxib, mavacoxib and meloxicam in cockatiels (*Nymphicus hollandicus*). Sci Rep 2017;7(1):12043.
63. Hameed SS, Guo J, Tizard I, et al. Studies on immunity and immunopathogenesis of parrot bornaviral disease in cockatiels. Virology 2018;515:81–91.

Moving?

Make sure your subscription moves with you!

To notify us of your new address, find your **Clinics Account Number** (located on your mailing label above your name), and contact customer service at:

Email: journalscustomerservice-usa@elsevier.com

800-654-2452 (subscribers in the U.S. & Canada)
314-447-8871 (subscribers outside of the U.S. & Canada)

Fax number: 314-447-8029

Elsevier Health Sciences Division
Subscription Customer Service
3251 Riverport Lane
Maryland Heights, MO 63043

*To ensure uninterrupted delivery of your subscription, please notify us at least 4 weeks in advance of move.

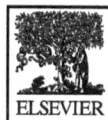

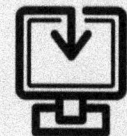

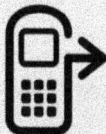

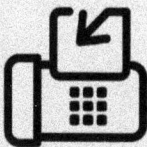

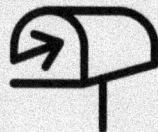

ELSEVIER

www.ingramcontent.com/pod-product-compliance
Lightning Source LLC
Chambersburg PA
CBHW050454190326
41458CB00005B/1285